Local Flaps in Facial Reconstruction

Velupillai Ilankovan • Madan Ethunandan
Tian Ee Seah

Local Flaps in Facial Reconstruction

A Defect Based Approach

Second Edition

Springer

Velupillai Ilankovan
Bournemouth University
Poole, UK

Head and Neck Surgery
Pekingese Union Medical College
Beijing, China

Tian Ee Seah
Oral and Maxillofacial Surgeon
TES Clinic for Face and Jaw
Singapore, Singapore

Madan Ethunandan
Oral and Maxillofacial Surgeon
University Hospital Southampton
Southampton, UK

SRIHER
Chennai, India

ISBN 978-3-031-49463-5 ISBN 978-3-031-49464-2 (eBook)
https://doi.org/10.1007/978-3-031-49464-2

This Springer imprint is published by the registered company Springer Nature Switzerland AG
The registered company address is: Gewerbestrasse 11, 6330 Cham, Switzerland

Paper in this product is recyclable.

To my parents for providing me with the opportunity to become a surgeon and my wife Regina, children Christopher and Victoria, for their support and tolerance over the years.

— Velupillai Ilankovan

To my parents for being excellent role models and giving me the opportunities and my wife Annie and daughter Tanuvi for all their support, sacrifices, love and friendship.

— Madan Ethunandan

To my parents whose unwavering care and support laid the foundation of my journey. To my wife, VicPearly, whose love and understanding have been my anchor throughout my career. To my daughter, Rachel, who is the love of our lives.

— Tian Ee Seah

Preface

The first edition of the *Local Flaps in Facial Reconstruction—A Defect Based Approach* was published almost 7 years ago and has been well received across the world and translated into other languages. It was designed to help in the decision-making process and provide practical step-by-step information for reconstructing specific defects in the facial region.

The frequency of skin cancer continues to increase across the globe and clinicians from various backgrounds are involved in the care of these patients. Medical and surgical management of these conditions are rapidly changing, with targeted and patient-specific practices coming into the forefront. Reconstruction techniques should also be patient specific and "personalised". The current edition has been "completely" updated with new text, excellent surgically relevant colour drawings and clinical photographs, to provide comprehensive practical solutions to facial defects confronted by the clinicians in day-to-day practice. New innovative solutions and modifications to established practices to facilitate individualised patient care have been described and descriptions of epidermal cell harvesting and nano fat stem cell injections have been included. The philosophy remains a problem-solving exercise using current knowledge and applications. The original ethos of a book that can be used in everyday practice, with scope for inclusion of personal comments is maintained.

Poole, Dorset, UK — Velupillai Ilankovan
Southampton, UK — Madan Ethunandan
Singapore, Singapore — Tian Ee Seah

Acknowledgements

We would like to thanks Dr Anna Sayan, Dr Chiew Ying Chieng and Mrs Jane Potter for all their help with the preparation of the manuscripts. We would also like, to thank the team at Springer Nature and Daniela Heller, Mahalakshmi Sathisbabu, Rosemarie Unger and Shaif Jainul Safha in particular for their valuable insight, patience and support. All illustrations were done by Dr Tian Ee Seah.

Contents

Part I Foundations

1 **Local Anaesthesia** . . . 3
Types of Anaesthesia. . . . 3
Important Common Steps . . . 3
Deciphering Drug Concentrations and Dilutions . . . 4
Tumescent Solution. . . . 5
Sensory Nerve Supply to the Skin of Head and Neck . . . 5
Anaesthesia for Specific Areas . . . 7
Forehead . . . 7
Temple. . . . 9
Cheek . . . 11
External Nose . . . 13
Lips . . . 14
External Ear/Pinna . . . 16
Scalp . . . 18
Neck . . . 20

2 **Facial Units and Subunits**. . . . 23
Forehead . . . 27
Cheek . . . 29
Nose . . . 31
Lips . . . 33
Chin. . . . 35
Pinna . . . 37
Eyelids. . . . 39
Scalp . . . 41
Neck . . . 43

3 **Basic Flaps**. . . . 45
Advancement Flaps. . . . 45
Rotation Flap. . . . 48
Transposition Flap. . . . 51
Interpolated Flap. . . . 54
Bilobed Flap . . . 56

Island Flap. 59
Rhombic Flap 63
Dog Ear Correction (Standing Cutaneous Deformity) 67

4 Decision-Making Process 69

Part II Reconstruction of Specific Defects

5 Scalp Reconstruction 73
Subunits and Anatomical Considerations 73
Central (Vertex) Defects 78
Small Defects 78
Medium-Sized Defects 78
Rotation Flap. 78
O-Z Closure 81
Multiple Rotation Flap (Pin Wheel Flap) 84
Multiple Rhomboid Flaps 87
Skin Graft (Full Thickness). 89
Split Skin Graft 93
Integra® and Skin Grafting 96
Pericranial Flap and Skin Grafting 100
Transposition Flap/Skin Grafting of Secondary Defect 104
Recell 108
Lateral Defects 110
Small Defects 110
Medium-Sized Defects 110
Bilateral Advancement Flap 112
Rotation/Transposition Flaps 114
Suggested Algorithm. 117
Central (Vertex) Defects 117
Lateral Defects 117

6 Forehead Reconstruction 119
Subunits and Anatomical Considerations 119
Central Defects (Between the Medial End of the Eyebrows) 122
Elliptical Excision. 122
M & W Flaps. 124
Upper Forehead. 126
Lower Forehead 128
Upper and Lower Forehead. 130
Bilateral Advancement Flap 132
Paramedian Defects (Between Medial End of the Eyebrow and Lateral Orbital Rim). 134
Elliptical Excision. 134
Unilateral/Bilateral Advancement Flaps 136

Lower Forehead ... 138
Upper Forehead ... 142
Lateral Forehead/Temple (Between the Lateral Orbital Rim and Zygomatic Arch) ... 142
V-T Flap ... 142
Rotation/Transposition Flap ... 145
Rhombic Flap (Limberg Flap) ... 147
Unilateral/Bilateral Advancement Flaps ... 150
Forehead Rotation Flap ... 152
Cervical/Cheek Rotation Flap ... 154
Multiple Transposition Flaps ± Skin Grafts ... 156
Skin Graft ... 159
Suggested Algorithm ... 161
Forehead ... 161
Large Defects ... 162

7 Nose ... 163
Subunits and Anatomical Considerations ... 163
Nasal Dorsum Defects ... 165
Primary Closure (Vertical) ... 165
Primary Closure (Horizontal) ... 167
Glabellar Advancement Flap ... 169
Glabella Transposition Flap ... 172
Nasal Tip Defects ... 174
Primary Closure ... 174
Skin Graft ... 174
Bilobed Flap ... 176
Sidewall Defects ... 180
Primary Closure ... 180
Skin Grafts ... 180
Glabella Transposition Flap ... 180
Bilobed Flap (Laterally Based) ... 184
Bilobed Flap (Medially Based) ... 187
Apron Flap ... 190
Ala Defects ... 195
Island Advancement Flap ... 195
Bilobed Flap (Laterally Based) ... 198
Bilobed Flap (Medially Based) ... 200
Nasolabial Flap (Inferiorly Based) ... 202
Two-Stage Melolabial Flap ... 204
Paramedian Forehead Flap ... 207
Apron Flap ... 211
Columella ... 211
Primary Closure (Vertical/Horizontal) ... 211

Skin Graft . . . 211
Two-Stage Melolabial Flap . . . 213
Suggested Algorithm . . . 213
Dorsum . . . 213
Nasal Tip . . . 213
Columella . . . 213
Side Wall . . . 213
Ala . . . 214
Paramedian Forehead Flap . . . 214

8 **Eyelids** . . . 215
Subunits and Anatomical Considerations . . . 215
Upper Eyelid . . . 218
Anterior Lamella Defects . . . 218
Full-Thickness Defects . . . 231
Lower Eyelid . . . 235
Anterior Lamella Defects . . . 235
Full-Thickness Defects . . . 241
Suggested Algorithm . . . 258
Upper Eyelid . . . 258
Lower Eyelid . . . 258

9 **Auricular Reconstruction** . . . 261
Subunits and Anatomical Considerations . . . 261
Special Considerations . . . 264
Concha (Cymba and Cavum) . . . 264
Antihelix . . . 282
Helical Rim/Antihelix Extending to Helical Rim . . . 286
Triangular Fossa . . . 304
Tragus . . . 308
Posterior Surface of Pinna . . . 312
Lobule . . . 322
Suggested Algorithm . . . 324
Concha . . . 324
Antihelix/Helix . . . 324
Triangular Fossa . . . 324
Tragus . . . 324
Posterior Surface of Pinna . . . 325
Lobule . . . 325

10 **Cheek Defects** . . . 327
Subunits and Anatomical Considerations . . . 327
Medial Subunit . . . 330
Primary Closure . . . 330
Island Advancement Flap . . . 334
Buccal Subunit . . . 339

Primary Closure 339
Rhombic Flap 341
Laterally Based Rotation/Transposition Flap 343
Inferiorly Based Rotation Advancement Flap. 347
Zygomatic Subunit 350
Primary Closure 350
Rhombic Flap 352
Rotation/Transposition Flap 355
Island Advancement Flap 358
Mandibular Subunit. 360
Primary Closure 360
Rhombic Flap 360
Rotation/Transposition Flap 364
Lateral Subunit 367
Primary Closure 367
Asymmetric Primary Closure 367
Rhombic Flap 370
Bilobed Flap 370
Suggested Algorithm. 373
Medial 373
Buccal 373
Zygomatic Unit. 373
Mandibular 373
Lateral Unit. 374

11 Lips/Chin 375
Lips 375
Subunits and Anatomical Considerations 375
Lower Lip 378
Skin Only 378
Mucosa Only. 387
Full-thickness Defects. 390
Bilateral Advancement Flap 404
Bilateral Commissurotomy and Advancement of Skin, Muscle, and Mucosal Flaps. 406
Upper Lip (Philtrum/Lateral) 413
Skin Only (Consider Converting to Full Thickness). 413
Full-Thickness Defects 432
Philtrum/Lateral Defects. 432
Chin Defects 443
Suggested Algorithm. 455
Lips 455
Upper/Lower Lip (Chronic Ulcers/Atrophy) 456

12 Neck Defects 457
Subunits and Anatomical Considerations 457
Central Neck 460
Lateral Neck 467
Posterior Neck. 474
Suggested Algorithm. 481
Central Neck 481
Lateral Neck 481
Posterior Neck. 481

Algorithms for Specific Sites. 483
Scalp 483
Forehead 484
Nose 485
Eyelids. 487
Ear. 488
Cheek 489
Lips 491
Neck 493

Index 495

Part I

Foundations

1 Local Anaesthesia

Types of Anaesthesia

Topical, infiltration, field block, nerve block.

Important Common Steps

Prepare skin using sterile technique.

Always aspirate before injecting local anaesthetic solution.

Aware of maximum doses (Table 1.1).

Knowledge of recognising and managing toxicity/complications.

Table 1.1 Duration of action and maximum doses of common local anaesthetic agents

Anaesthetic	Duration without adrenaline/ vasoconstrictor (min)	Duration with adrenaline/ vasoconstrictor (min)	Maximum dose without adrenaline/ vasoconstrictor (mg/kg)	Maximum dose with adrenaline/ vasoconstrictor (mg/kg)
Esters				
Cocaine	45	–	2.8	–
Procaine	15–30	30–90	7.1	8.5
Chloroprocaine	30–60	–	11.4	14.2
Tetracaine	120–240	240–480	1.4	–
Amides				
Lignocaine	30–120	60–240	4.5	7
Mepivacaine	30–120	45–180	4.5	7
Bupivacaine	120–240	240–480	2.5	3.2
Etidocaine	200	240–360	4.2	5.7
Prilocaine	30–120	60–400	5.7	8.5

V. Ilankovan et al., *Local Flaps in Facial Reconstruction*,
https://doi.org/10.1007/978-3-031-49464-2_1

Deciphering Drug Concentrations and Dilutions

Concentrations: Drug concentration is expressed as a percentage (e.g. Bupivacaine 0.25%, Lignocaine 1%).

Percentage is measured in grams per 100 mL (i.e. 1% is 10 mg/mL, 1 g/100 mL, 1000 mg/100 mL).

Calculate the mg/mL concentration quickly from the percentage by moving the decimal point 1 place to the right, as follows:

Bupivacaine 0.25% = 2.5 mg/mL
Tetracaine 0.5% = 5 mg/mL
Lignocaine 1% = 10 mg/mL
Lignocaine 2% = 20 mg/mL
Benzocaine 20% = 200 mg/mL

Dilutions: When adrenaline is combined with an anaesthetic solution, the result is expressed as a dilution (e.g. 1:100,000).

1:1000 means 1 mg per 1 mL (i.e. 0.1%)
1:10,000 means 1 mg per 10 mL (i.e. 0.01%)
1:2000 means 1 mg per 2 mL (i.e. 0.05%)
1:20,000 means 1 mg per 20 mL (i.e. 0.005%)
0.1 mL of 1:1000 adrenaline added to 10 mL of anaesthetic solution = 1:100,000 dilution, or 0.01 mg/mL

Adrenaline content examples: From the information provided in Table 1.2 below, 50 mL of 1% lignocaine with adrenaline 1:100,000 contains 500 mg of lignocaine and 0.5 mg of adrenaline.

Table 1.2 Adrenaline content in solution

Solution volume	1:100,000 (1 mg/100 mL)	1:200,000 (1 mg/200 mL)
1 mL	0.01 mg	0.005 mg
5 mL	0.05 mg	0.025 mg
10 mL	0.1 mg	0.05 mg
20 mL	0.2 mg	0.1 mg

Tumescent Solution

Various combinations are described in the literature. The aim is to make the tissue planes "turgid" and to offer anaesthesia and haemostasis over a large area, while using the least amount of anaesthetic solution and minimising the systemic side effects. Our combination is as follows:

1. Normal saline—500 mL
2. 1% plain lignocaine—50 mL
3. 1:1000 adrenaline—1 mL
4. 10% sodium bicarbonate—6 mL

Sensory Nerve Supply to the Skin of Head and Neck

The cutaneous sensory nerve supply of the head and neck region is principally by the branches of the trigeminal nerve and cervical plexus, with smaller contributions from the other cranial nerves (Figs. 1.1 and 1.2).

Most of these nerves can be anaesthetised by nerve blocks, enabling surgical procedures to be carried out under local anaesthesia in addition to helping with post-operative analgesia.

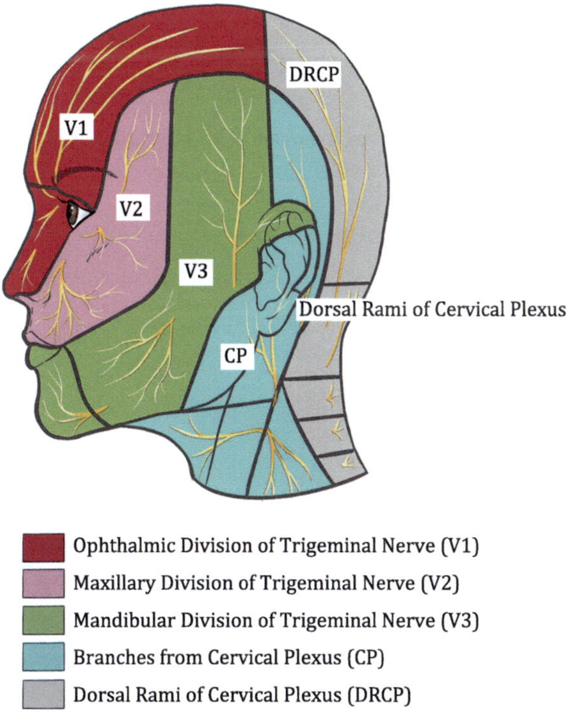

Fig. 1.1 Sensory nerve supply of the head and neck

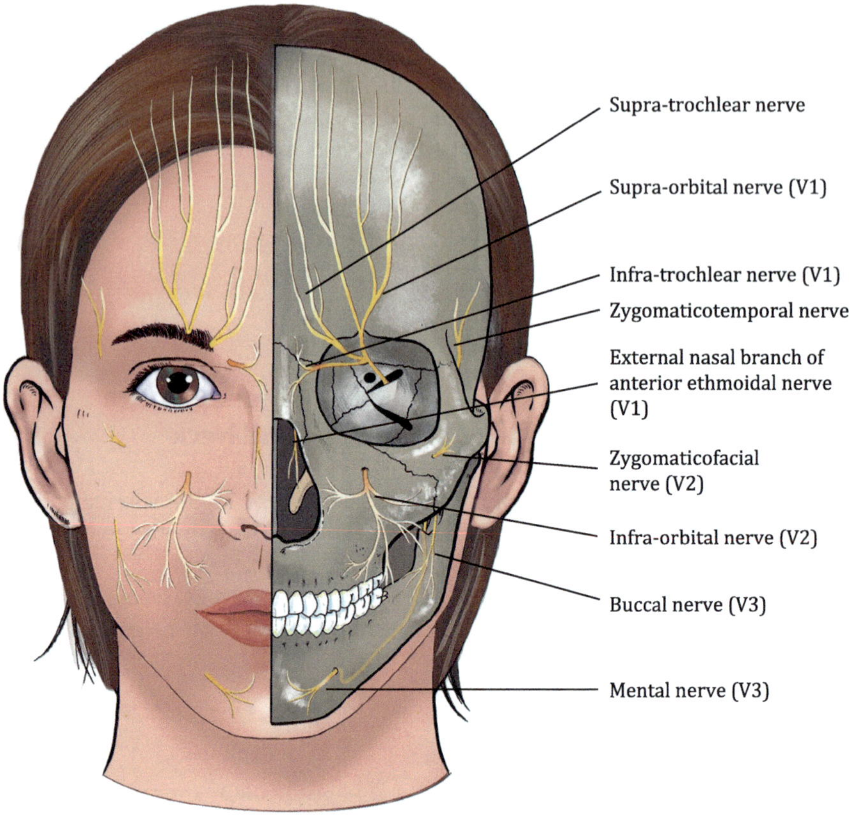

Fig. 1.2 Sensory nerves of the skin of the head and neck region and its relationship with the facial skeleton

Anaesthesia for Specific Areas

Forehead

Nerves: Supra-orbital, Supra-trochlear (Figs. 1.2 and 1.3).

Landmarks

Supra-orbital N: Emerges from the supra-orbital foramen along the vertical plane of the pupil.

Supra-trochlear N: Medial end of eyebrow, about 1.5 cm from midline.

Technique

Supra-orbital Nerve: Prepare skin using sterile technique. Request patient to look straight forward, palpate supra-orbital ridge and locate supra-orbital notch/foramen along vertical plane of pupil. Insert needle and raise a small skin wheal, advance needle 3–4 mm and deposit solution superior to foramen in a supra-periosteal location (±2 mL).

Supra-trochlear Nerve: Insert needle medial end of eyebrow, 1.5 cm from the midline and infiltrate anaesthetic in the subcutaneous tissues. Advance needle across the midline and deposit solution in a similar location to anaesthetise the contralateral nerve.

Area of Anaesthesia

Forehead: Up to lateral canthus, anterior scalp up to coronal plane.

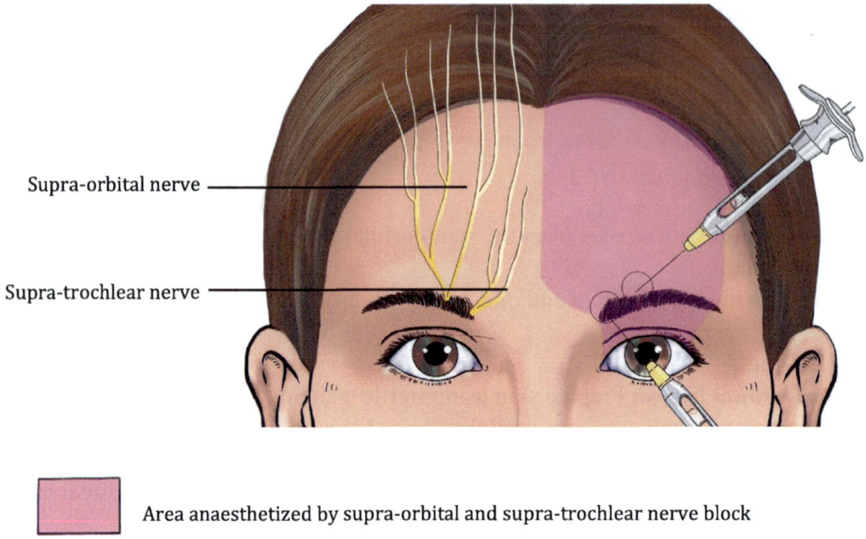

Fig. 1.3 Supra-orbital, supra-trochlear nerve block

Temple

Nerves: Zygomaticotemporal, Auriculotemporal (Figs. 1.2 and 1.4).

Landmarks
Zygomaticotemporal N: Emerges from the zygomaticotemporal foramen and pierces the temporal fascia 2.5 cm above the medial end of the zygomatic arch.

Technique
Prepare skin using sterile technique. Insert needle 2.5 cm above the medial end of the zygomatic arch, lateral to the lateral orbital rim and deposit solution into the subcutaneous tissues.

Area of Anaesthesia
Lateral forehead, medial temple.

Landmarks
Auriculotemporal N: Arises from the mandibular division of the trigeminal nerve, passes posterior to the neck of the condyle, runs superiorly crossing the root of zygomatic arch.

Technique
Prepare skin using sterile technique. Insert needle 2 cm above the tragus, just anterior to the superior attachment of the helix to the scalp and deposit solution into the subcutaneous tissues.

Area of Anaesthesia
Lateral temple, tragus, superior helix.

Caution
Avoid intra-vascular injection into superficial temporal vessels.

Risk of bruising, haematoma.

Paralysis: Temporal branch of facial nerve.

Image—Also see ear anaesthesia

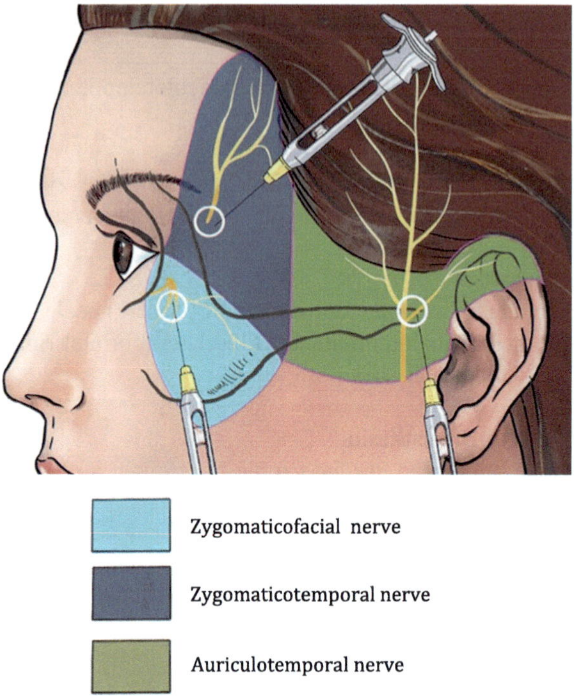

Fig. 1.4 Zygomaticotemporal, zygomaticofacial, auriculotemporal nerve block

Cheek

Nerves: Zygomaticofacial, infra-orbital (Figs. 1.2, 1.4, and 1.5).

Landmarks
Infra-orbital N: Emerges from the infra-orbital foramen along the vertical plane of the pupil, 1.5 cm below the bony infra-orbital rim.

Technique
Prepare skin using sterile technique. Ask patient to look straight ahead, palpate infra-orbital rim and insert needle 2 cm below infra-orbital rim along the vertical plane of the pupil. Deposit solution above periosteum, close to infra-orbital foramen.

Area of Anaesthesia
Cheek, lower eyelid, lateral nose, upper lip.

Landmark
Zygomaticofacial Nerve (Figs. 1.2 and 1.4)**:** Emerges from the zygomaticofacial foramen, 2 cm below and lateral to the lateral canthus.

Technique
Prepare skin using sterile technique. Insert needle 2 cm below and lateral to the lateral canthus. Deposit solution above periosteum, close to the nerve.

Area of Anaesthesia
Skin overlying zygomatic prominence, lateral lower eyelid.

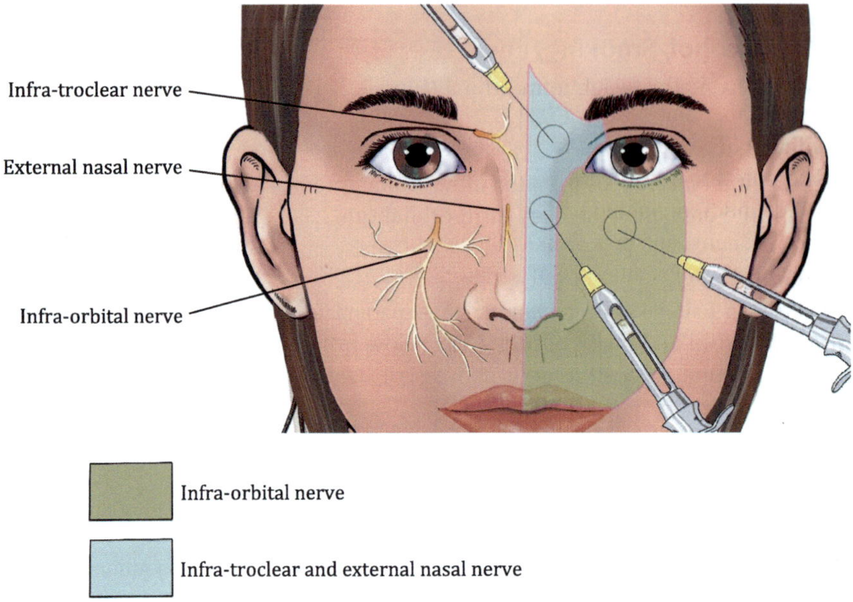

Fig. 1.5 Infra-orbital, infra-trochlear and external nasal nerve block

External Nose

Nerves: Infra-orbital, infra-trochlear, external nasal (Figs. 1.2 and 1.5).

Landmarks

Infra-trochlear N: Branch of the nasociliary nerve and emerges from the upper eyelid, 1 cm above the medial canthus.

Technique

Prepare skin using sterile technique. Insert needle 1 cm above medial canthus and infiltrate anaesthetic into the subcutaneous tissues.

Area of Anaesthesia

Upper nose, medial upper eye lid.

Landmark

External nasal N: Terminal branch of ethmoid nerve, emerges from the lower margin of the nasal bone, run on the surface of the upper lateral/alar cartilage, to the tip of nose, 1 cm from the midline.

Technique

Prepare skin using sterile techniques. Insert needle 1 cm lateral to midline, just inferior to the junction of nasal bone and upper lateral cartilage and deposit anaesthetic in the subcutaneous tissues.

Area of Anaesthesia

Mid, lower nose.

Landmark

Infra-orbital N: Emerges from the infra-orbital foramen along the vertical plane of the pupil, 1.5 cm below the bony infra-orbital rim.

Technique

Prepare skin using sterile technique. Ask patient to look straight ahead, palpatein-fra-orbital rim and insert needle 2 cm below infra-orbital rim along the verticalplane of the pupil. Deposit solution above periosteum, close to infra-orbital foramen.

Area of Anaesthesia

Cheek, lower eyelid, lateral nose, upper lip.

Lips

Upper Lip

Nerves: Infra-orbital (see Fig. 1.5).

Landmark

Infra-orbital N: Emerges from the infra-orbital foramen along the vertical plane of the pupil, 1.5 cm below the bony infra-orbital rim.

Technique

Prepare skin using sterile technique. Ask patient to look straight ahead, palpatein-fra-orbital rim and insert needle 2 cm below infra-orbital rim along the verticalplane of the pupil. Deposit solution above periosteum, close to infra-orbital foramen.

Area of Anaesthesia

Cheek, lower eyelid, lateral nose, upper lip.

Lower Lip/Chin

Nerves: Mental nerve (Fig. 1.6).

Landmark

Mental N: Emerges from the mental foramen, 2 cm above the lower border of mandible, along the vertical plane of pupil.

Technique

Prepare skin using sterile techniques. Ask patient to look straight ahead. Palpate lower border of mandible and insert needle 2 cm above lower border, along the vertical plane of the pupil. Deposit solution in the supra-periosteal plane close to the mental foramen.

Area of Anaesthesia

Lower lip, chin.

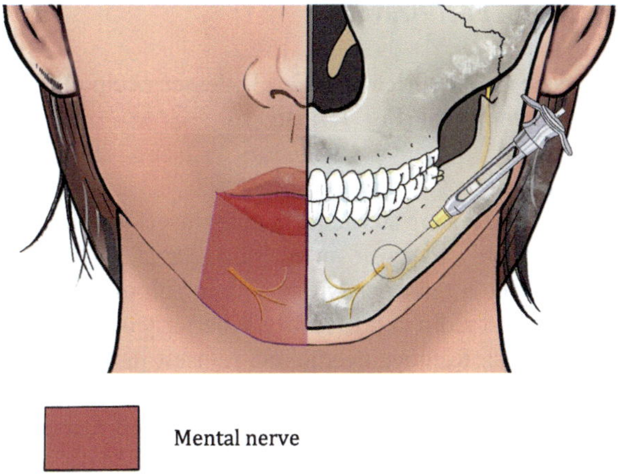

Fig. 1.6 Mental nerve block

External Ear/Pinna

Nerves: Great auricular (C2,C3), lesser occipital (C2), auricular branch of vagus, auriculotemporal (Fig. 1.7a and b).

Technique

Prepare skin using sterile technique. Insert needle into skin below the attachment of the earlobe and raise small skin wheal. Advance needle anteriorly/superiorly towards the tragus, depositing solution along the way. Withdraw needle, but do not remove and redirect posteriorly/superiorly along auriculocephalic sulus and deposit anaesthetic. Remove needle and reinsert just above attachment of helix and direct needle anteriorly/inferiorly towards tragus, depositing solution along the way. Withdraw needle, but do not remove and redirect posteriorly/inferiorly along auriculocephalic sulcus and deposit anaesthetic. Make sure that the solution is deposited all around the base of the pinna. Additional infiltration is required in the concha, to anaesthetise the area supplied by the auricular branch of vagus (Fig. 1.7c–e).

Area of Anaesthesia

Great auricular: Skin overlying angle of mandible, lower/middle cranial surface of pinna and ear lobe.

Lesser occipital: Posterior scalp adjacent to pinna and upper/middle cranial surface of pinna.

Auriculotemporal: Upper part of lateral surface of pinna and part of meatal skin.

Auricular branch of vagus: Part of meatal and adjacent conchal skin.

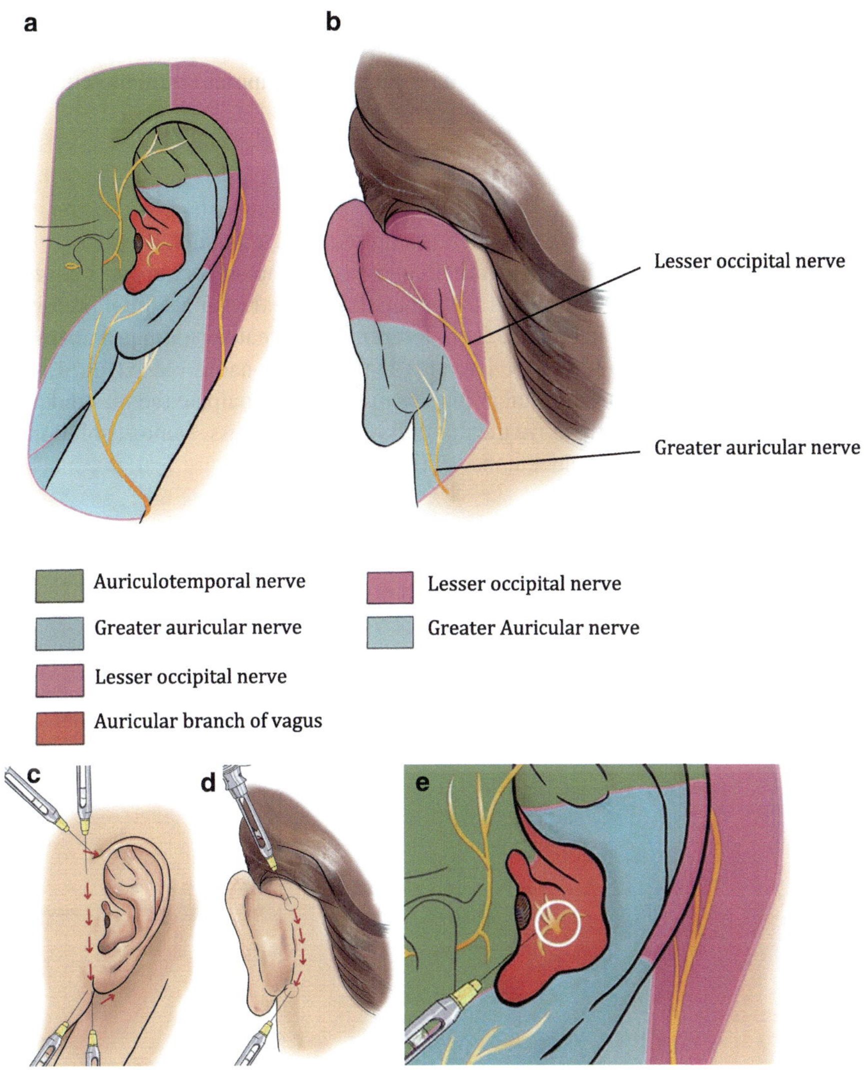

Fig. 1.7 (**a**) Nerve supply external ear/pinna, (**b**) Nerve supply external ear/pinna—posterior surface, (**c**) Local anaesthesia for pinna, (**d**) Local anaesthesia for pinna, (**e**) Vagus branch block for conchal area

Scalp

Nerves: Supra-trochlear, supra-orbital, zygomaticotemporal, auriculotemporal, lesser occipital (C2), greater occipital (C2), third occipital (C3) (Figs. 1.1, 1.2, 1.3, 1.4, and 1.8a, b).

Technique

For anaesthesia of the anterior and lateral scalp see Figs. 1.3 and 1.4.

Greater Occipital/Third occipital: Request patient to sit forward and slightly flex head. Prepare skin using sterile technique. Palpate external occipital protuberance. Insert needle 2 cm lateral and 2 cm inferior to external occipital protuberance and deposit solution in a fan-shaped manner in the subcutaneous plane (Fig. 1.8a).

Lesser occipital: With the patient in the same position, palpate the mastoid process and insert needle 2 cm above the tip of the mastoid process. Deposit solution in a fan-shaped manner in the subcutaneous tissue (Fig. 1.8b).

Area of Anaesthesia

Great occipital: Majority of posterior scalp up to vertex.

Third occipital: Small area of lower part posterior scalp.

Lesser occipital: Scalp posterior and superior to pinna.

Caution

Intra-vascular injection/damage to occipital artery.

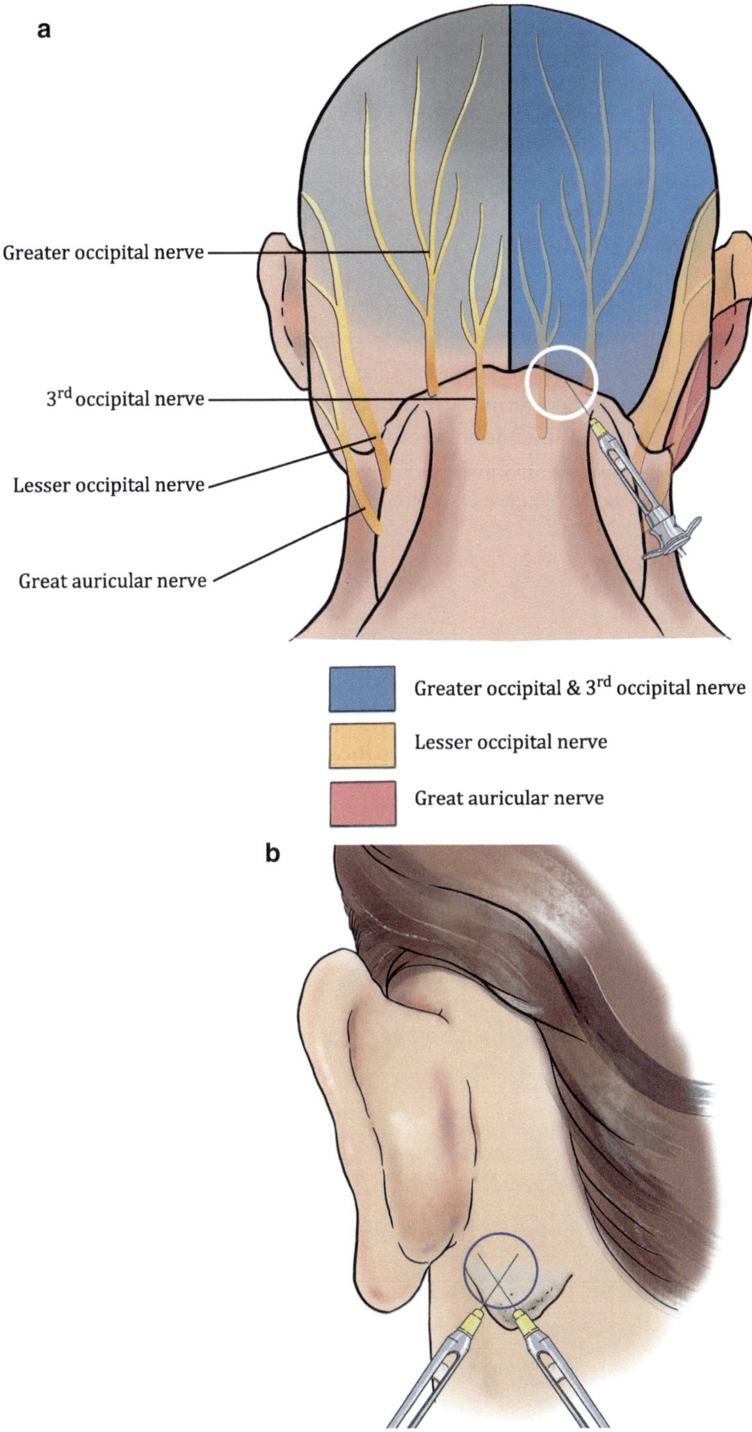

Fig. 1.8 (**a**) Local anaesthesia of posterior scalp, (**b**) Local anaesthesia of posterior scalp

Neck

Nerves: Great auricular, transverse cervical, supra-clavicular, lesser occipital (anterior primary rami of C2–C4) (Fig. 1.9a and b).

Landmark
The nerves emerge as individual nerves at the midpoint of the posterior border of the sternocleidomastoid muscle.

Technique
Turn the patients head to the opposite side to define the SCM. Confirm the position of the mastoid process and the Chassaignac's tubercle (CT) of C6. The fingers are stretched to outline the posterior border of SCM, mastoid process and CT. The site of needle insertion is at the midpoint of the line connecting the mastoid process to the CT. Deposit solution subcutaneously, 2–3 cm around the midpoint to achieve anaesthesia of all the four nerves. Avoid deep needle penetration.

Area of Anaesthesia
Anterior/lateral neck.

Caution
Haematoma (aspiration and avoid multiple injection).

Phrenic and accessory nerve blockade (avoid deep injections and bilateral blockade in patients with significant respiratory disease).

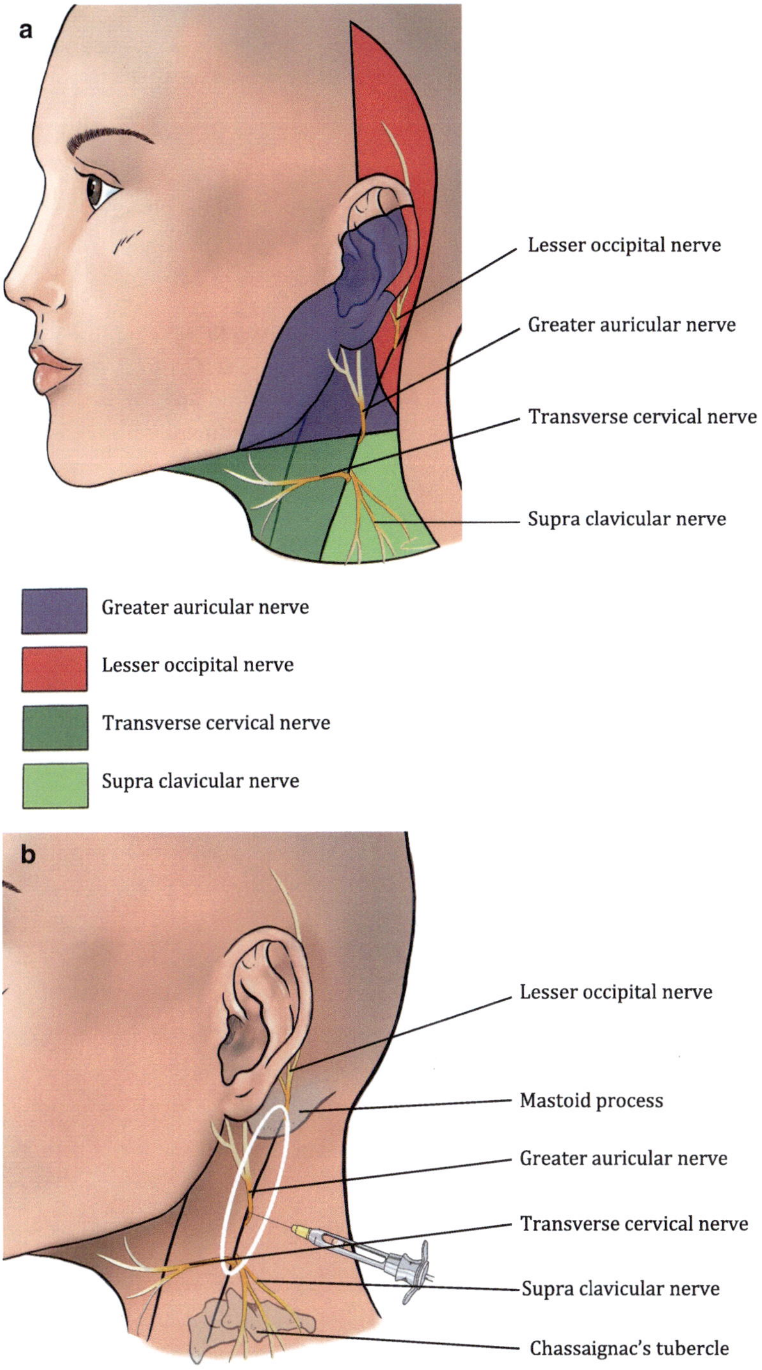

Fig. 1.9 (**a**) Sensory nerve supply of anterior/lateral neck. (**b**) Local anaesthesia of anterior/lateral neck

Facial Units and Subunits

2

The decision to reconstruct facial defects needs to take into account various factors, which includes the final aesthetic outcome. Aesthetic aspects are more important in the face than almost any other part of the body. An understanding of the concept of facial aesthetic units and subunits and the factors influencing the placement of incisions/scars can help the clinician obtain the most cosmetically pleasing outcome.

Relaxed skin tension lines (RSTL) described by Borges result from the orientation of the collagen fibres in the skin (Fig. 2.1). They are manifested as furrows/creases when the skin is relaxed and can be made more prominent by pinching. The furrows extend for longer and are made with greater ease when the skin is pinched at right angles to the RSTL. Wrinkle lines described by Kraissl are formed at right angles to the underlying muscle fibres and are made more prominent in response to differing facial expressions. They often, though not always, follow the RSTLs. The above should not be confused with Langer's lines, who described "cleavage lines" in a cadaver and were never intended to delineate the ideal lines for incisions.

RSTLs are perpendicular to the *lines of maximum extensibility (LME),* which are dependent on the orientation and stretching of the elastic fibres. Where possible, the excisions and flaps repair should be made parallel to the RSTL as this will place the maximum closure tension to be parallel to the LME and perpendicular to the RSTL. There are exceptions (e.g. lower eyelid), and these will be discussed in the relevant chapters.

The face can be divided into specific areas, designated as *"aesthetic units,"* within which the skin has similar characteristics. These characteristics include colour, thickness, amount of subcutaneous fat, texture and presence of hair. These "units" are separated from each other by relatively well-defined ridges and creases, designated as *"aesthetic borders."* The borders include easily discernable landmarks such as the hair line, eyebrows, nasolabial fold, philtrum, vermillion border and labiomental fold.

V. Ilankovan et al., *Local Flaps in Facial Reconstruction*,
https://doi.org/10.1007/978-3-031-49464-2_2

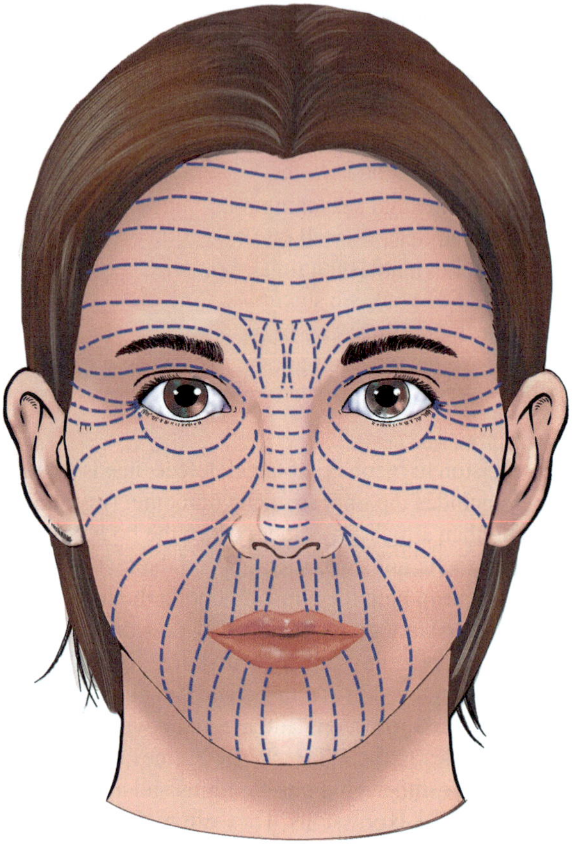

Fig. 2.1 Orientation of RSTLs

The principle aesthetic units of face are the forehead, eyelids, nose, cheek, lips, chin and pinna. To this can be added the scalp and the neck, to encompass the "head and neck" region (Fig. 2.2).

Some of the principle aesthetic units can be further subdivided into smaller areas designated *"aesthetic subunits,"* which are separated by less discrete borders than that which separate the aesthetic unit (Fig. 2.3).

Some publications refer to the aesthetic units as aesthetic regions. In this book, the term aesthetic unit will be used as defined above. Similarly, some publications refer to the aesthetic subunits as aesthetic units, topographical subunits, etc. In this book, the term aesthetic subunit will be used as defined above.

The aesthetic units can be further categorised for reconstructive purposes, and these will be discussed in greater detail in the next few pages.

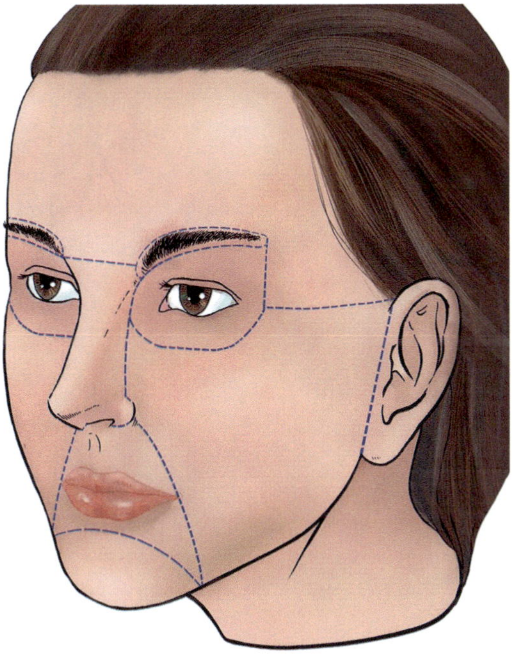

Fig. 2.2 Aesthetic units

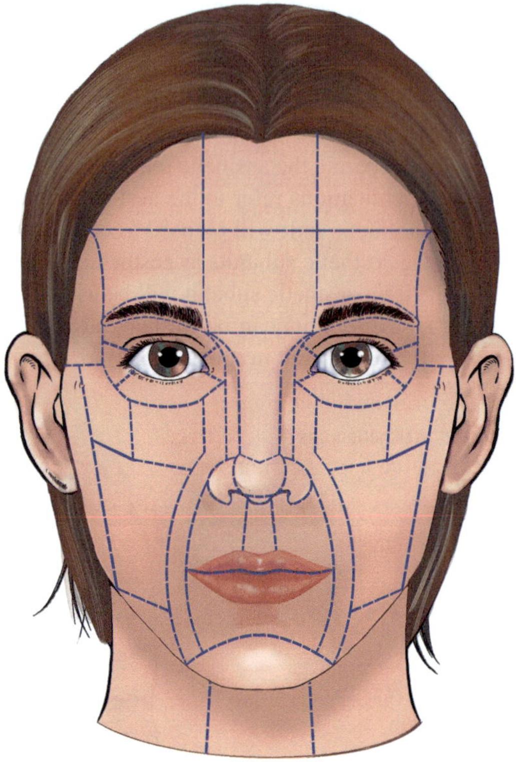

Fig. 2.3 Aesthetic subunits

Forehead

The aesthetic unit of the forehead is defined by the frontal hairline superiorly, temple and temporal hairline laterally and the eyebrow and glabella inferiorly. It is immediately obvious that hair loss can affect the superior extent of the forehead, which can be modified by hair styling!

The unit can be further subdivided vertically into central, lateral and temporal subunits and in addition, from the reconstructive point of view, horizontally into lower and upper forehead (Fig. 2.4). The central subunit represents the area between the medial ends of the eyebrow. The lateral subunit extends from the medial eyebrow to the lateral orbital rims. The temple subunit extends from the lateral orbital rim to the zygomatic arch.

The principal skin creases are horizontally oriented across the forehead, except for its vertical orientation in the glabella region and an obliquely radiating orientation from the lateral canthus in the temporal region (crow's foot) (Fig. 2.1).

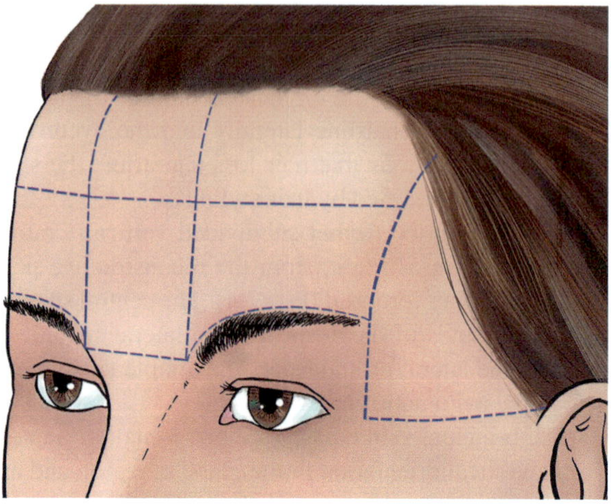

Fig. 2.4 Subunits of the forehead

Cheek

The cheek is the largest aesthetic unit in the face. It has an undulating contour and is defined by the nasofacial, melolabial and mentolabial folds medially, infra-orbital rim and zygomatic arch superiorly, pinna and angle of the mandible posteriorly and the lower border of the mandible inferiorly.

It can be divided into medial, infra-orbital, buccal, lateral, zygomatic, and mandibular subunits for reconstructive purposes (Fig. 2.5).

The medial subunit consists of skin adjacent to the nasofacial, nasolabial and mentolabial folds. The infra-orbital unit lies below the orbital rim, between the medial and zygomatic units. The buccal subunit encompasses the central cheek area lateral to the medial unit. The lateral subunit is the area adjacent to the pinna and angle of the mandible. The zygomatic subunit is between the buccal unit and temple, and the mandibular subunit is the area overlying the body of the mandible.

The skin in the subunits of the cheek varies in their characteristics. Reconstructive options should take into account adjacent tissue laxity and the likelihood of distorting the surrounding landmarks (eyelids, nose, lips and pinna).

Scars are best placed along the aesthetic borders, and consideration should be given to extending the defect, especially in the medial and lateral subunits. When this is inappropriate, scars are best designed to be parallel to the RSTL. The RSTLs in the cheeks are curvilinear or radially fan out from the lateral canthus area (crow's foot) and offer excellent camouflage for the scars. The skin creases are more prominent in the elderly and can be made more obvious by requesting the patient to smile and shut their eyes tight (Fig. 2.1).

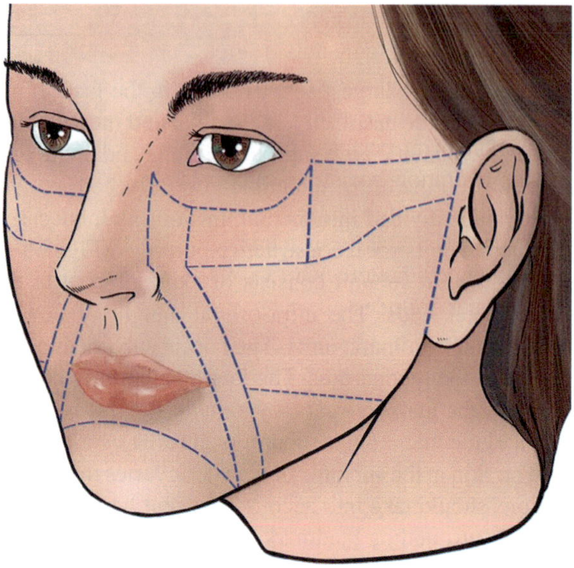

Fig. 2.5 Cheek subunits

Nose

The nose is a complex structure and lends itself to being divided into further subunits, separated by less discrete borders. It is typically divided into nine subunits; columella, tip, dorsum and paired sidewalls, ala and nasal facets (Fig. 2.6).

The complex three-dimensional shape is supported by a bony and cartilaginous framework. The overlying skin is of varying thickness and mobility, and the deep surface is lined by mucous membrane. The concept of "subunit" reconstruction was initially popularised for the nose and often involves altering the size, shape and depth of the defect to reconstruct a "full subunit" so that the scars lie in the most advantageous positions and deceive the eye. There are exceptions to these guidelines and these, along with the other aspects will be discussed further in the chapter on nasal reconstruction.

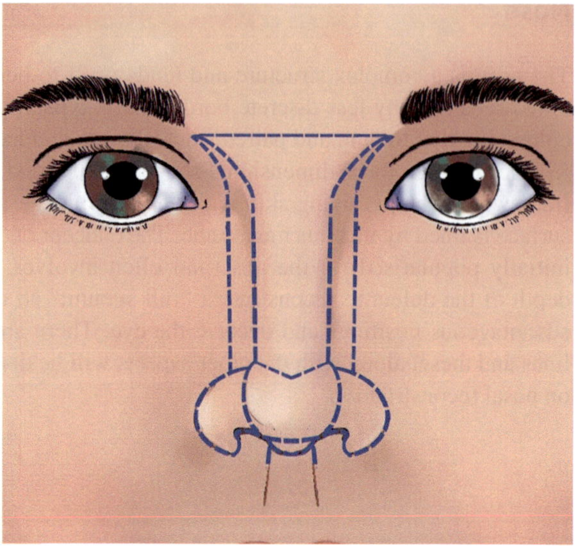

Fig. 2.6 Nasal subunits

Lips

The upper and lower lips have prominent aesthetic and social connotations and form a distinct facial aesthetic unit. The lip unit is defined by the base of the nose superiorly, nasolabial fold laterally and mentolabial fold inferiorly. The lip aesthetic unit can be divided into the cutaneous upper lip, cutaneous lower lip and the vermillion subunits. The upper lip can be further divided into a philtrum and two lateral subunits (Fig. 2.7).

The lip is a composite structure made up of skin, muscle and mucosa. The mucocutaneous junction is defined by the vermillion border and represents a very important facial landmark. The RSTLs are oriented radially around the oral stoma and are vertical in the central region and oblique in the lateral aspects.

Lip reconstruction needs to address both aesthetics and function. Satisfactory function requires the presence of intact sensory and motor nerves and restoration of the orbicularis oris muscle sphincter.

Ideally tissue mobilised from within the lip complex provides the best match. Incisions should be placed parallel to the perioral rhytides for simple excisions. It is extremely important not to distort the vermillion border, and its precise approximation is mandatory. Flaps mobilised from the adjacent areas should ideally have their incisions along the aesthetic borders (base of nose, vermillion, nasolabial and mentolabial folds). Consideration should be given to modifying the defect, to place the scar in the most advantageous position.

The specific reconstructive options will depend on a multitude of factors, including the presence of full and partial thickness defects. These will be discussed in greater detail in the session on lip reconstruction.

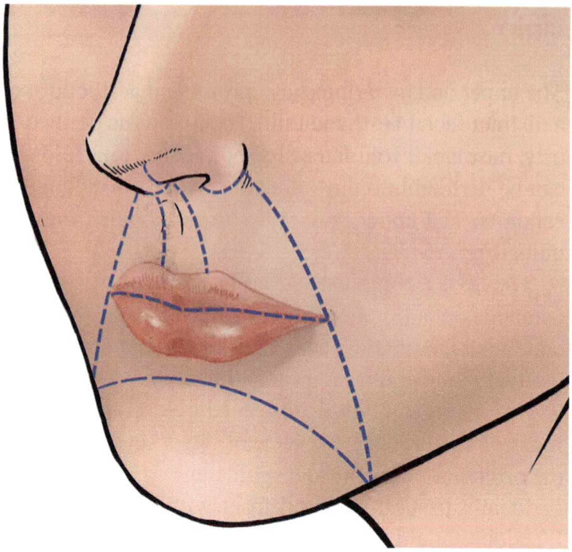

Fig. 2.7 Lip subunits

Chin

The chin unit is defined by the mentolabial fold superiorly and laterally and the lower border of the mandible inferiorly (Fig. 2.8). The RSTLs are arranged in a curvilinear pattern, and scars are ideally designed to lie parallel to these.

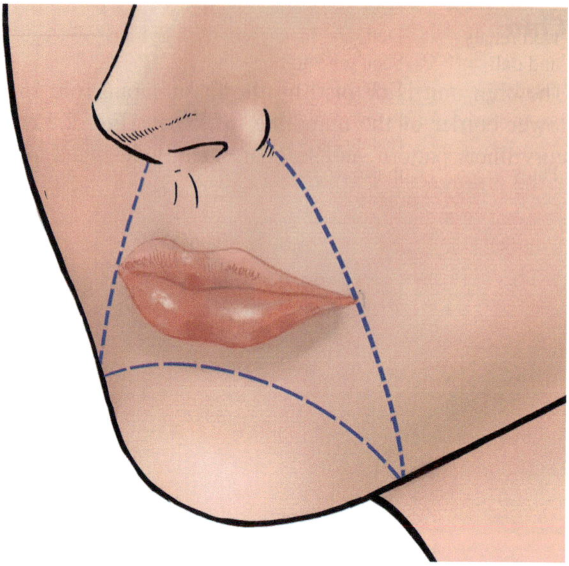

Fig. 2.8 Chin subunits

Pinna

The pinna is a structure made up of a complex three-dimensional cartilaginous framework and draped by skin on the lateral and medial aspects. The goal of reconstruction is to try and preserve the shape, size and position of the pinna. Knowledge of the different parts of the pinna is essential for reconstruction (Fig. 2.9).

The pinna lies between horizontal lines drawn from the superior orbital rim and the nasal spine. It protrudes from the scalp at an angle of 25°–35°.

The skin on the lateral surface is thin and densely adherent to the underlying cartilage, whereas the posterior skin in thick and more mobile. The auricular cartilage is supple and can be easily deformed by wound tension and scar contracture. Scars can be camouflaged in the many undulations of the pinna. Local flap reconstruction often results in a decreased height of the pinna, but when the shape is maintained, is surprisingly inconspicuous.

The specific aspects of ear reconstruction will be discussed in the session on ear reconstruction.

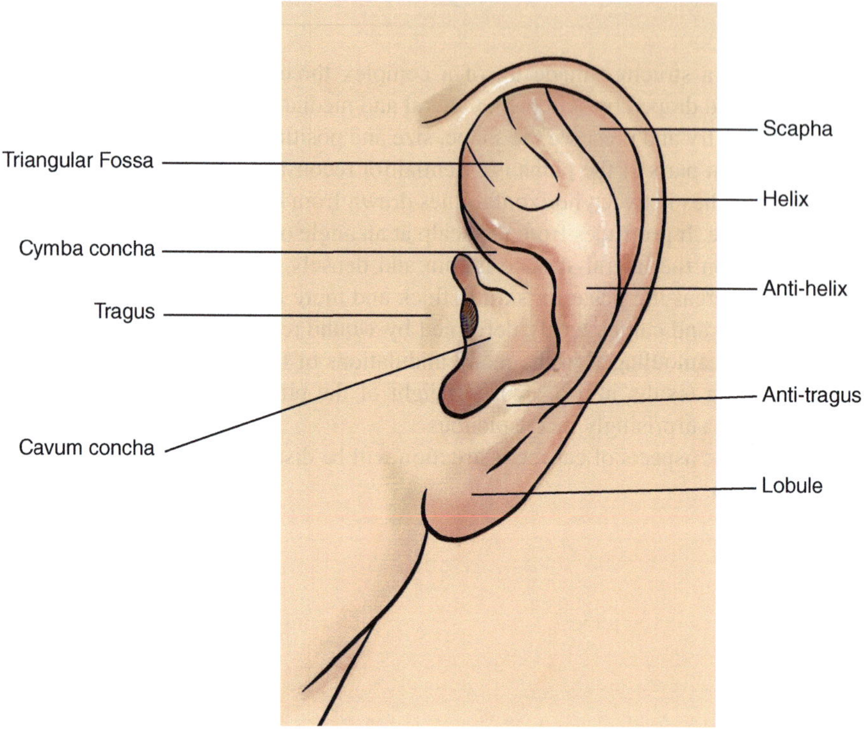

Fig. 2.9 Pinna—Landmarks

Eyelids

Eyelids perform many important functions, which include protection of the eye and maintaining an adequate tear film. The aesthetic eyelid unit is defined by the lower margin of the eyebrow, lateral and inferior orbital rims and the nasojugal fold. A sound understanding of anatomy and function is essential for eyelid reconstruction and should only be attempted by an appropriately trained clinician.

The eyelids are complex multi-layered structures supported by cartilaginous tarsal plates. The free lid margin contains eyelashes and secretory glands, and the extension of the tarsal plates forms the medial and lateral canthal tendons.

Reconstruction could be more easily understood if the eyelids were considered to consist of an **anterior lamella** composed of skin and orbicularis oculi and a **posterior lamella** composed of conjunctiva, tarsal plate, orbital septum and the lid retractors. The orbital septum is occasionally considered the middle lamella, and the "grey line" along the lid margin represents the junction between the anterior and posterior lamellae.

The eyelid aesthetic unit can be further subdivided from a reconstructive point of view into upper lid, lower lid, medial canthus and lateral canthus subunits (Fig. 2.10).

The skin of the eyelid is the thinnest in the body, and the RSTLs around the eyelids are horizontally oriented. However, excision parallel to the RSTLs, especially in the lower lid, runs the risk of eyelid retraction and ectropion. It is therefore preferable to orient excisions to be perpendicular to the lid margins unless there is significant skin redundancy. Excisions along the RSTL in the adjacent lateral and medial canthus, eyebrow and glabella regions can be performed and will provide relatively unobtrusive scars.

Full-thickness defects require reconstruction of both the anterior and posterior lamella, in which case it is mandatory that at least one of the reconstructed lamella should contain its own blood supply.

There are many factors to be considered before a decision is made to reconstruct an eyelid defect and these will be described in more detail in the session on eyelid reconstruction.

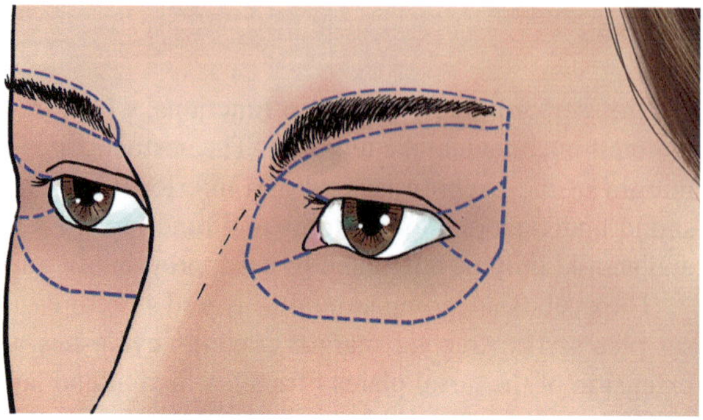

Fig. 2.10 Eyelid subunits

Scalp

The anatomical layers of the scalp are well described by the acronym "SCALP." The layers of the scalp in the temporal region are more complex and will be described in greater detail in the session on scalp reconstruction.

The extent of the "scalp" unit varies with the presence of hair. As scars can often be hidden, it is easier to consider the subunits of the scalp in terms of its differential mobility. It can be divided into relatively tight and loose areas (Fig. 2.11a, b).

Scalp mobility varies according to its location and constituent structures. Above the temporal line, the scalp is tight, contains a dense galeal layer, has no underlying muscle and poorly distensible. Below the temporal line, the scalp is relatively mobile, were the galea becomes the temporo-parietal fascia, which is thinner, overlies muscles and is more distensible.

The thickness of the scalp varies with the presence of hair and becomes thinner with hair loss. The nerves and vessels run within the galeal layer. The first three layers are firmly adherent to each other.

A detailed knowledge of anatomy and variations in the mobility is essential for scalp reconstruction. The scalp has a rich blood supply, which enables large random pattern flaps to be raised, which is often necessary due to the relative inelasticity of the scalp tissue.

The size, location, thickness (full/partial) of the defect and the necessity to preserve hair and the hair line are some of the factors that needs to be taken into account, when deciding on the most appropriate reconstructive option.

Primary closure and small local flaps can be used in the mobile regions of the scalp, but larger flaps and other means of reconstruction are often required to reconstruct defects in the tight regions of the scalp.

The reconstructive options and the factors to be considered will be discussed in greater detail in the session on scalp reconstruction.

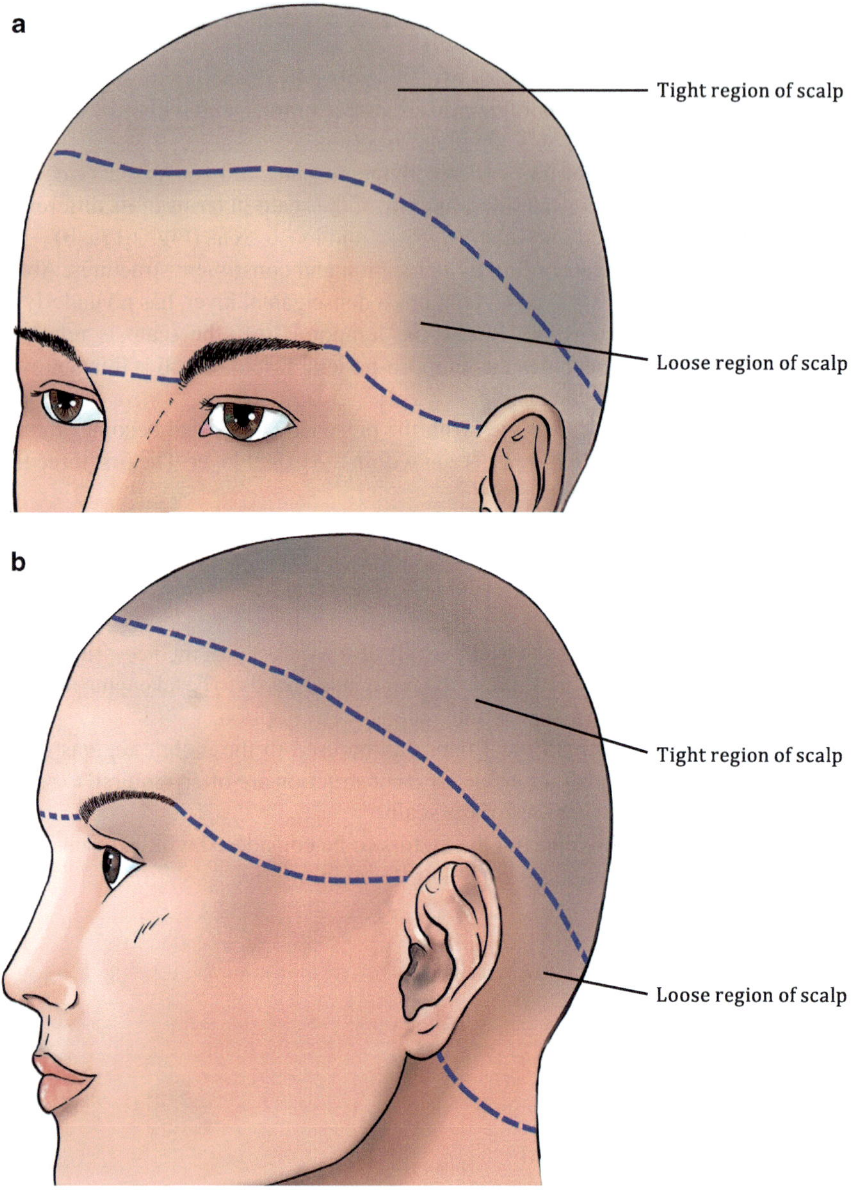

Fig. 2.11 (**a**) Scalp, oblique view (loose and tight regions). (**b**) Scalp, profile view (loose and tight regions)

Neck

The circumferential neck unit can be defined superiorly by the lower border of the mandible anteriorly and the hair line posteriorly. The inferior limits are the clavicle anteriorly and the upper border of the scapula posteriorly. The neck can be divided into anterior and posterior subunits, with the anterior subunit, being further divided into a midline and two lateral units (Fig. 2.12).

The thickness and mobility of the neck skin vary with the location and are often defined by the age of the person and general body habitus. The RSTLs are obliquely and transversely oriented in the neck.

The skin redundancy and the RSTLs allow flaps to be raised in the neck to reconstruct a variety of neck and adjacent defects, with good aesthetic outcomes. It also enables relatively large defects to be closed primarily.

A detailed knowledge of the anatomy, especially of the underlying nerves and vessels is essential to avoid damaging these structures. The various factors to be considered and the reconstructive options for neck defects will be discussed in the session on neck reconstruction.

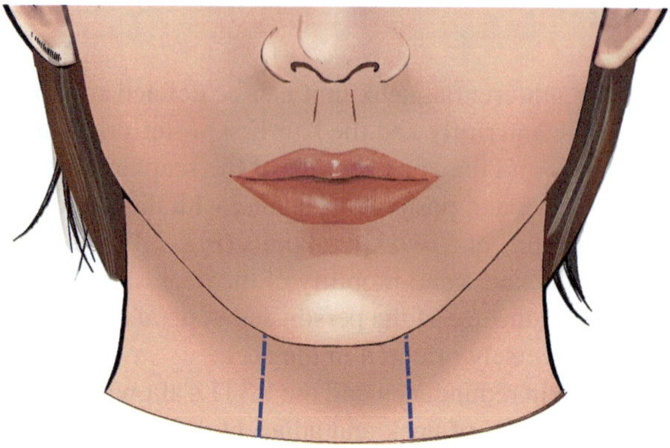

Fig. 2.12 Neck sub units

Basic Flaps

3

Advancement Flaps

These are flaps that are moved forward (advanced) into the defect by primarily a sliding and stretching movement. One of the margins of the defect will form the leading edge of the flap. They are most useful where there is tissue laxity immediately adjacent to the defect. The most common types of advancement flaps are unilateral and bilateral advancement flaps, island advancement flaps and less common V-Y and Y-V advancement.

In unilateral and bilateral advancement flaps, two parallel incisions are made from the base of the defect, preferably along RSTLs and the surrounding tissues widely undermined and the defect closed in layer (Fig. 3.1a–g). The defect is often modified to obtain parallel edges. The length of the defect to flap ratio is preferably restricted to 1:3, and it is vitally important to avoid tension during closure. A combination of a long thin flap closed under tension is a recipe for wound breakdown.

In the case of bilateral advancement flaps (Fig. 3.1h–n), one flap is first raised to assess the necessity and if required, the dimensions of the second flap.

Tips: The margins of the flap and the adjacent tissue are of unequal length due to its design. In addition, the flap is often thinner. These have to be taken into account during closure, which can be accommodated by differential suturing and excision of Burrow's triangle.

The incisions, though often parallel, can diverge slightly to obtain a broader pedicle and more appropriate placement of the scars.

The primary defect is closed initially and the adjacent margins subsequently. It is often easier to place all the sutures along the advancing margins, prior to tying of the sutures. The location Burrow's triangle can be placed anywhere along the margins for best placement of the scars.

V. Ilankovan et al., *Local Flaps in Facial Reconstruction*,
https://doi.org/10.1007/978-3-031-49464-2_3

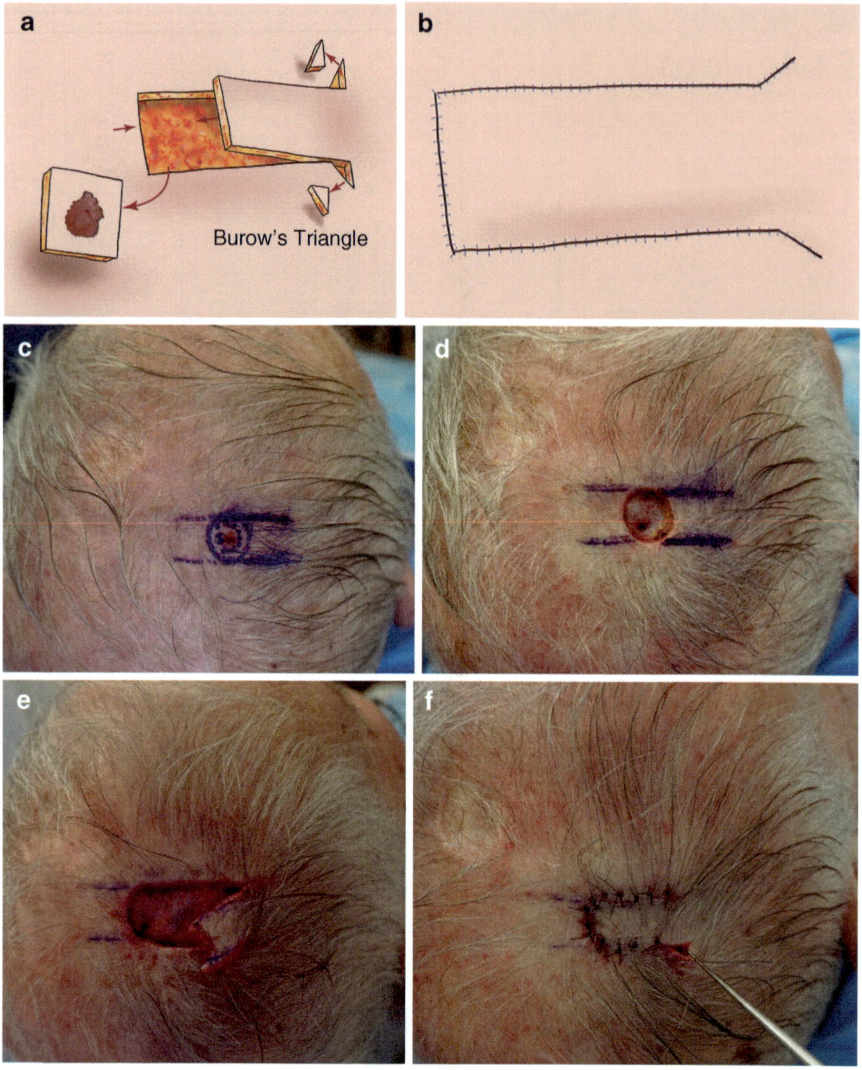

Fig. 3.1 Advancement flaps. (**a–g**) Unilateral advancement flap, (**h–n**) Bilateral advancement flap. (**a**) Excision defect and flap raised, (**b**) Final closure, (**c**) Excision and flap marking, (**d**) Defect following excision, (**e**) Flap raised in sub-galeal flap, (**f**) Flap advanced into defect with dog ear, (**g**) Final result follwing excison of dod ear, (**h**) Excison and flap marking, (**i**) Excison defect and flaps raised, (**j**) Final closure, (**k**) Skin markings, (**l**) Excision defect and flap incisions, (**m**) Flaps raised in subgaleal plane, (**n**) Final closure

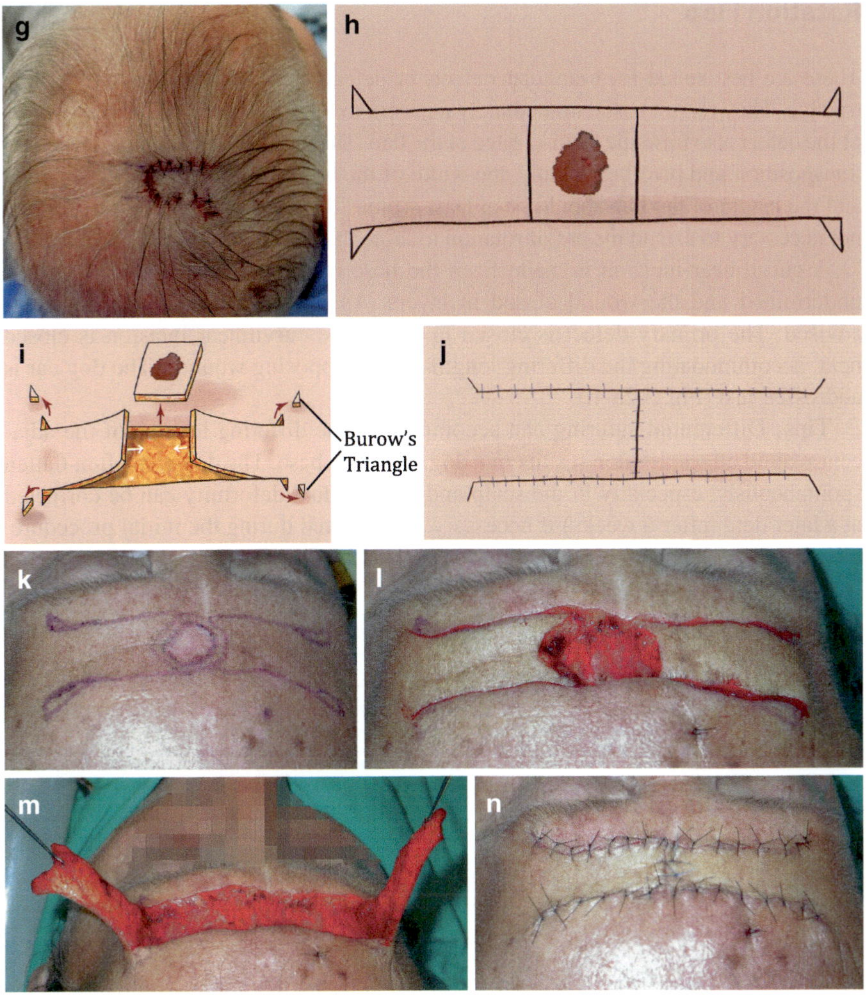

Fig. 3.1 (continued)

Rotation Flap

These are best suited for triangular defects or defects that could be converted into a triangle. They recruit tissue immediately adjacent to the defect, and one of the borders of the defect also form the leading edge of the flap. The principal movements are lateral transposition and pivoting. Ideally, the width of the defect should be twice the height and the length of the flap should be at least 4 times the width of the defect. It is often not necessary to extend the arc of rotation to more than 90° to the axis of the defect.

A curvilinear incision is made from the base of the defect, the tissues widely undermined and the wound closed in layers. An orderly sequence of closure is advised. The primary defect is closed first, and the curvilinear incision is closed next, accommodating the differing lengths of the opposing wounds. The dog ear is addressed last (Fig. 3.2a–h).

Tips: Differential suturing can accommodate the differing lengths of the adjacent wound edges. It often results in a dog ear at the base. The dog ears often flatten spontaneously, especially in the scalp and any residual deformity can be corrected at a later date (after 6 weeks) if necessary. If corrected during the initial procedure, this should be done outside the circumference of the flap, to avoid compromising its vascularity.

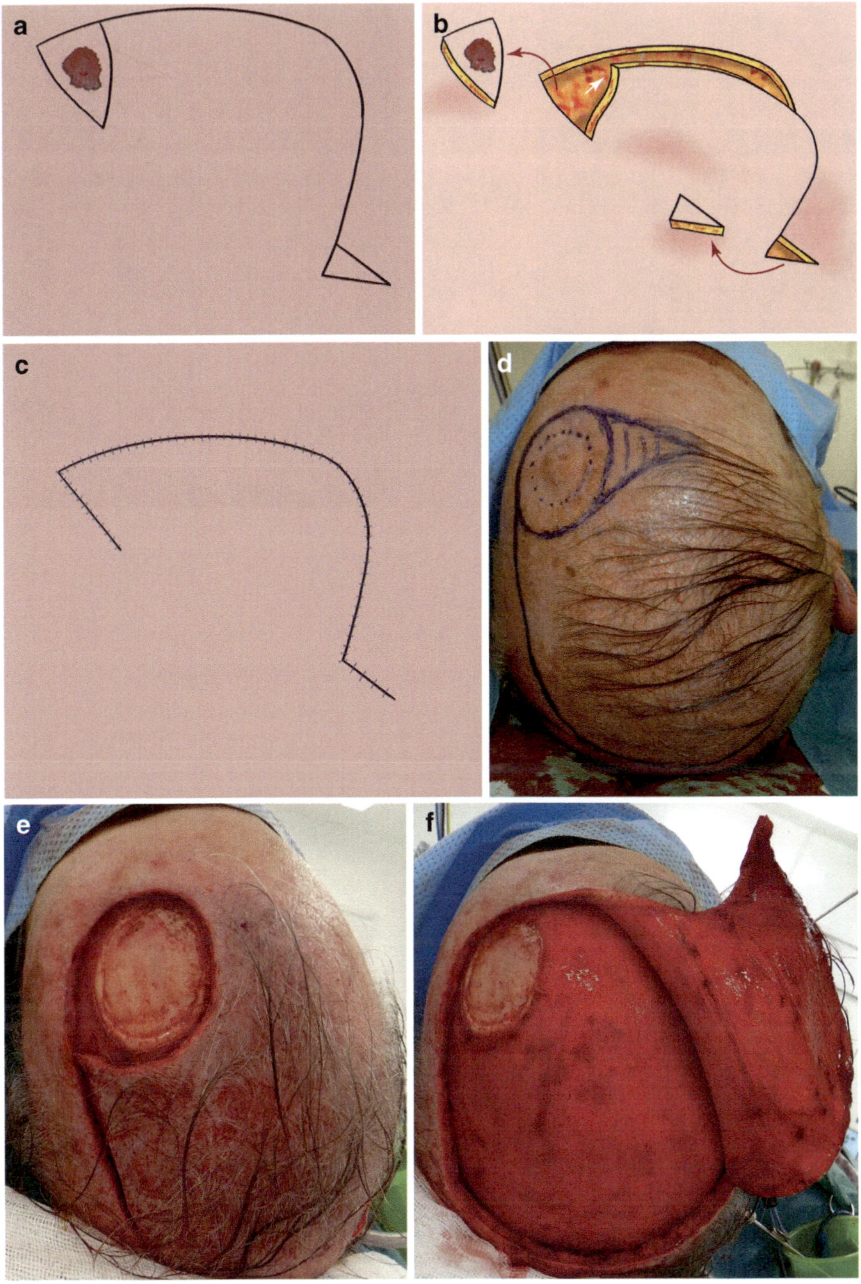

Fig. 3.2 Rotation flap. (**a**) Skin markings of excison and flap, (**b**) Excison defect and flap raised, (**c**) final closure, (**d**) Skin marking for excision and flap, (**e**) Excision defect and flap incision, (**f**) Flap raised with galeal scoring, (**g**) Closure with dog ears insitu, (**h**) Late result with spontaneous settling of dog ear

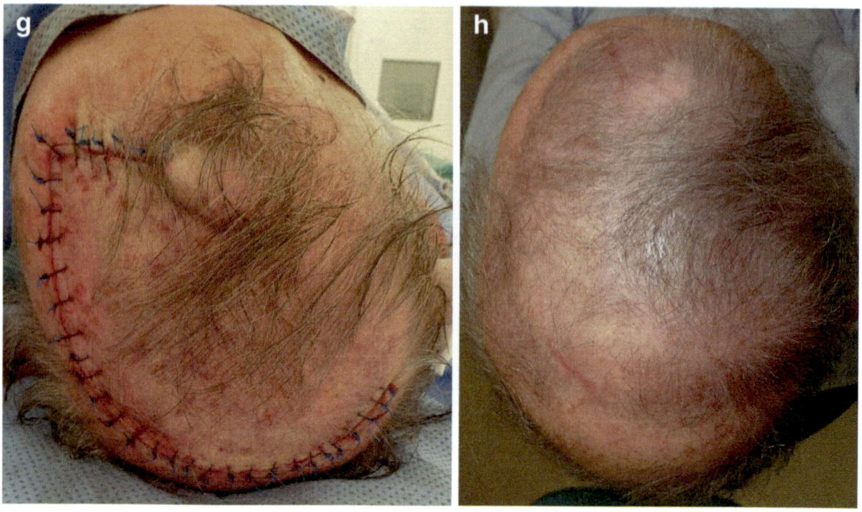

Fig. 3.2 (continued)

Transposition Flap

Transposition flaps can be used to reconstruct defects of various shapes. The principal movement is lateral, and the flap recruits tissue immediately adjacent to or distant to the defect. One of the margins of the defect will form one of the margins of the flap. This could be along most of the length of the flap or just the base, depending on whether the tissue is recruited immediately adjacent or distant (with intervening tissue) to the defect.

Unlike rotation and bilobed flaps, transposition flaps have a linear configuration, which enables the scar to be more easily placed along RSTLs and aesthetic borders. The lateral transposition leads to a decrease in the effective length of the flap and this will have to be taken into account when designing the flap. Similarly, the greater the arc of movement the greater the size of the dog ear.

In the case of the standard transposition flap, two parallel incisions are made along the proximal edge of the defect, the width of which is equal to the width of the defect. The length of the flap should be longer than the defect, to account for the decrease in effective length and pointed ends to facilitate linear closure. The flap is often raised in the subcutaneous plane and mobilised into the defect. The adjacent margins are undermined, and the wound is closed in layers. An orderly sequence of closure is advised, with closure of the secondary defect carried out initially followed by appropriate trimming of the flap and closure of the primary defect. The dog ear is addressed last (Fig. 3.3a–j).

Tips: The length of the flap can be up to three times the width, though this could be marginally exceeded in the face, provided there is no tension. Dog ears are excised away from the base of the defect to avoid vascular compromise. The thickness of the flap might have to be reduced to accommodate the defect characteristics (Fig. 3.3i).

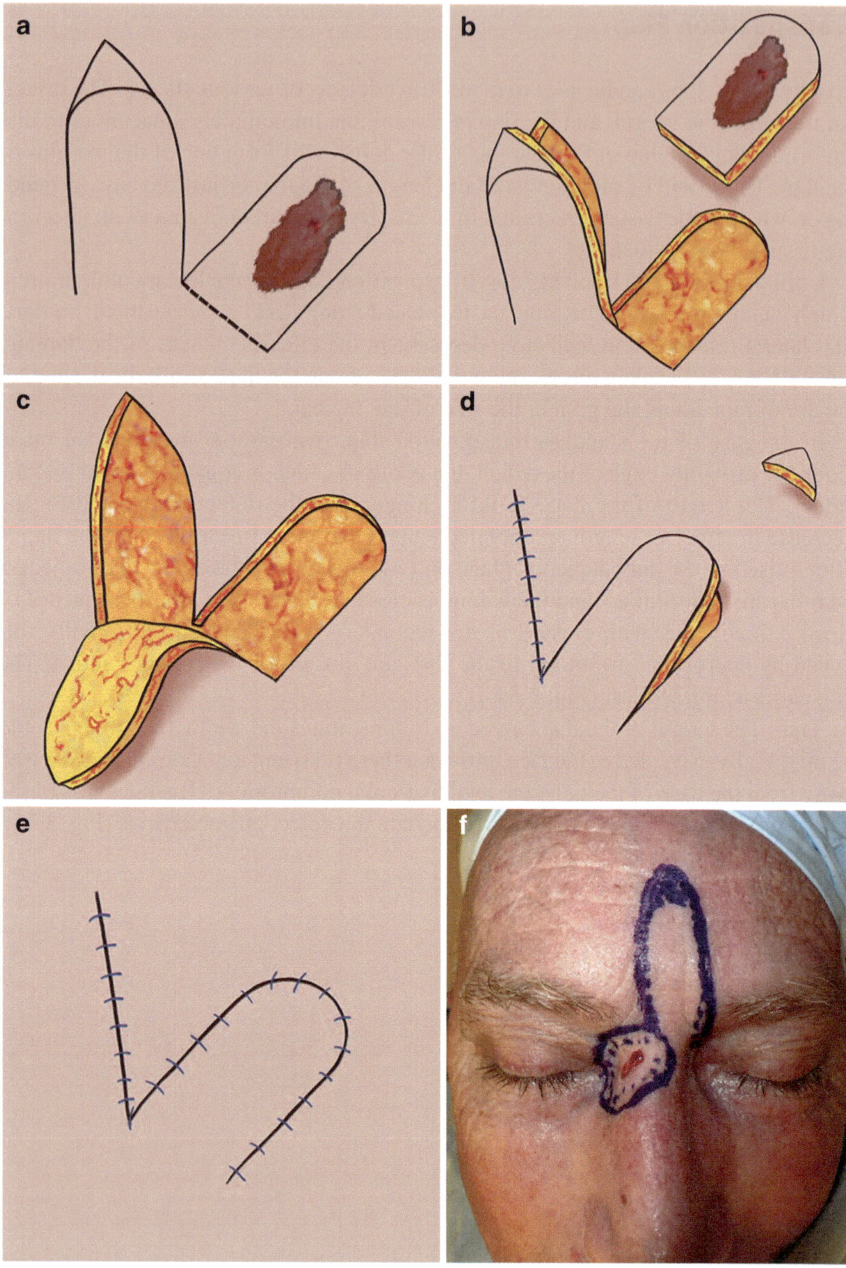

Fig. 3.3 Transposition flap. (**a**) Markings for excision and flap, (**b**) Excision defect and flap incisions, (**c**) Flap raised, (**d**) Closure of secondary defect and flap insitu, (**e**) Final closure, (**f**) Markings for excision and flap, (**g**) Excision defect and flap raised, (**h**) Trial flap transposition, (**i**) Closure of secondary defect and "thining" of flap, (**j**) Final closure

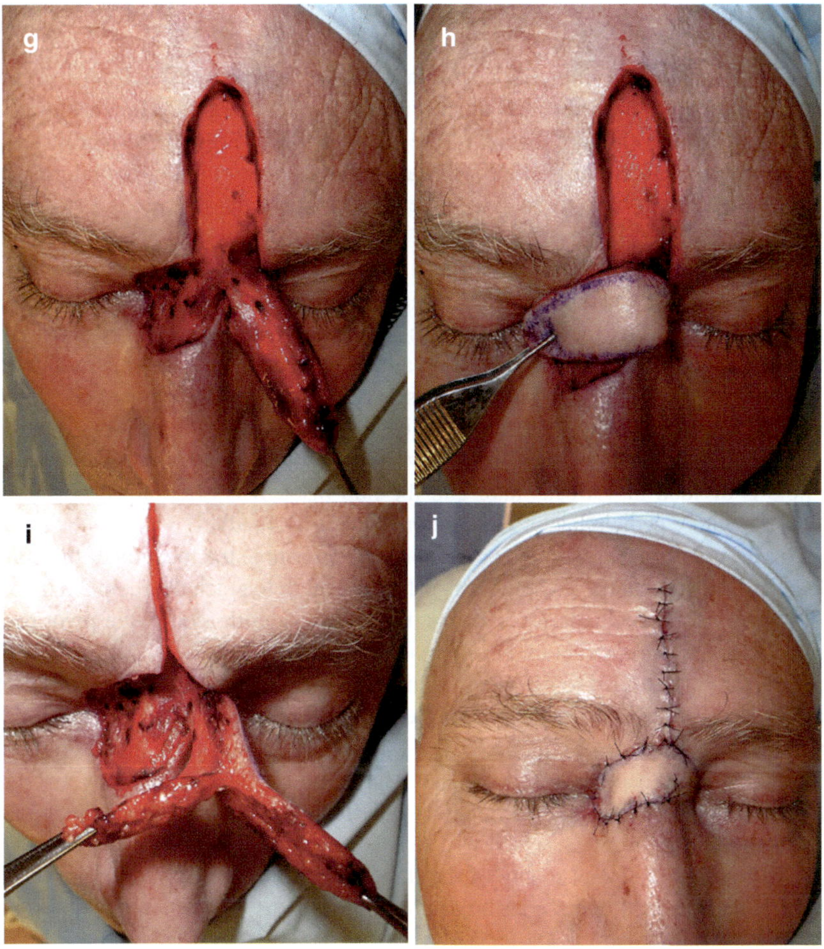

Fig. 3.3 (continued)

Interpolated Flap

These are similar in configuration to transposition flaps, but differ from it in that none of the flap margins is in contact with the defect margins. They are used to reconstruct defects that are distant to the donor site and are able to recruit tissue away from the defect. The pedicle will have to cross over or under the intervening tissue, which might have to be disconnected at a later date, making it a two-stage procedure.

The flap can be utilised to reconstruct defects of various shapes. A template is made of the defect and trial transfer carried out with a piece of string or length of gauze, to confirm that the flap will reach the defect. The flap is raised, with care being taken to avoid damage to its vascular supply. Depending on whether the flap is an axial pattern (based on a named vessel) or random pattern (no named vessel), the base of the pedicle can be narrow or of adequate width. The flap is sutured in place and the donor site closed primarily, by undermining the wound edges. The pedicle is divided in 4 weeks later and the flap inset. It is often not necessary to return the whole pedicle back to the donor site (Fig. 3.4a–d).

Tips: A trial transfer should be carried out to determine the location of the donor site and to ensure that the pedicle is of sufficient length to reach the recipient defect. Allowance should be made for loss of effective flap length around the pivot point and necessity to cross structure before reaching the defect.

If the flap is designed to go under the intervening tissue, a section of the pedicle can be de-epithelised to make it a single-stage procedure. The tunnel created to accommodate the pedicel will have to be of sufficient dimensions, not to compromise the vascular pedicle, which will also have to take into account any swelling that is likely to occur in the post-operative period. The tunnelled pedicle can also lead to contour deformities, which will have to be taken into account.

As the defect is distant to any of the flap margins, it is possible to preserve the aesthetic margins and boundaries adjacent to the defect.

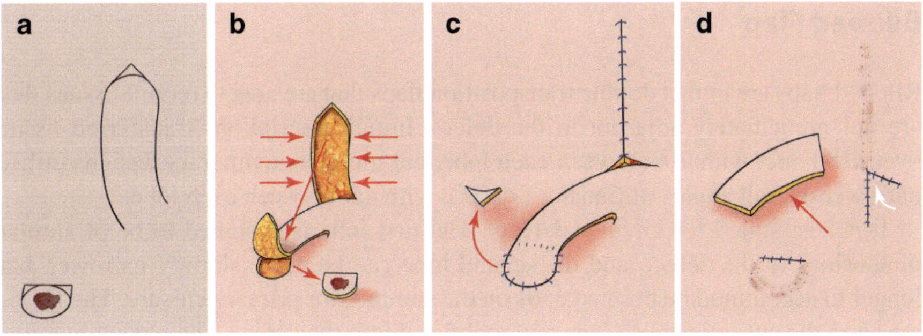

Fig. 3.4 Interpolated flap. (**a**) Markings for excison and flap, (**b**) Flap raised and transposed into defect, over bridge of intact skin, (**c**) Closure of secondary defect followed by flap inset, (**d**) Delayed division of pedicle and final closure

Bilobed Flap

Bilobed flaps are in fact double transposition flaps that are able to recruit tissues that are not immediately adjacent to the defect. Initial descriptions transferred tissue over a180° arc, with 90° between each lobe, but more contemporary designs utilise narrower overall angles of transfer ($<100^{\circ}$), with 45° between each lobe.

It is best suited for circular defects. The first lobe is designed to be of similar dimensions to the defect, and the second lobe can be made slightly narrower, but longer to accommodate pointed ends on the summit, for primary closure. The flap is raised in the subcutaneous plane and mobilised into the defect. The wound margins are widely undermined and the defect closed in layers. Closure is best carried out in an orderly sequence; the tertiary defect is closed first, followed closure of the primary defect. The flap covering the secondary defect is appropriately trimmed and closed next, and the dog ear is addressed last (Fig. 3.5a–n).

Tips: The flap is designed to best utilise the tissue laxity, avoid distorting adjacent structures and placement of scars. Due to curvilinear incisions, it is not possible to accommodate all the scars along RSTLs and there is a tendency for "pin cushioning" of the flap. This can be partly mitigated by modifying the defect and flap margin to include right-angled corners and parallel wound margins.

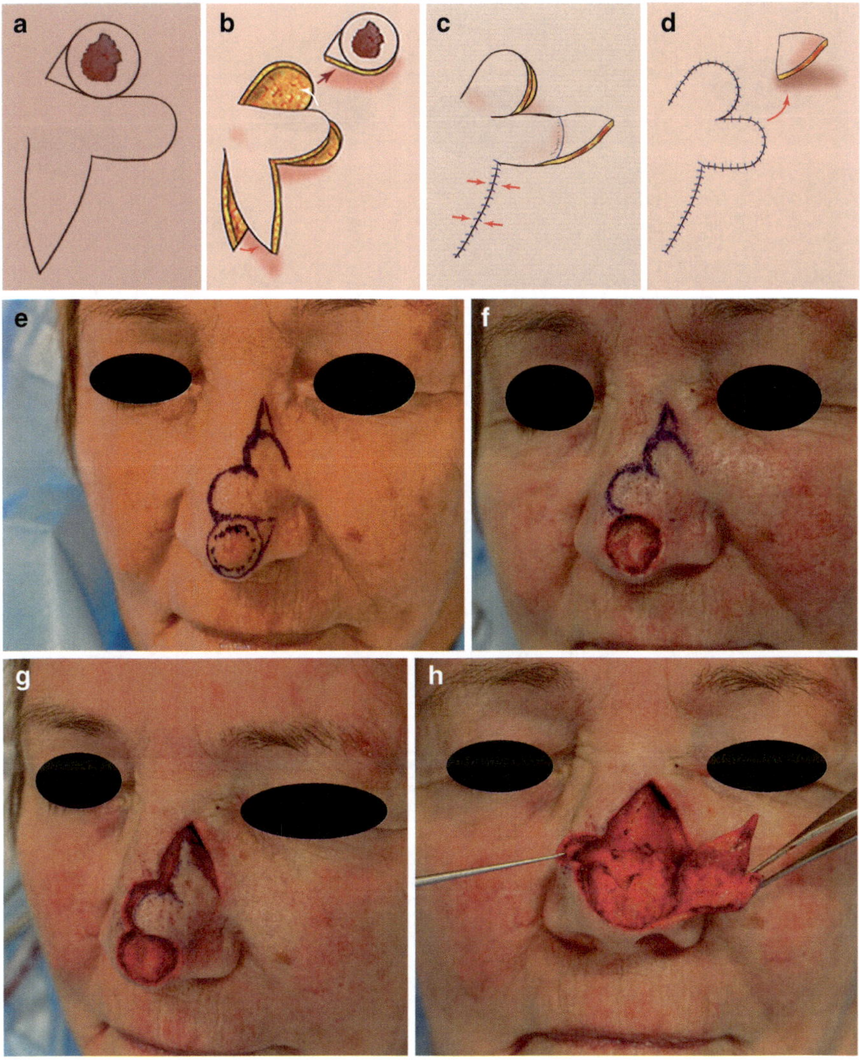

Fig. 3.5 Bilobed flap. (**a**) Markings for excision and flap, (**b**) Excision defect and flap incisions, (**c**) Closure of tertiary defect and flap contoured into the primary defect, (**d**) Final closure after contouring of secondary defect and dog ear, (**e**) Markings for excision and flap, (**f**) Excision defect, (**g**) Flap incisions, (**h**) Flaps raised and wide undermining, (**i**) Closure of tertiary defect, (**j**) Flap inset into primary defect, (**k**) Revision and inset of flap into secondary defect, (**l**) Dog ear, (**m**) Final closure after correction of dog ear, (**n**) Late result with no further revisions

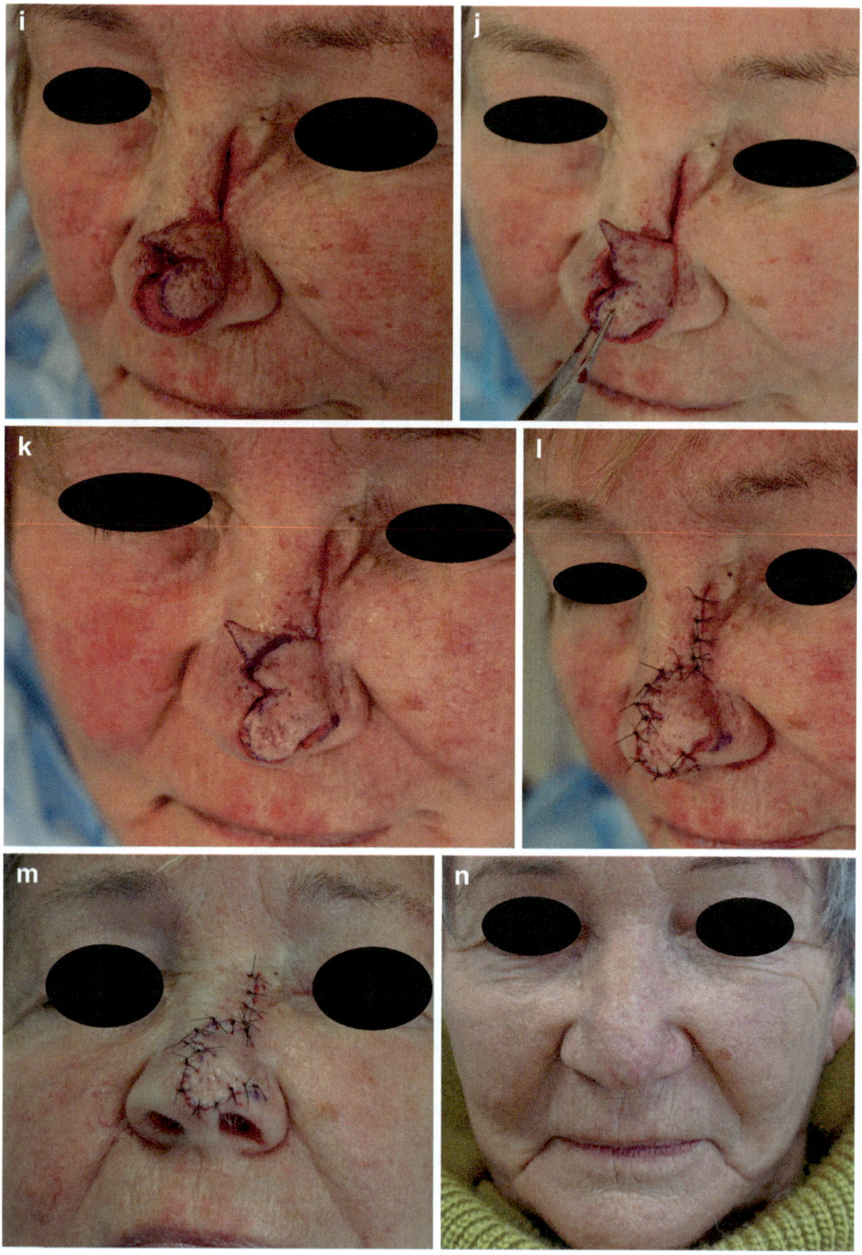

Fig. 3.5 (continued)

Island Flap

These flaps can be used to reconstruct defects of a variety of shapes. The flap recruits tissue immediately adjacent or distant to the defect. When tissue is harvested immediately adjacent to the flap, one of the defect margins commonly forms the leading edge of the flap. When harvested from a distant site, the pedicle has to traverse a bridge of skin (over or under), which might have to be divided at a later date, making it a two-stage procedure.

The skin around all the borders of the flap is incised, and the sub-cutaneous tissue beneath is preserved to act as the pedicle. The flap devoid of marginal skin attachments is then moved into the defect to aid reconstruction. The wound edges are undermined widely, taking care to preserve an adequate amount of subcutaneous pedicle. The wound is closed in layers, and an orderly sequence of closure is advised. The primary defect is closed initially, followed by the secondary defect, which can be closed primarily. The principal movements are advancement or transposition (Fig. 3.6a–k).

Tips: The dimensions of flap harvested immediately adjacent to the defect will have to be larger than the defect to account for loss of effective length during transfer and to maintain a sufficient amount of sub-cutaneous pedicle to aid vascularity. The flap margin away from the defect is triangulated to aid primary closure.

In the case of harvesting a flap from a distant site, the pedicle can be tunnelled under the intervening bridge of skin to make it a single stage procedure or over it for a two-staged procedure. The tunnel created to accommodate the pedicel will have to be of sufficient dimensions, not to compromise the vascular pedicle, which will also have to take into account any swelling that is likely to occur in the post-operative period. The tunnelled pedicle can also lead to contour deformities, which will have to be taken into account.

In selected cases, it may be necessary to incise the skin (only) outside the confines of the flap, as a relieving incision and the required undermining of the surrounding tissue can be performed with adequate retraction (Fig. 3.6l–q)

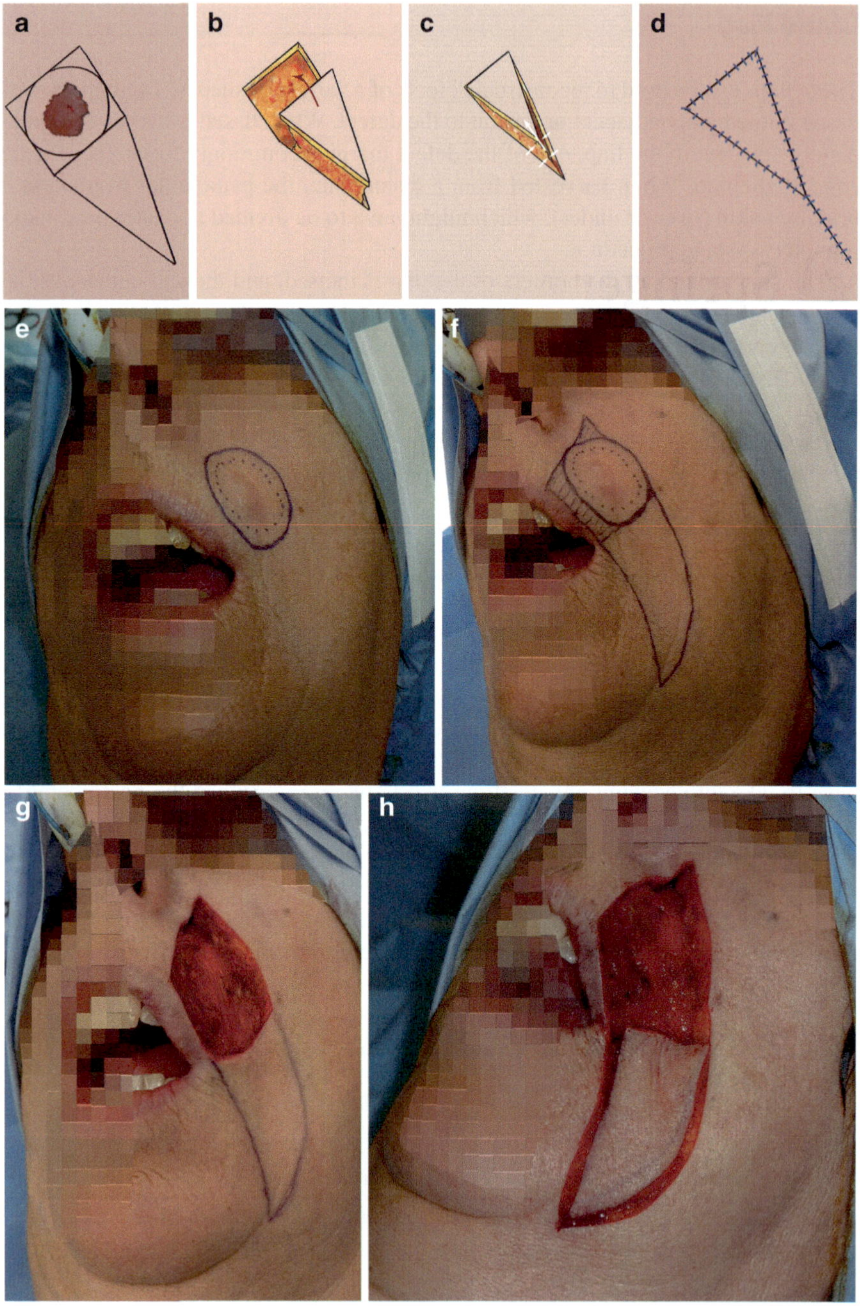

Fig. 3.6 Island flaps. (**a**) Markings for excision and flap, (**b**) Excision defect and flap incisions, (**c**) Flap moved into defect maintaining subcutaneous pedicle, (**d**) Final closure, (**e**) Markings for excision, (**f**) Markings of flap and modification of excision margins, (**g**) Excision defect, (**h**) Flap incisions, (**i**) Maintaing a subcutaneous pedicle, (**j**) Flap moved into defect, (**k**) Final closure, (**l**) Markings for excision and flap, (**m**) Excision defect and flap incisions of varying depth, (**n**) Flap moved into defect, (**o**) Final closure, (**p**) Markings for excision and flap, (**q**) Final closure

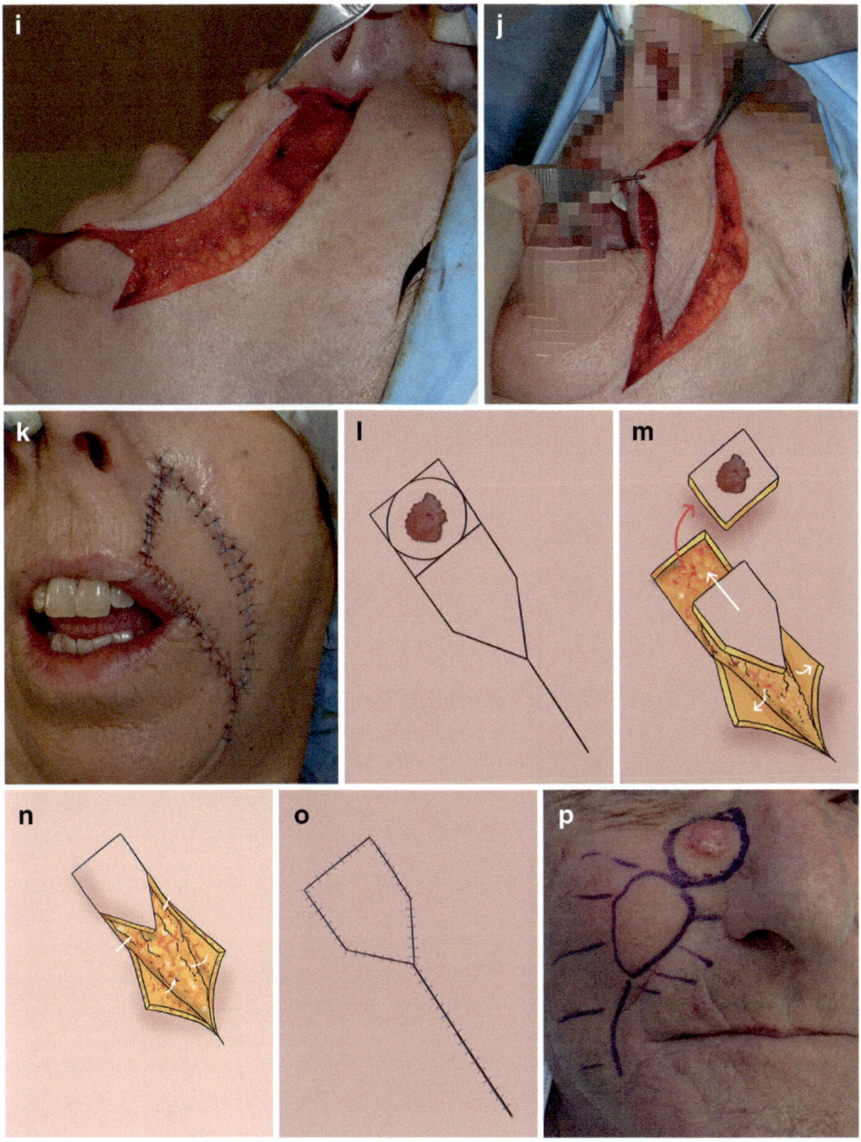

Fig. 3.6 (continued)

Fig. 3.6 (continued)

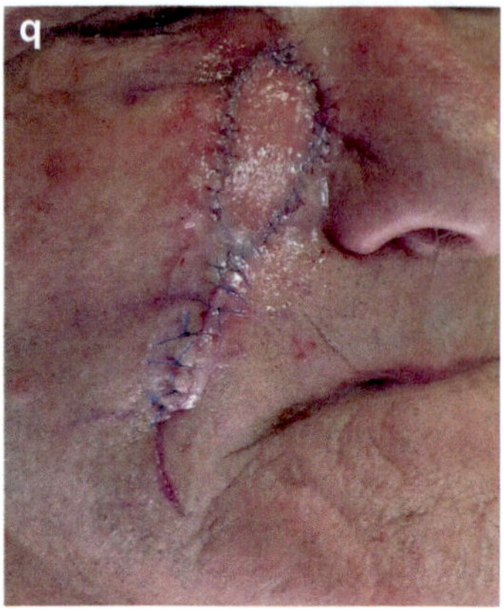

Rhombic Flap

The rhombic flap is a type of transposition flap, first described by Limberg following work on paper models. The defect and the flap are based on very specific geometric designs.

The defect is converted into a rhombus, with 60° and 120° internal angles. A rhombus is similar to two equilateral triangles, whose bases are placed on each other. This results in a defect in which all the sides and the short diagonal are of equal length. The flap is designed by extending the short diagonal to a distance equal to one of the sides, and a further line is drawn from its extremity, parallel to the adjacent side of the defect, again of equal length. It is possible to harvest four flaps for each rhombic defect. The flap is raised in the subcutaneous plane and mobilised into the defect. The wound margins of the wound are undermined and the defect closed in layers. An orderly sequence of closure is advised, with closure of the secondary defect carried out initially followed by that of the primary defect. The dog ear is corrected last (Fig. 3.7a–q).

Tips: For any rhombic defect, four potential flaps can be harvested. The final decision is based on the availability of tissue laxity, the best placement of scars and avoiding distortion of the adjacent structures. In practice, it is often possible to minimise or avoid excision of additional tissue to achieve the rhombic configuration, when using this flap. This often results in a dog ear at the base that might have to be corrected. Similarly, angulating the short diagonal can increase the tissue availability to cover the distal end of the defect.

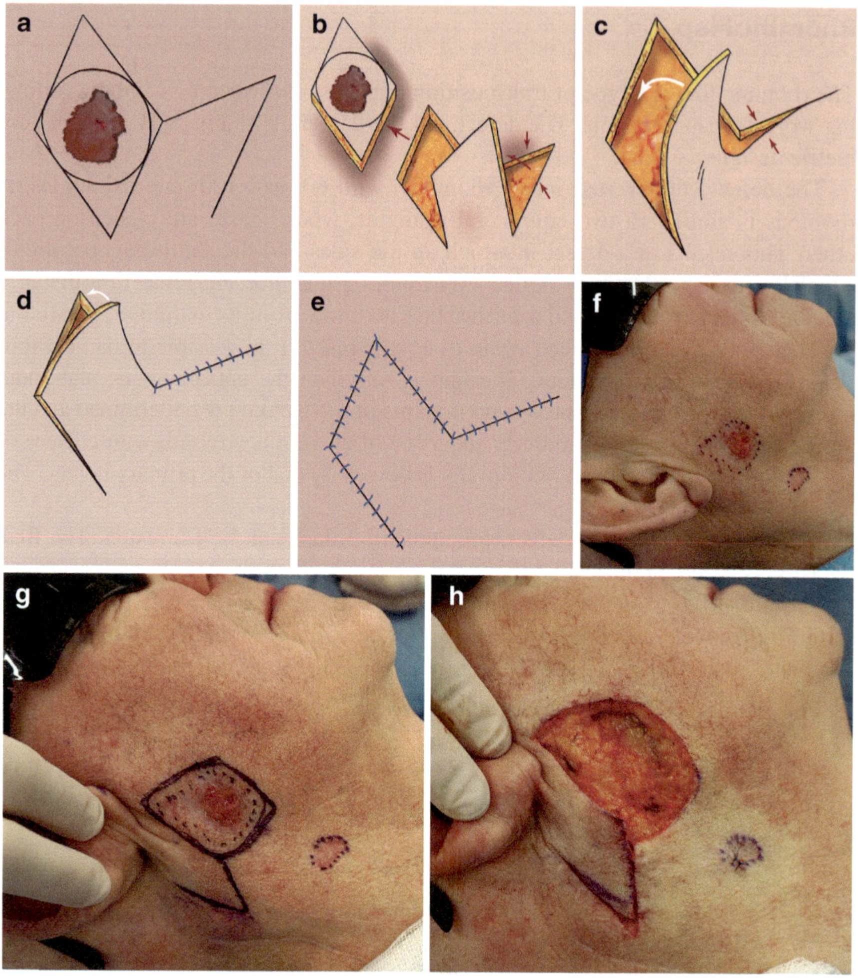

Fig. 3.7 Rhombic (Limberg) flap. (**a**) Markings following modification of excision margings and flap design, (**b**) Excision defect and flap incisions, (**c**) Flap raised and closure od secondary defect, (**d**) Sequentail closure of primary defect, (**e**) Final closure, (**f**) Lesion marked with excision margins, (**g**) Markings with modification of excision margins and planned flap, (**h**) Excision defect and flap incisions, (**i**) Trial transfer of flap into defect, (**j**) Wide undermining of surrounding tissues, (**k**) Closure of secondary defect, (**l**) Sequential closure of primary defect, (**m**) Resultant dog ear, (**n**) Marking for excision of dog ear, (**o**) Dog ear elevated, (**p**) Dog ear delineated for excision, (**q**) Final closure

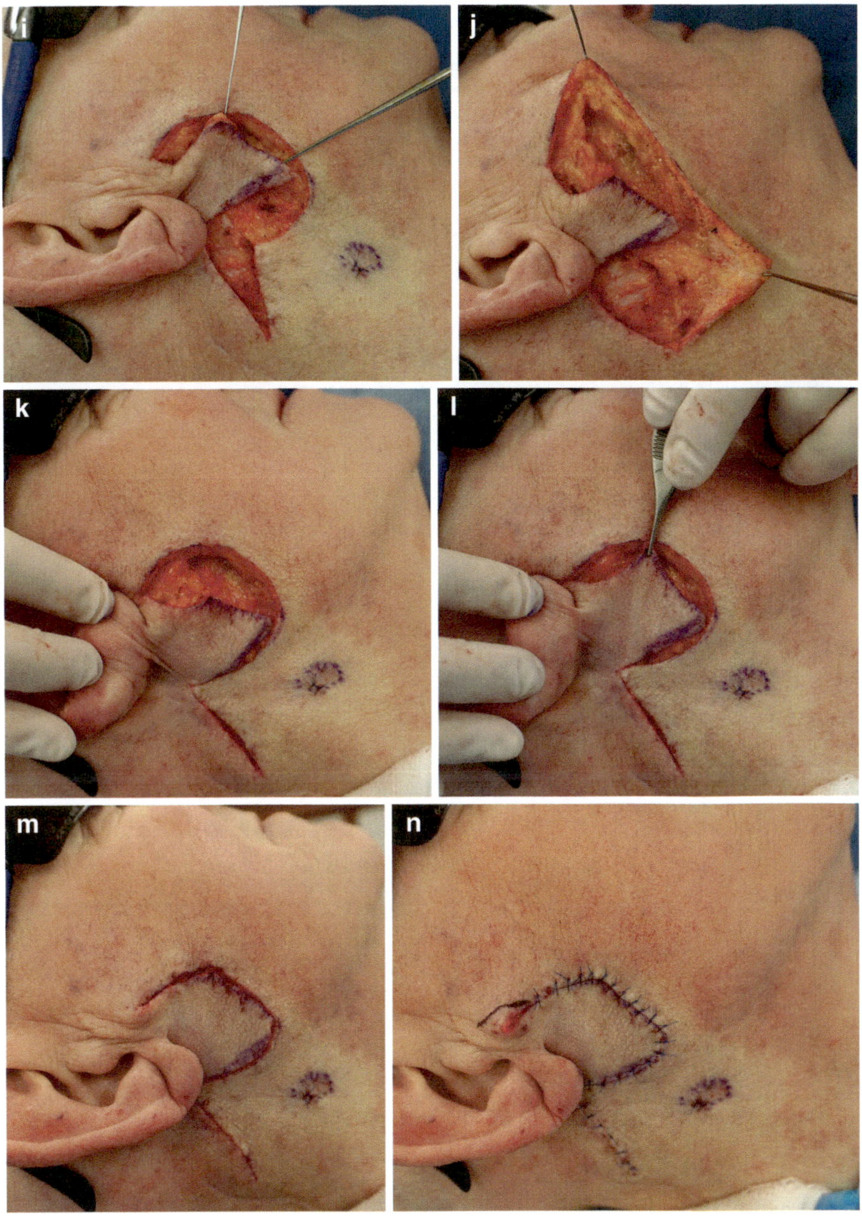

Fig. 3.7 (continued)

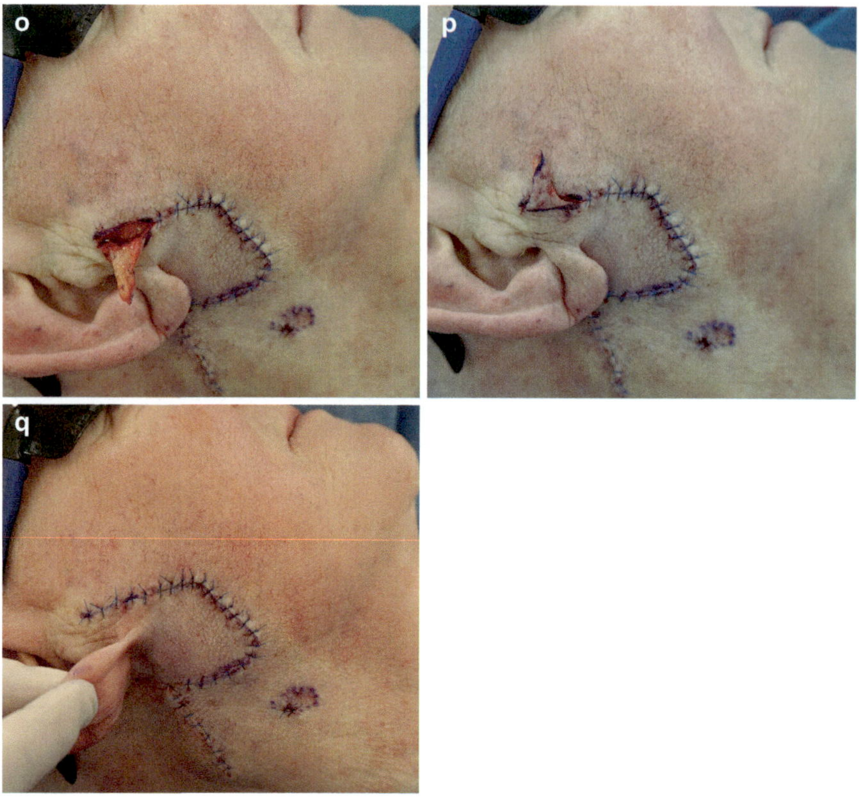

Fig. 3.7 (continued)

Dog Ear Correction (Standing Cutaneous Deformity)

A dog ear (standing cutaneous deformity) often develops at the base of a transposition, rotation flap and at the extremity following excision of lesion planned for primary closure.

Excision of the dog ear should follow an orderly sequence. The wound is sutured till the dog ear appears. A skin hook/toothed forceps is placed into the summit of the dog ear to define it fully. An incision is made along the one of the bases of the dog ear and the tissue brought across the wound, to accurately define the excess. The excess tissue is then removed, and the wound is closed in layers. The excess tissue to be removed is designed to be on the "away" rather than on the "flap" side, to avoid compromising the vascularity of the flap pedicle (Fig. 3.8a–h).

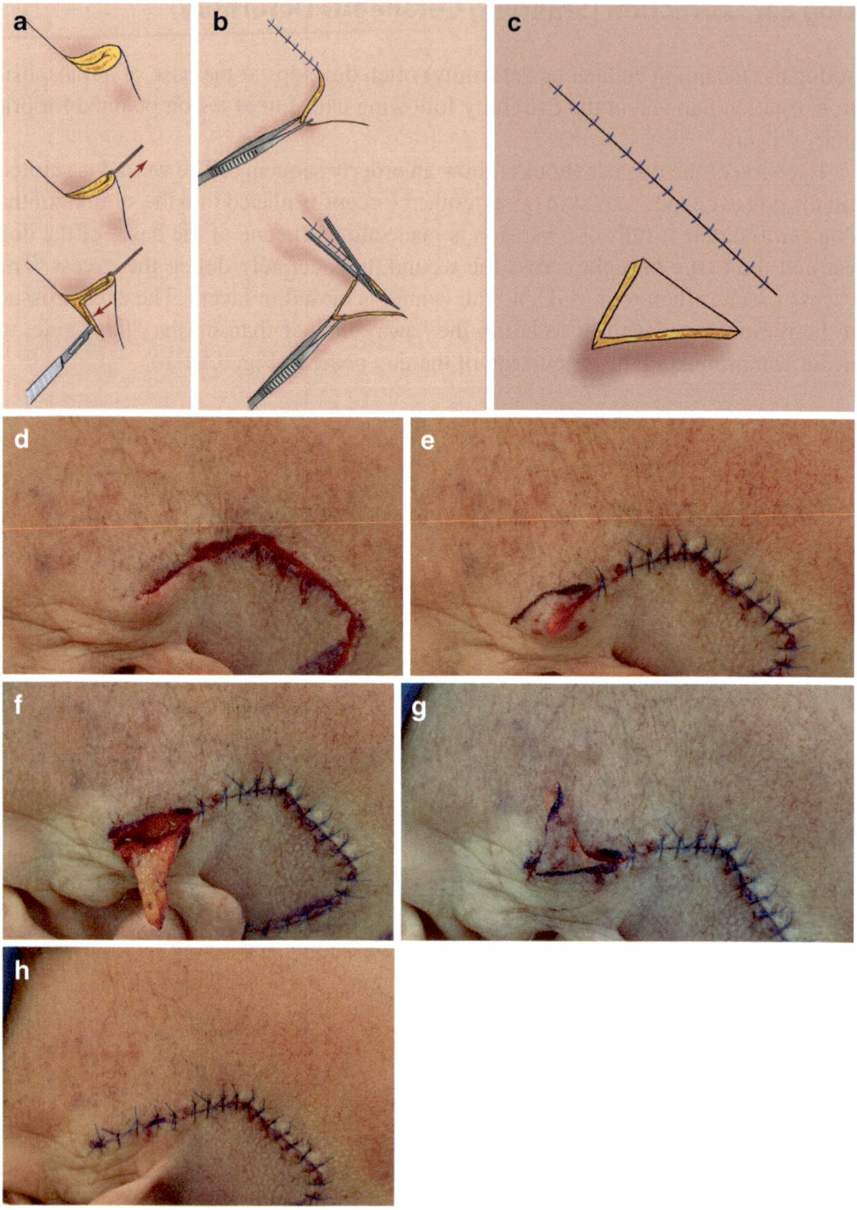

Fig. 3.8 Dog ear correction. (**a**) Dog ear delineated with a skin hook and an incison made along its base, (**b**) The excess tissue is spreadover the incision line and the excess trimmed appropriately, (**c**) Final closure, (**d**) Dog ear following developing with closure, (**e**) Excision of dog ear marked along its base, away from flap, (**f**) Excess dog ear tissue delineated, (**g**) Tissue laid across the incision to delineate appropriate excision, (**h**) Final closure

4 Decision-Making Process

The principal aim of reconstruction is to replace lost tissue with tissue with the best match in terms of size, shape, contour, colour and if possible function. This will require the flap/graft to be harvested from a site, which fulfils the above characteristics and places the secondary defect in the most advantageous position.

In the head and neck region, the flap is often harvested from a site adjacent to the defect for the "best" match. This requires sourcing flaps from areas with adequate tissue laxity and placement of scars along RSTLs, without causing distortion of the adjacent structures and landmarks.

The assessment of the defect will have to take into consideration the.

1. Size of defect
2. Site of the defect
3. Shape of the defect
4. Thickness of defect
5. Components of the defect (skin, cartilage, bone, mucosa, combinations)
6. Vascularity of the base (in case a graft)

Assessment of the flap, in addition will have to take into consideration.

1. Vascularity
2. Tissue laxity to facilitate closure of the secondary defect
3. Placement of scar along RSTL/aesthetic boundaries
4. Avoid distorting adjacent landmarks
5. One/multi-stage reconstruction
6. Injury to adjacent neurovascular structures

V. Ilankovan et al., *Local Flaps in Facial Reconstruction*,
https://doi.org/10.1007/978-3-031-49464-2_4

Tips

1. The best placement of scars might require "enlarging" the defect to place the eventual suture lines in the most appropriate position.
2. A more distant flap might have to be harvested to avoid distortion of the structures and landmarks adjacent to the defect.
3. For defects encompassing more than one unit, consideration should be given to reconstructing each unit individually, to place the scars in the most advantageous position.
4. The patient's expectations, surgeon's capabilities and resources available should be taken into consideration.
5. There are often "compromises/price to be paid" to be made to achieve the desired results, and these will have to be discussed with the patient in detail prior to undertaking the procedure.
6. In case of multi-stage procedures, the patient co-operation and the "temporary inconveniences" will have to be discussed in detail.

Part II

Reconstruction of Specific Defects

Scalp Reconstruction

5

Subunits and Anatomical Considerations

Skin of scalp is among the thickest in the body and relatively inelastic. It is hair bearing and covers a convex area, which can all add up to difficulties in reconstruction. The acronym "SCALP" represents S—skin, C—subcutaneous tissue, A—galea aponeurotica, L—loose areolar tissue, P—pericranium (Fig. 5.1). The blood vessels and nerves run within the galeal layer, which connects the frontalis and occipitalis muscles. In the temple region (below the temporal line), the terminology of the scalp layers becomes potentially confusing (Fig. 5.2). This can be more easily appreciated, if one was to consider the temporalis fascia (deep temporal fascia) to be an extension of the pericranium and the overlying galea, as the temporoparietal fascia (superficial temporal fascia, suprazygomatic (SMAS)). Not surprisingly, the

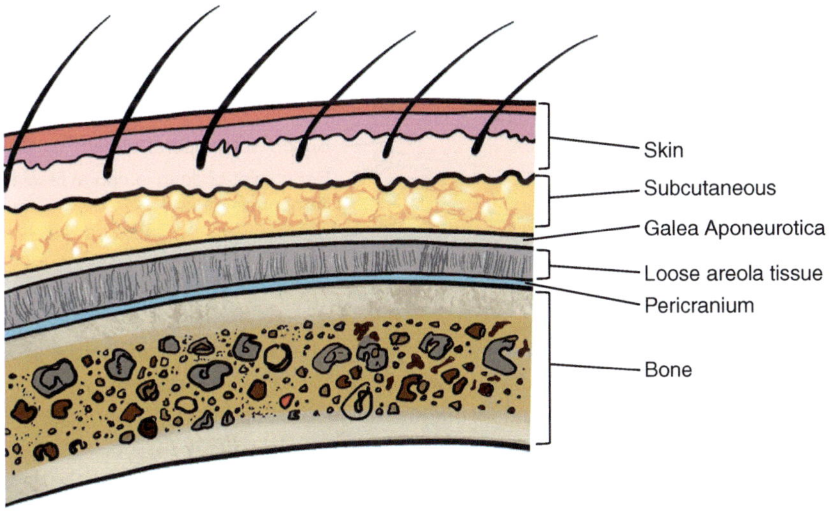

Fig. 5.1 Layers of the scalp

V. Ilankovan et al., *Local Flaps in Facial Reconstruction*,
https://doi.org/10.1007/978-3-031-49464-2_5

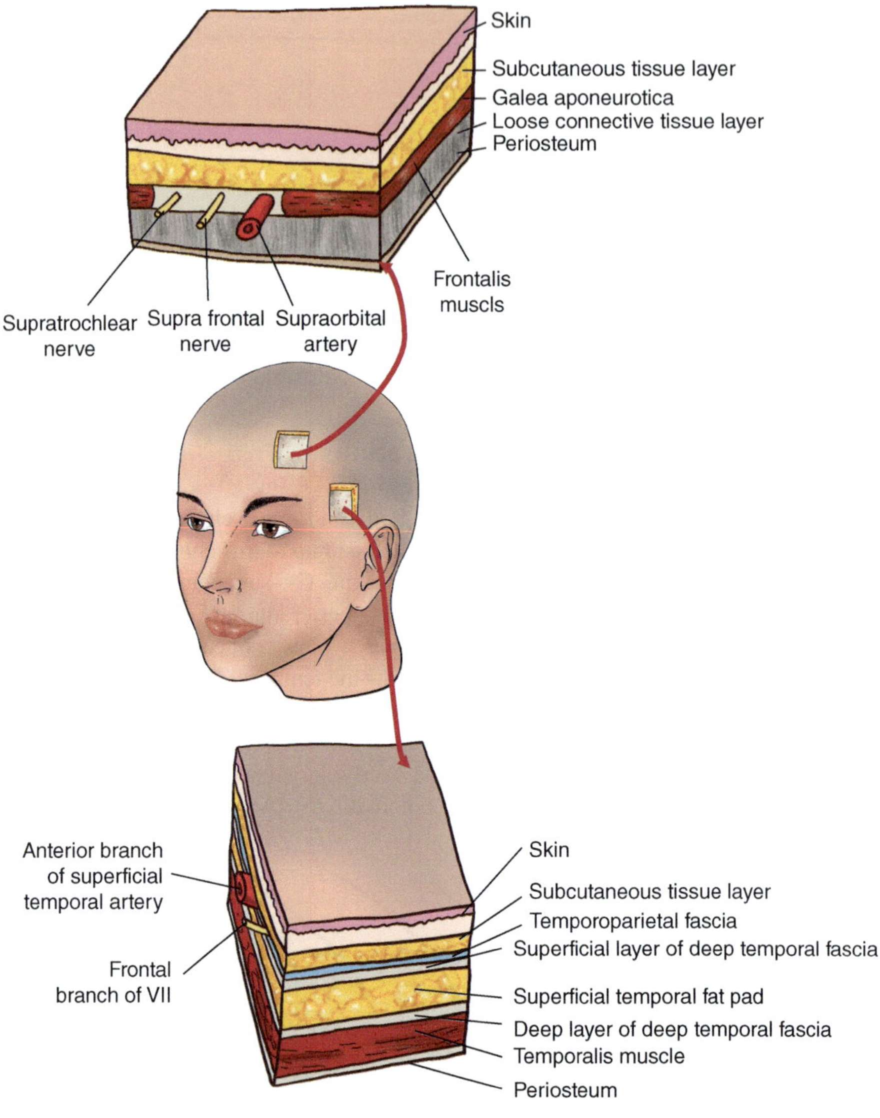

Fig. 5.2 Scalp layers in the central and temporal region

vessels and nerves lie within the temporoparietal fascia. A few centimetres above the zygomatic arch, the temporalis fascia divides into two layers (superficial and deep layers of the deep temporal fascia) enclosing the superficial temporal fat pad. The temporoparietal fascia fuses with the superficial layer of the deep temporal fascia and the periosteum of the zygomatic arch. The frontal branch of the facial nerve present in the temporoparietal fascia, crossing the zygomatic arch is liable to damage, if its location is not appreciated.

The scalp covering the vertex (central) is tight and poorly distensible. This is thought to be due to the thick galea and no underlying muscle. Whereas the scalp overlying the temporal and parietal regions (lateral) is relatively mobile and is thought to be due to the thin galea and the presence of an underlying temporalis muscle (Figs. 5.3 and 5.4).

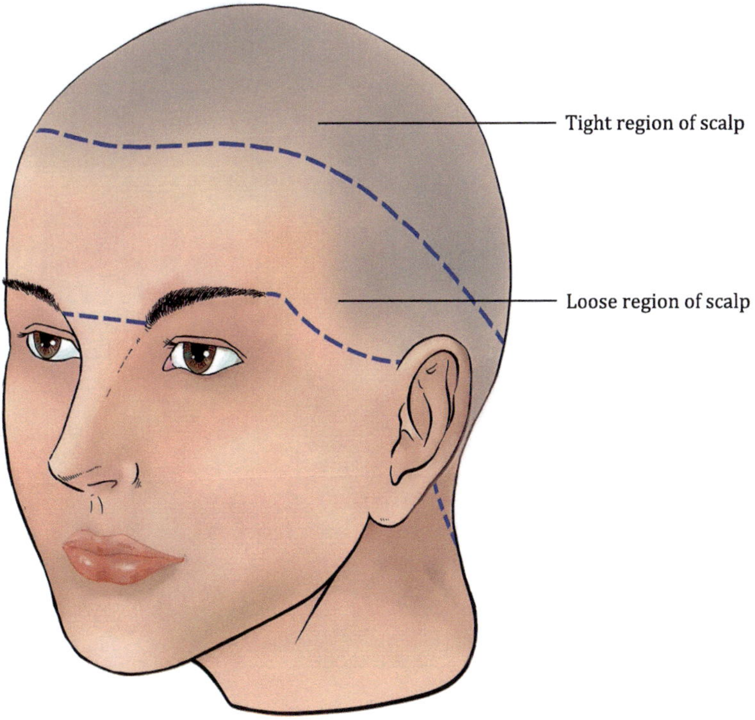

Fig. 5.3 Tight and loose areas of scalp - anterior view

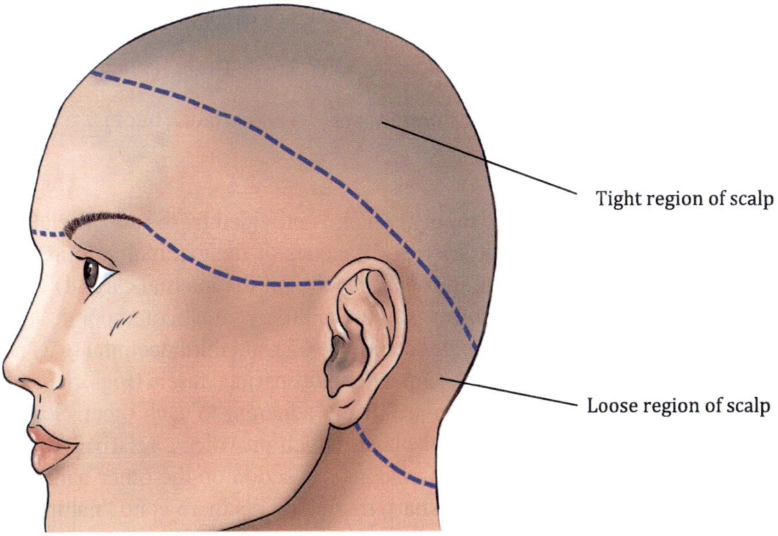

Fig. 5.4 Tight and loose areas of the scalp - lateral view

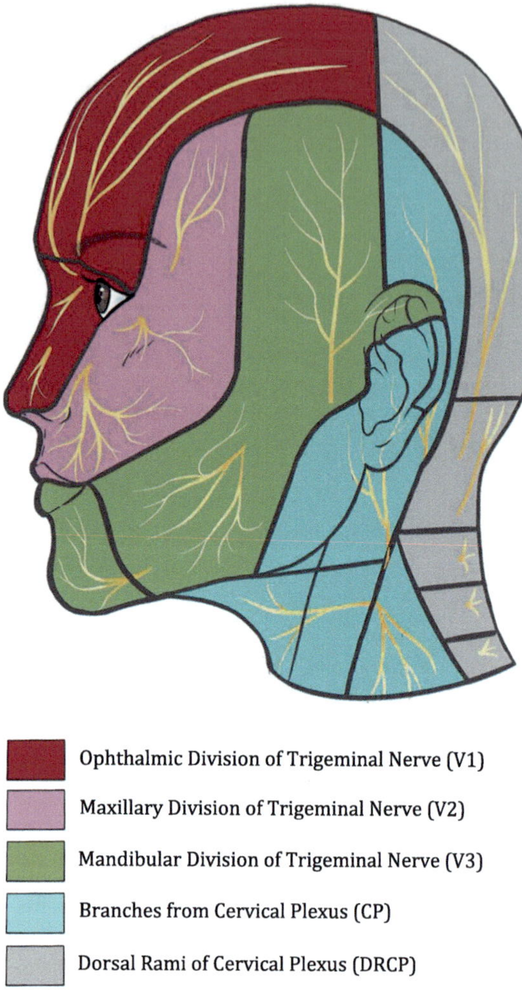

Fig. 5.5 Sensory nerve supply of scalp

The scalp has a rich vascular supply, which is provided by the superficial temporal, posterior auricular, occipital arteries (branches of the external carotid) and the supra-orbital and supra-trochlear arteries (branches of the internal carotid). The sensory supply is by the supra-trochlear, supra-orbital, zygomaticotemporal, auriculotemporal, lesser occipital (C2), greater occipital (C2) and third occipital (C3) nerves. The vessels and nerves run within the galea/temporoparietal fascia (Figs. 5.5 and 5.6).

The first three layers of the scalp are firmly adherent to each other. Scalp flaps can be raised easily in the sub-galeal plane, which provides a relatively avascular and quick layer for dissection. Subcutaneous dissection on the other hand is more difficult and must be carried out by sharp dissection, as there is no "natural" plane to work with. Incisions should be made parallel to the hair follicles and injudicious use of diathermy avoided, to minimise damage to the hair follicles and risk of alopecia. Because of their relative inelasticity, scalp flaps will have to be large in relation to the defect, to achieve closure without excessive tension.

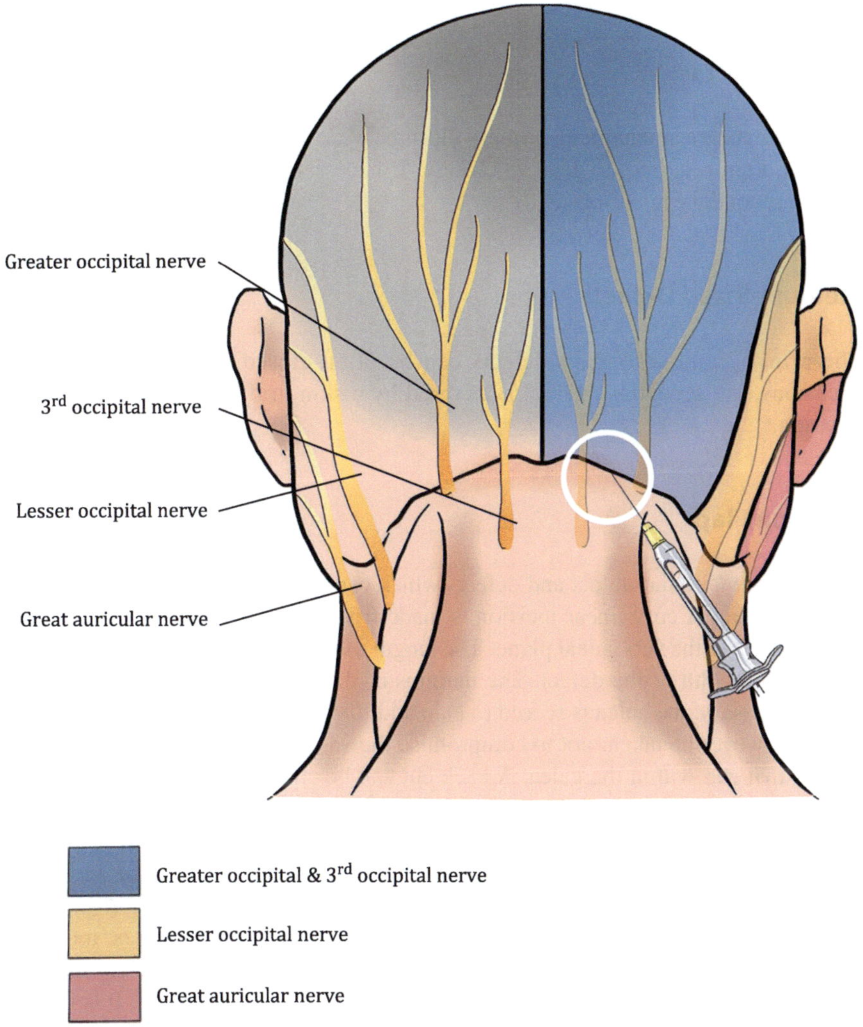

Fig. 5.6 Sensory nerve suppy for posterior scalp

Central (Vertex) Defects

Small Defects

Small defects are amenable to primary closure. Wide undermining in the sub-galeal plane is often required, to achieve closure. If necessary, small areas can be left to heal by secondary intention.

Medium-Sized Defects

The primary and secondary defects can be often closed primarily, though on occasions, the secondary defect is covered by a skin graft in a less conspicuous location.

Rotation Flap

Indications: Circular defect and defects which can be converted to a triangle.

Technique: A curvilinear incision is made from the base of the defect, and the flap is raised in the sub-galeal plane. The length of the flap is designed to be at least 6 times the width of the defect. The margins of the defect are widely undermined and if necessary, the galea is scored to gain additional extensibility of the flap. Care should however be taken, not to compromise the vascular supply, by damaging the vessels that run within the galea. A back cut can be employed to decrease the tension of closure, but again care must be taken to avoid vascular compromise. The dog ear often settles with time and can be corrected at a later date if necessary. The wounds are closed in layers, and a pressure dressing/drain employed as necessary (Fig. 5.7a–h).

Tips: For large circular defects, the orientation of the incision can be modified include named vessels in the flap to improve vascularity. The distribution of hair and hair line should also be taken into account, when planning the incision. It is important to appreciate the difference in length (outer greater than inner) and thickness (raised flap thinner than native lateral margins) of the two flap margins, and this would have to be accommodated in the suturing technique. The drain is ideally placed away from the base of the flap.

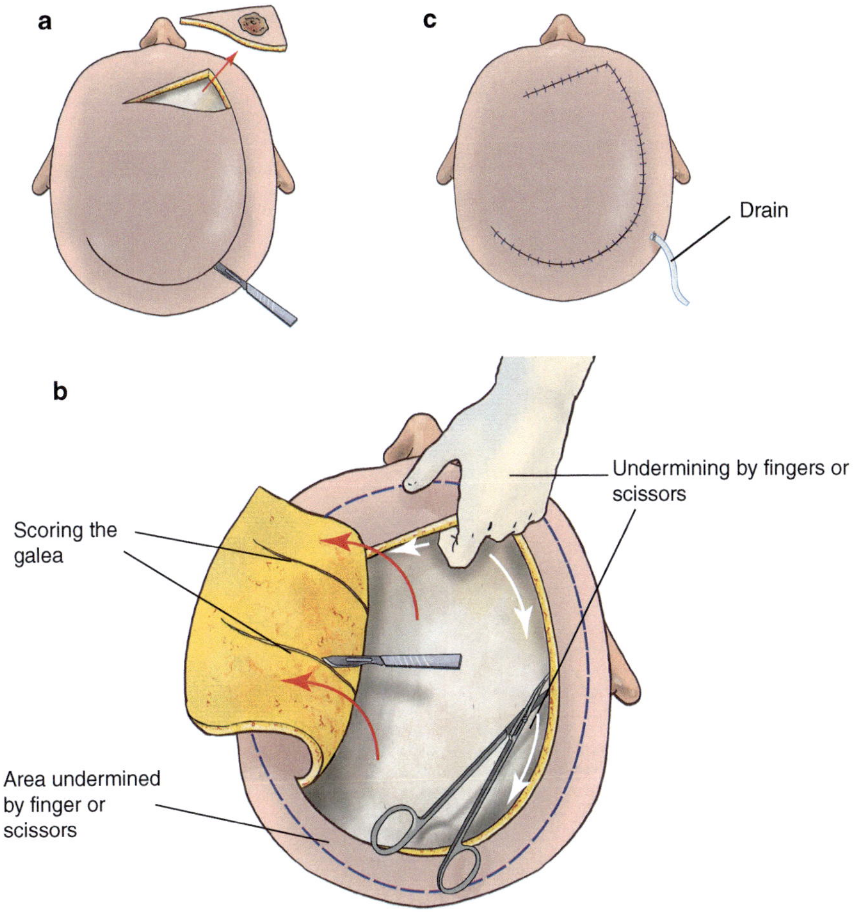

Fig. 5.7 Scalp rotation flap. (**a**) Defect following excision and flap incision, (**b**) Wide subgaleal undermining of surrounding tissue and scoring of galea, (**c**) Final closure and drains, (**d**) Marking of excision and flap, (**e**) Excision defect, (**f**) Flap raised with scoring of galea, (**g**) final closure with dog ear left in situ, (**h**) Late result with spontaneous flattening of dog ear

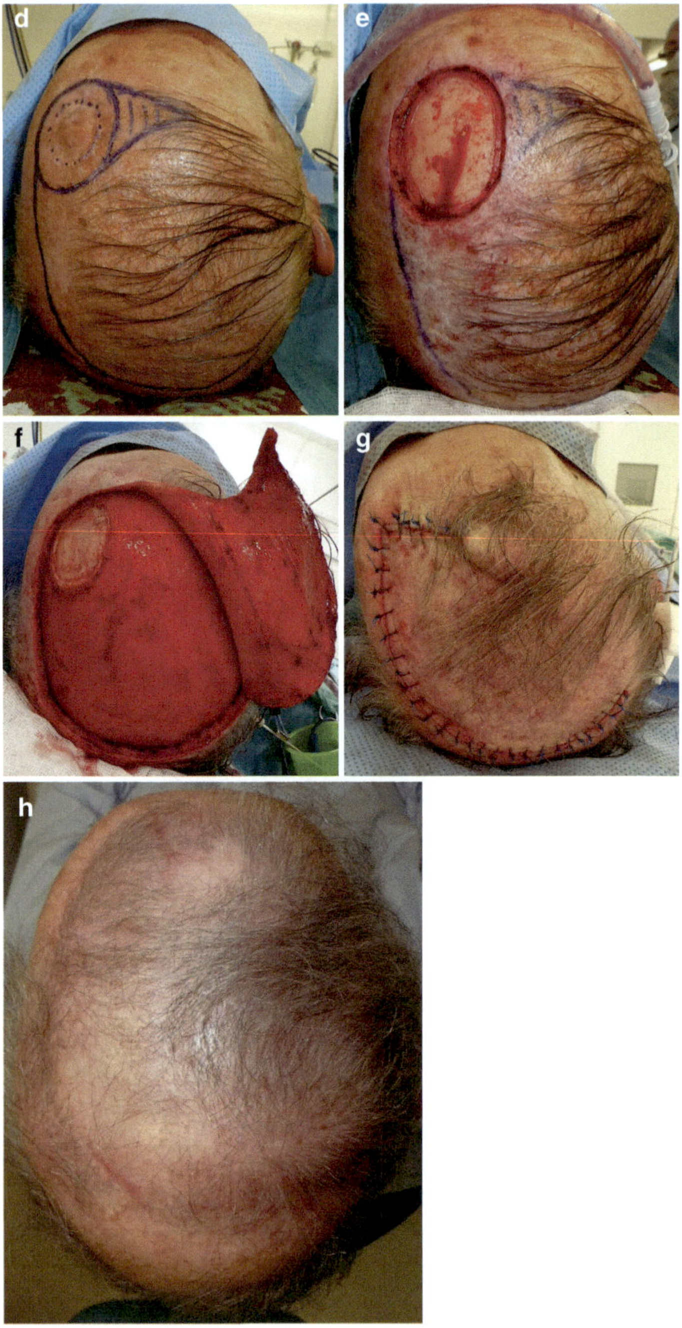

Fig. 5.7 (continued)

O-Z Closure

Indications: Circular or elliptical defects.

Technique: Two curvilinear incisions are made from the opposite ends of the defect. For circular defects, the placement of the incision can be determined according to the areas of maximum tissue laxity, scar position and neurovascular structures. In the case of elliptical defects, the incisions commence at the opposite poles. The incision is made through the galea, and the flap undermined widely in the sub-galeal plane. Similar to rotation flaps, the length of the incisions will have to be generous (around 4–6 times the size of the defect). The primary defect is sutured first, followed by the margins of the curvilinear incisions (Fig. 5.8a–i).

Tips: It is important to appreciate the difference in length (outer greater than inner) and thickness (raised flap thinner than native lateral margins) of the two flap margins and this would have to be accommodated in the suturing technique.

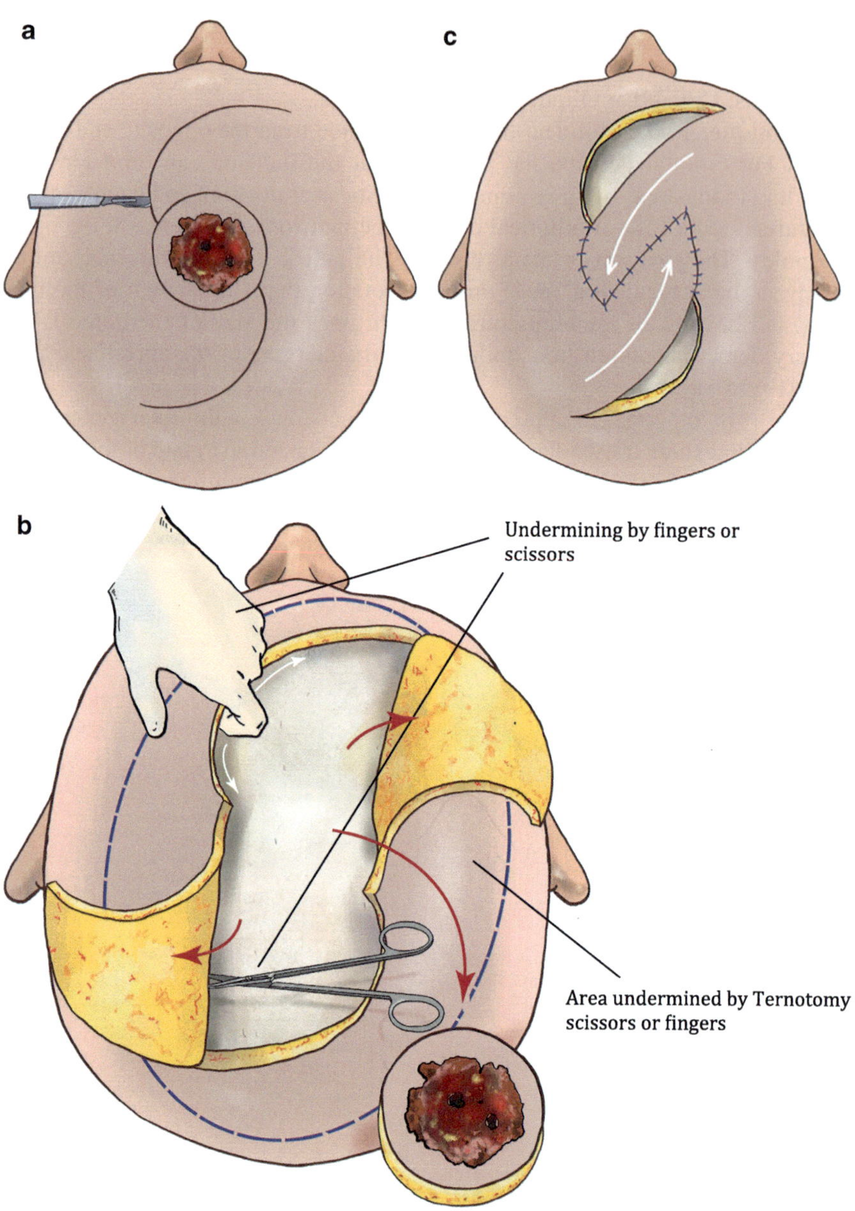

Fig. 5.8 O-Z closure. (**a**) Markings for excision and flap incision, (**b**) Excision defect and wide subgaleal undermining, (**c**) Initial closure of primary defect, (**d**) Final closure, (**e**) Markings of excision and planned flap, (**f**) Excision defect, (**g**) Flaps raised in a sub galeal plane with wide undermining, (**h**) Initial closure of primary defect, (**i**) Final closure

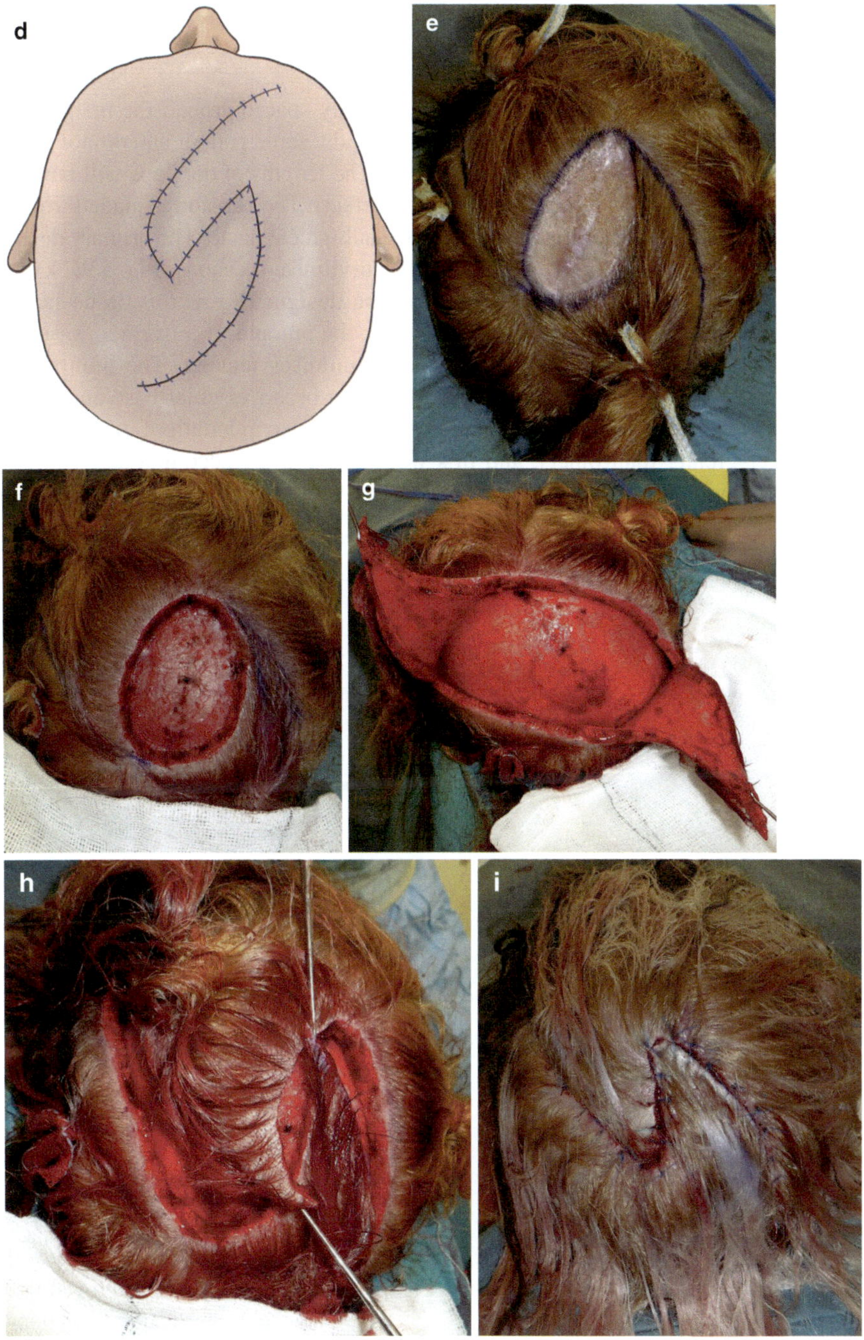

Fig. 5.8 (continued)

Multiple Rotation Flap (Pin Wheel Flap)

Indications: Circular defects in the vertex.

Technique: The curvilinear incisions are equally spaced around the margins of the flap. It is vitally important that they all follow the same pattern and do not compromise the blood supply of the adjacent flaps. The lengths of the flaps will have to be generous (around 2–3 times the size of the defect). The incision is made through the galea and the flap undermined widely in the sub-galeal plane. The primary defect is sutured first, followed by the margins of the curvilinear incisions (Fig. 5.9a–k).

Tips: The orientation of the flaps should be designed to recruit tissue laxity most efficiently. With the use of multiple flaps, the amount of movement of each individual flap component is decreased and minimises tension. The number of flaps should be kept to the minimum to maintain a broad vascular base and minimise scarring. It is important to appreciate the difference in length of the flap margins (outer greater than inner), and this would have to be accommodated in the suturing technique.

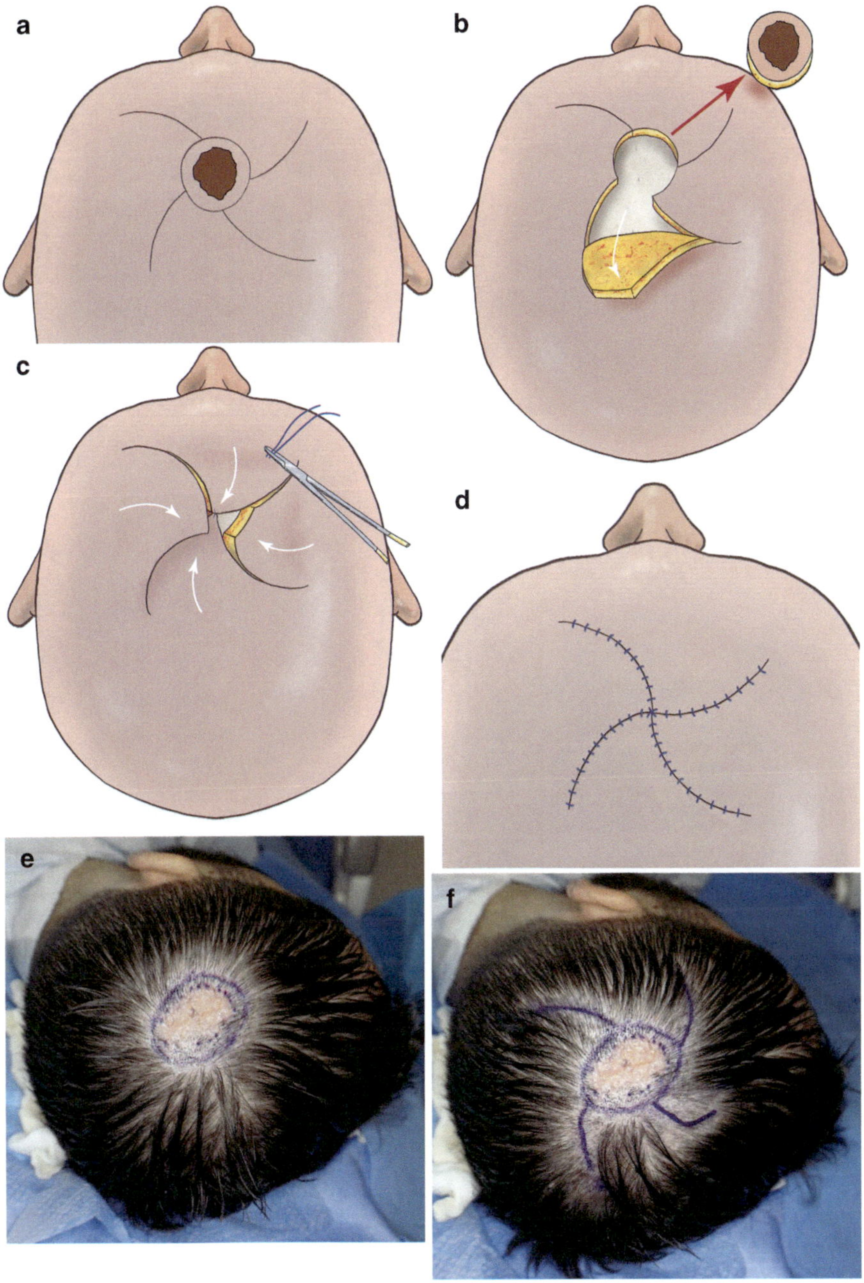

Fig. 5.9 Multiple rotation (Pin wheel) flap. (**a**) Markings for excision and flaps, (**b**) Excision defect and falps raised, (**c**) Closure of primary defect, (**d**) Final closure, (**e**) Markings for excision, (**f**) Flap markings, (**g**) Excision defect, (**h**) Flap incisions, (**i**) Flaps raised with subgaleal undermining, (**j**) Closure of primary defect, (**k**) Final closure

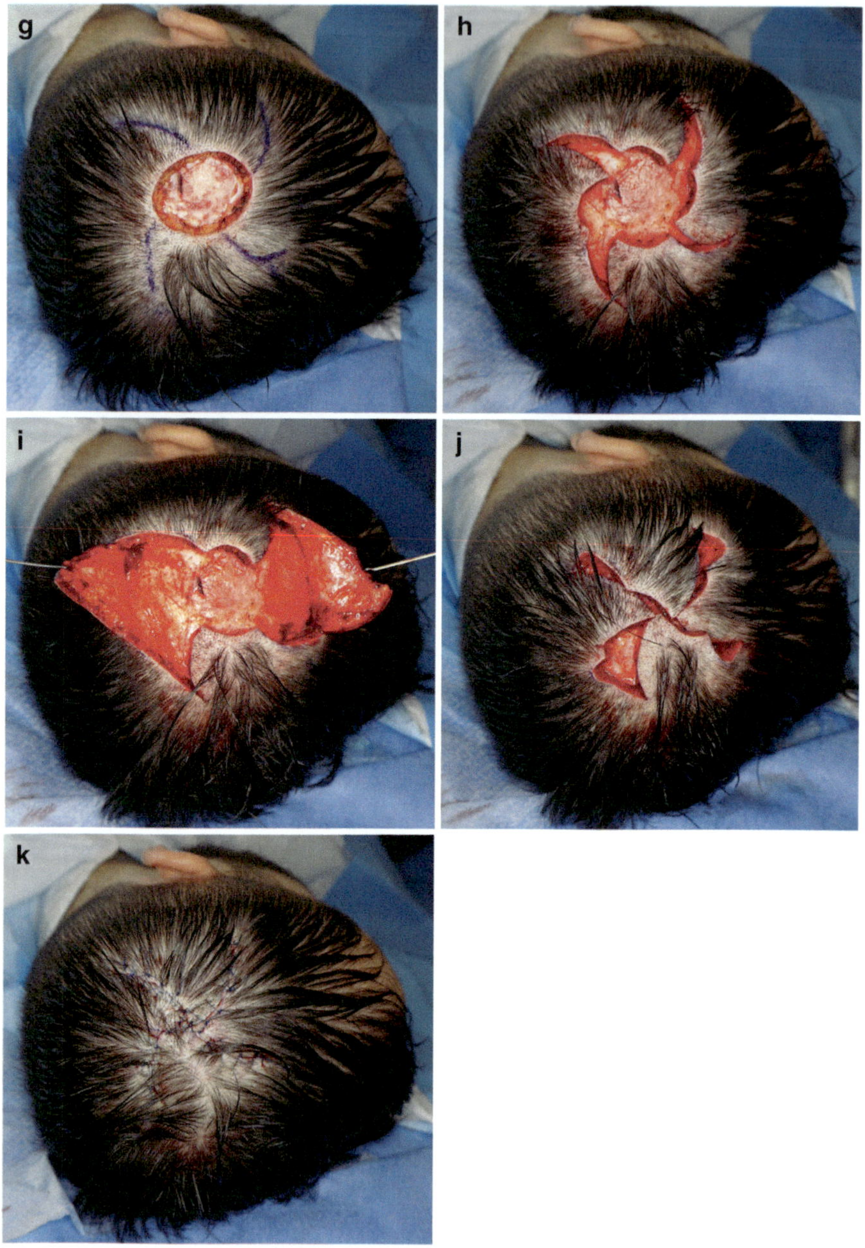

Fig. 5.9 (continued)

Multiple Rhomboid Flaps

Indication: Medium-sized defect vertex. This is useful for hexagonal defects or defects which could be converted to a hexagon.

Technique: The margins of the flap are converted to a hexagon, with equal sides. Three limberg flap are marked out from the corners of alternate facets, making sure that the length of the limbs are equal to that of each facet and the secondary limbs are parallel to the relevant facet. It is mandatory that the flaps are all oriented in the same direction to maintain the vascularity of the flaps. The flaps are raised in the sub-galeal plane, and the surrounding tissue is undermined geneorously. The secondary defects are closed intially, which decreases the tension and aids precise approximation of the flap margins (Fig. 5.10a–d).

Tips: It might be easier to place the sutures across the leading edges of the secondary defects before tying them. Time spent in designing the appropriate position of the individual flaps to take into account relative tissue laxity will make closure easier, without tension. It is a complicated flap to design and execute and similar defect can often be addressed with other flaps (pin wheel/O-Z).

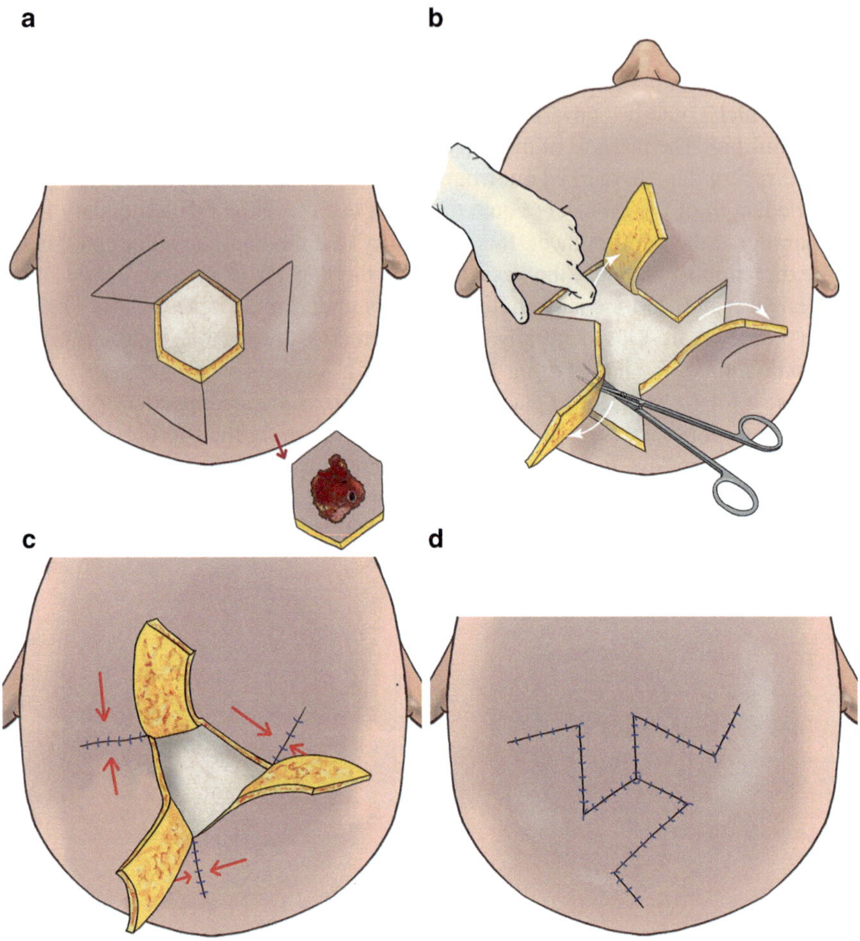

Fig. 5.10 Multiple Rhomboid flaps. (**a**) Defect following excision and flap markings, (**b**) flaps raised with wide subgaleal undermining, (**c**) Initial closure of secondary defect, (**d**) Final closure

Skin Graft (Full Thickness)

Indication: Medium/large scalp defects, when atleast the periosteum is preserved at the base of the defect.

Technique: A suitable template is made of the defect, which is transferred to the donar site to harvest the graft. The graft is sutured to the defect, with additional "long" sutures that can be used for "tying" over the bolus. If possible, the graft can be "quilted" to the base, to decrease the risk of heamatoma and dead space. A non-adherent dressing is laid over the sutured graft, over which a cotton wool ball/sponge soaked in proflavin or a suitable antibiotic ointment is paced. The tie-over bolus sutures are now used to hold the dressing in place. Alternatively the dressing could be held in place with skin staples (Fig. 5.11a–i).

Tips: The defect created can often be made smaller, by undermining around the periphery and using a "purse string" suture (Fig. 5.11a, b). The skin of the scalp is among the thickest in the body, and the native defect margins can be shelved to make the junction with the skin graft smoother. It is easier to suture from the graft to the native skin, which prevents displacement of the graft, when the suture is pulled through. Meticulous haemostasis is paramount, and the space between the skin graft and the defect can be flushed with saline on a blunt needle, prior to placement of the last few sutures to make sure there is no haematoma beneath the skin graft.

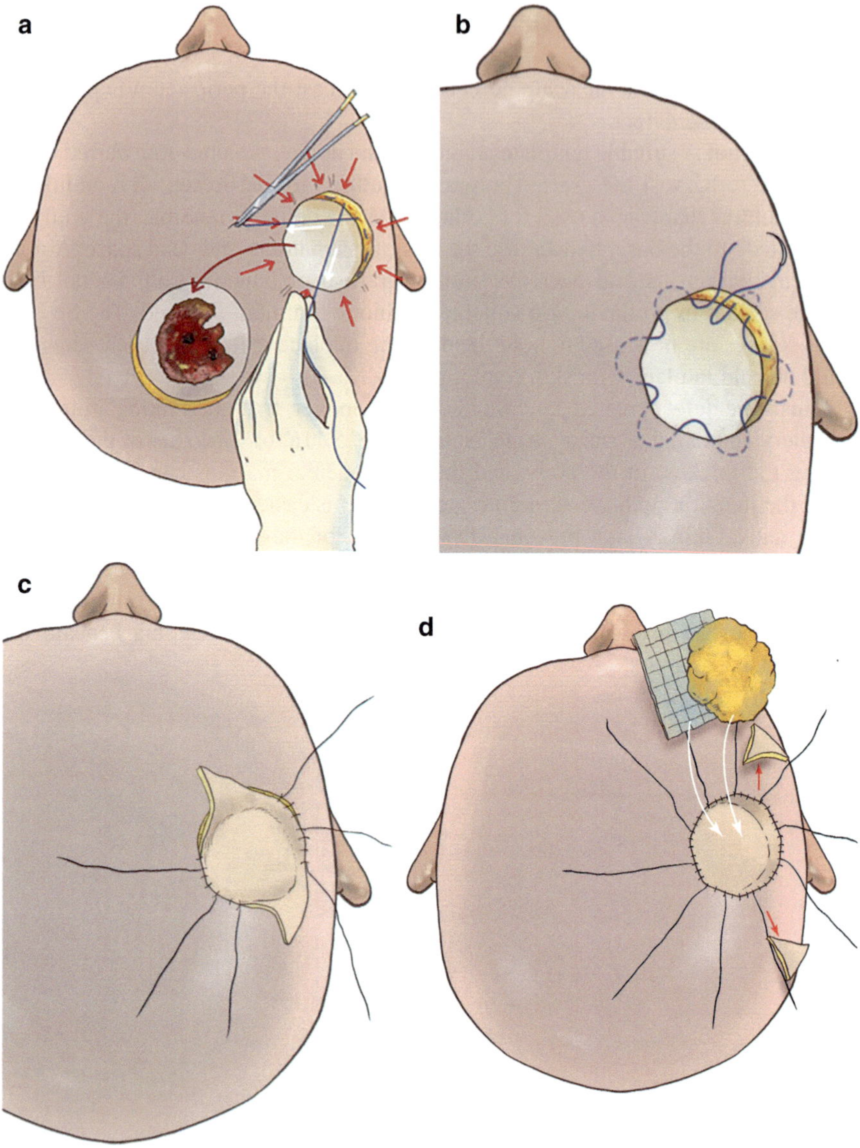

Fig. 5.11 Full thickness skin graft. (**a**) Defect following excision and purse string sutures to reduce size of defect, (**b**) Purse string sutures, (**c**) Skin graft sutured into place, (**d**) Non adherent and bolus dressing placed over graft, (**e**) Tie over bolus sutures and dressing is situ, (**f**) Dressing sutured in place, (**g**) Excision defect with intact pericranium, (**h**) Skin graft sutured in defect, (**i**) Dressing stapled in place

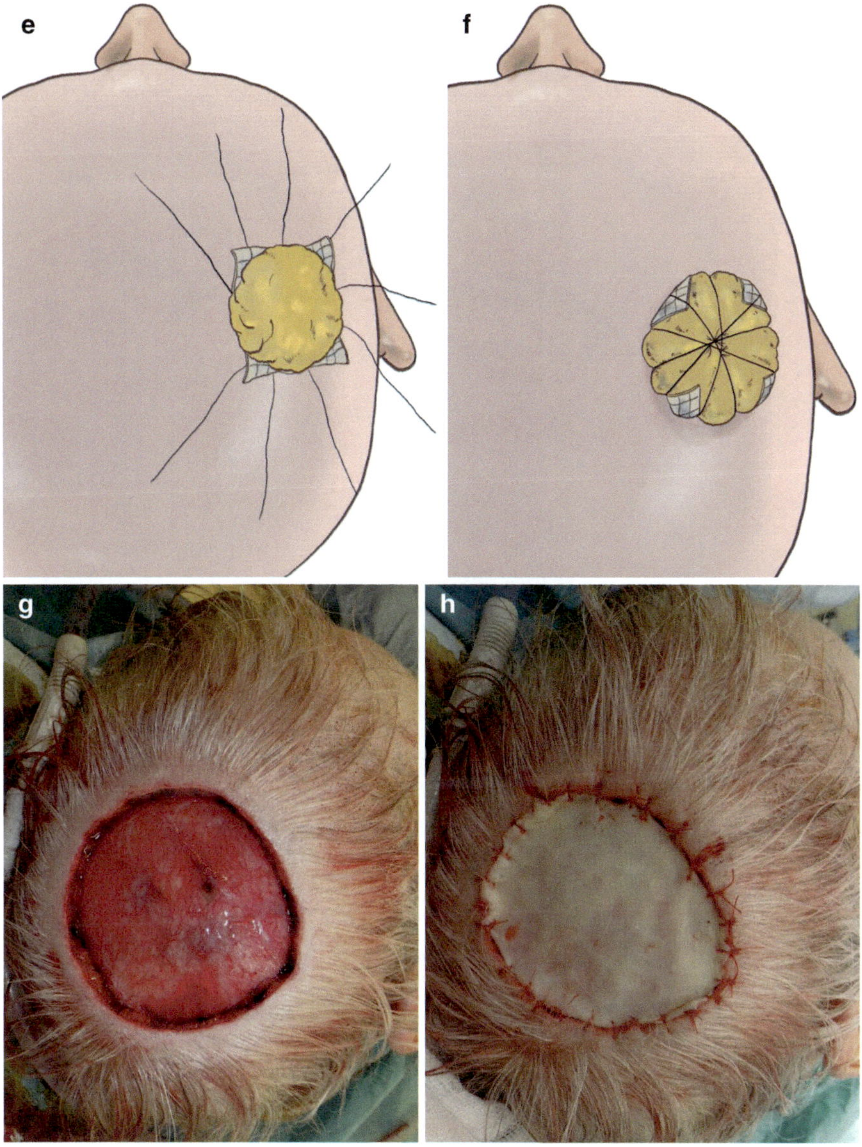

Fig. 5.11 (continued)

Fig. 5.11 (continued)

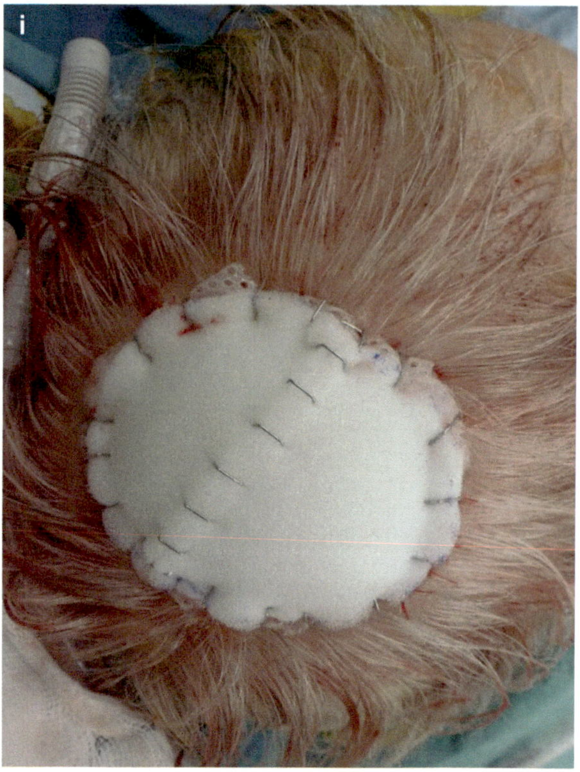

Split Skin Graft

Indication: Medium and large defects the vertex and lateral scalp. Could be considered when the native bed has a compromised blood supply (e.g. exposed bone), secondary defects.

Technique: A graft of suitable thickness and size is harvested with a dermatome from the donor site. It is vitally important that the surfaces are accurately oriented to avoid flap failure. The graft is laid in the defects, with the graft overlapping of the defect margins. The margins are sutured into place with a resorbable suture, with additional suture left long to be used for "tying" over the bolus dressing. A non-adherent dressing is laid over the sutured graft, over which a cotton wool ball/sponge soaked in proflavin or a suitable antibiotic ointment is paced. The tie-over bolus sutures are now used to hold the dressing in place. Alternatively, the dressing could be held with skin staples (Fig. 5.12a–g).

Tips: Deciding on the thickness of the graft depends on the vascularity of the bed, the stresses that it is likely to encounter in the recipient site and the size of the defect. A split skin graft can be considered when a pericranial flap is used to cover exposed bone prior to grafting and when the outer table is "burred" to expose the dipole and a transposition flap is not considered to cover the defect.

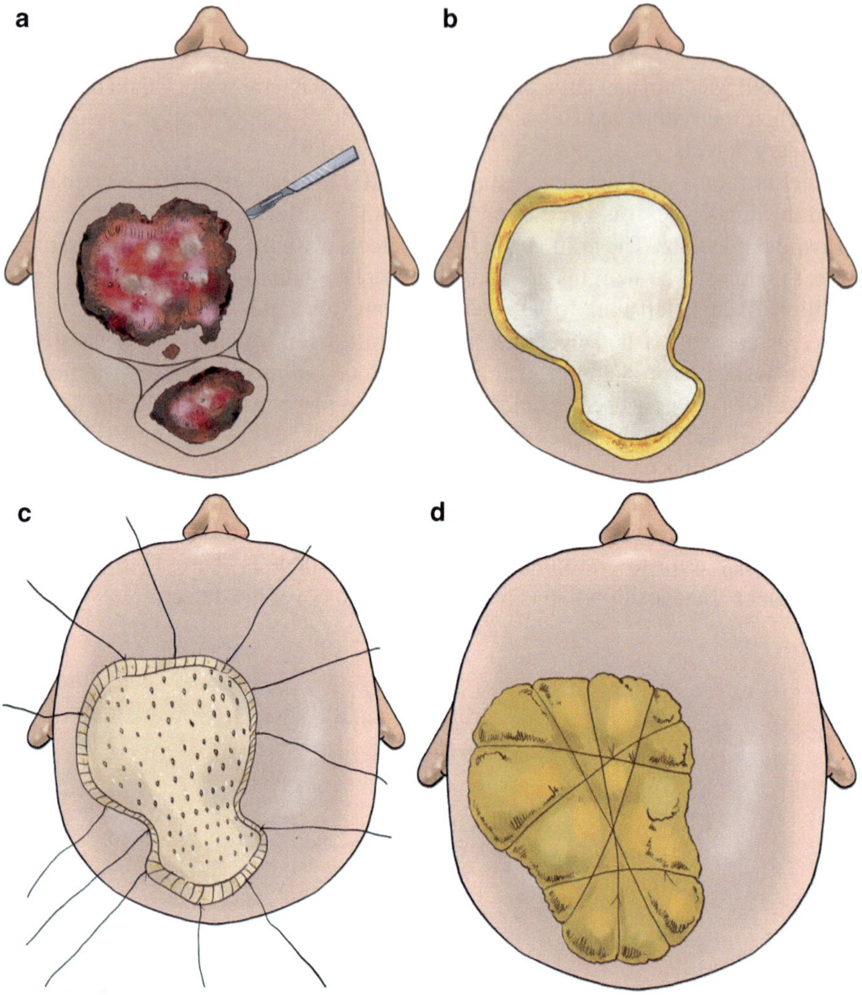

Fig. 5.12 Split skin graft. (**a**) Markings for excision, (**b**) Excision defect, (**c**) Skin graft sutured in situ with "stab" holes, (**d**) Tie over bolus dressing, (**e**) Secondary scalp defect, (**f**) Split skin graft (**g**) Split skin graft in situ

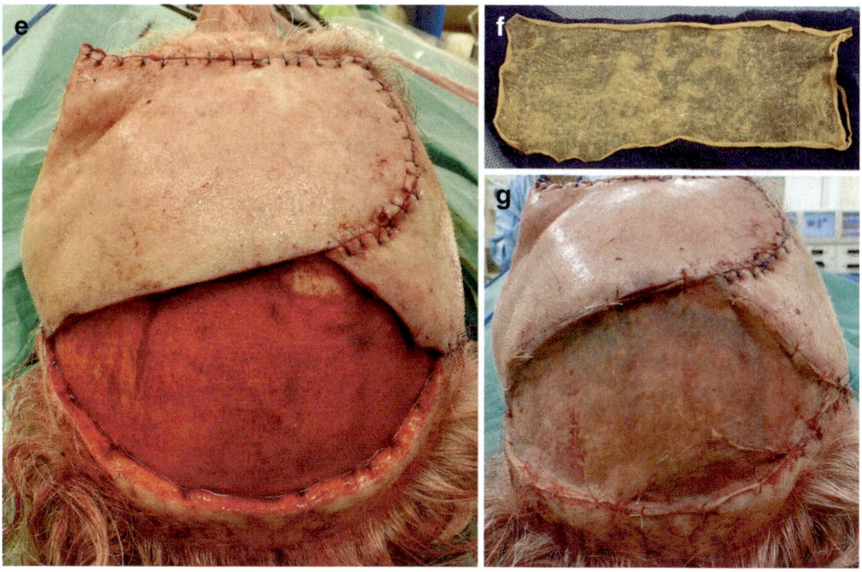

Fig. 5.12 (continued)

Integra® and Skin Grafting

Indications: Defects with exposed bone, unable to line base with pericranial flap, likely to receive radiotherapy following skin graft reconstruction.

Technique: A suitable template is made of the defect and an appropriate size of Integra® cut. The Integra® is prepared according to the manufactures instructions and sutured into the defect. Care is taken to place the Integra® the correct way over the defect. A tie-over dressing with sponge and antibiotic paste is used to hold the Integra in place. Wound care advice is provided, and the wound reviewed regularly for signs of infection. The dressing is removed in 4 weeks' time and the wound inspected for vascular ingrowth. If satisfactory, the superficial surface is gently scrubbed/curetted, and a split skin graft placed (Fig. 5.13a–j).

Tips: Meticulously follow the manufacturers instruction. Profusely irrigate and gently scrub the surface of the Integra® prior to skin grafting at the second stage.

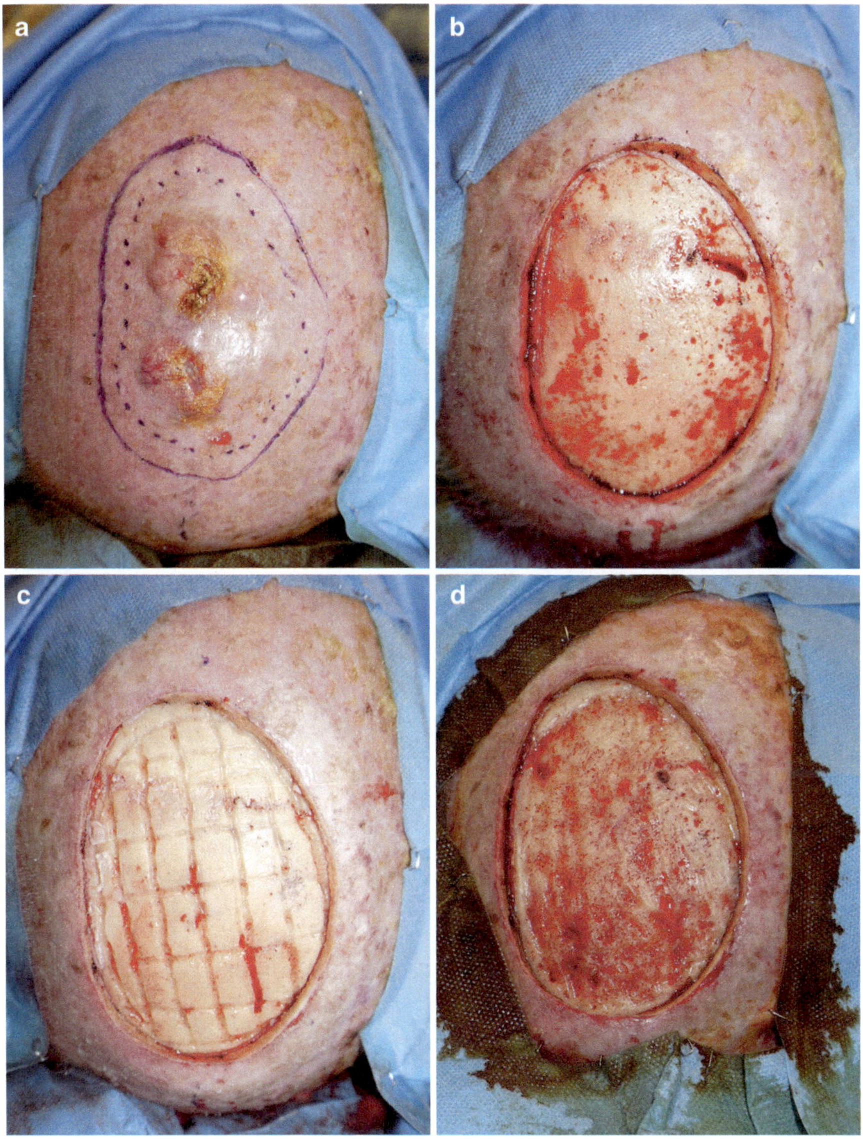

Fig. 5.13 Integra® with split skin graft. (**a**) Markings for excision, (**b**) Excision defect down to bone, (**c**) Depth orientation grooves for removal of outer cortex, (**d**) Defect following removal of outer cortex, (**e**) Integra® being prepared according to manufacturers instructions, (**f**) Sutured into place with silicone layer in situ, (**g**) Pressure dressing in situ, (**h**) Second stage - excellent vascular ingrowth of Integra®, (**i**) Split skin graft sutured in situ, (**j**) Complete "take" of skin graft

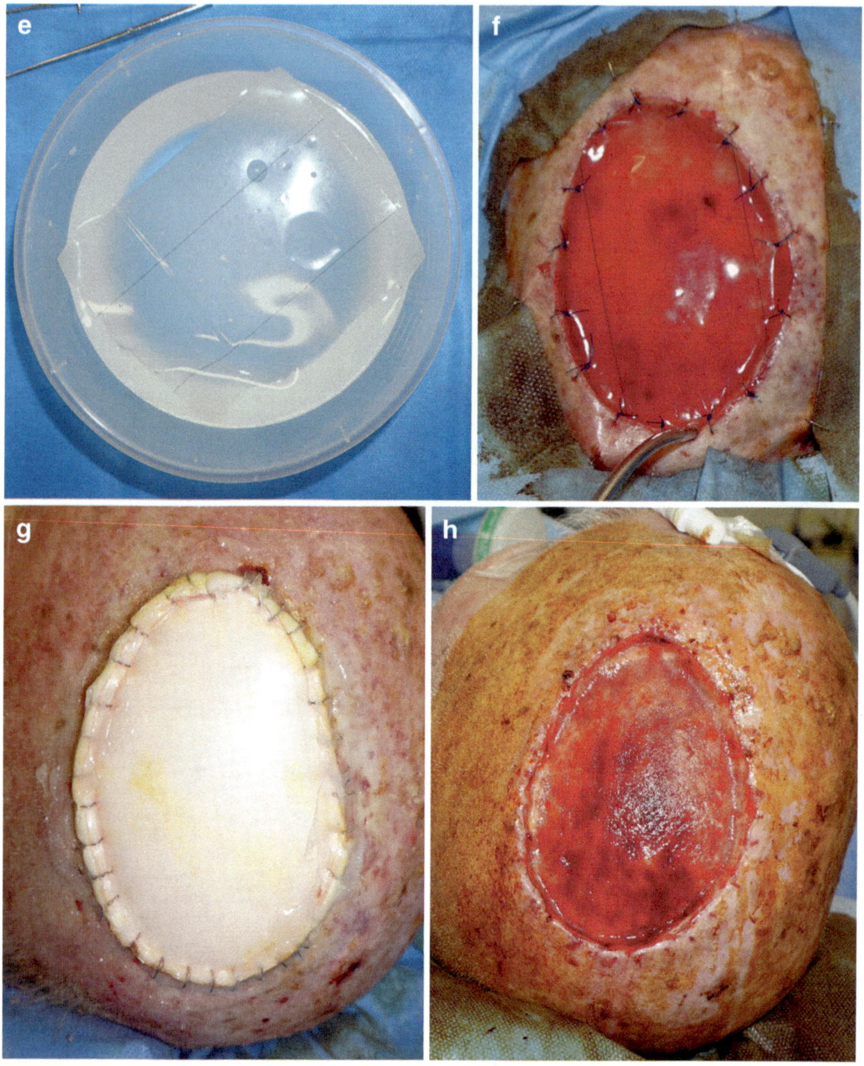

Fig. 5.13 (continued)

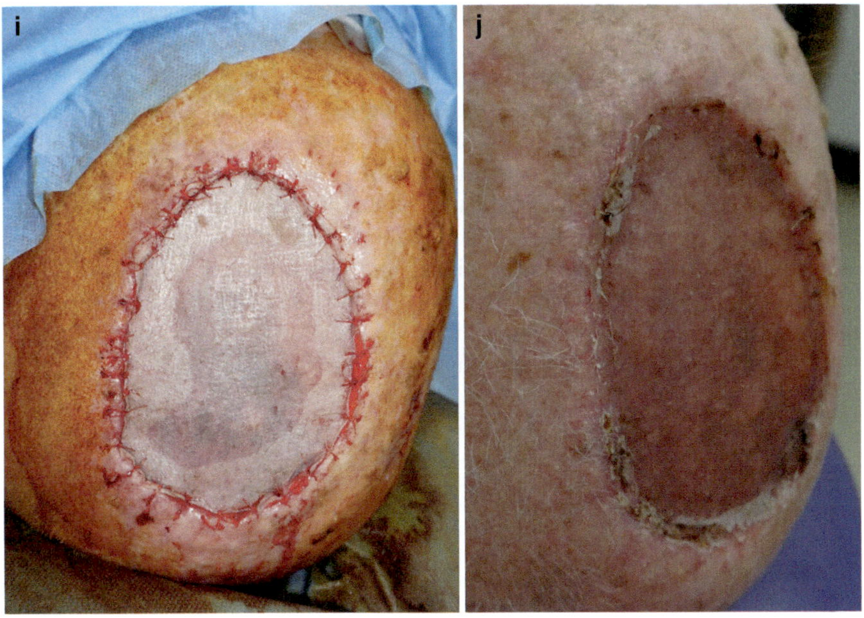

Fig. 5.13 (continued)

Pericranial Flap and Skin Grafting

Indications: Defect with exposed bone when a skin graft is planned.

Technique: The margins of the existing defect are widely undermined and/or additional incisions made and the scalp flap raised in the sub-galeal plane, taking care not to perforate the underlying pericranium. An appropriately oriented pericranial flap is raised on a broad base and transposed into the defect. The skin incisions are closed first, and residual defect lined by the pericranium, is covered with a split skin graft. The graft is held in place with appropriate dressing (Fig. 5.14a–o).

Tips: Try and orient the pericranial flap on known vascular pedicles and retain a broad base. Take care to avoid perforations. Do not allow the pericranium to dry out and use frequent irrigation while raising and securing the flap.

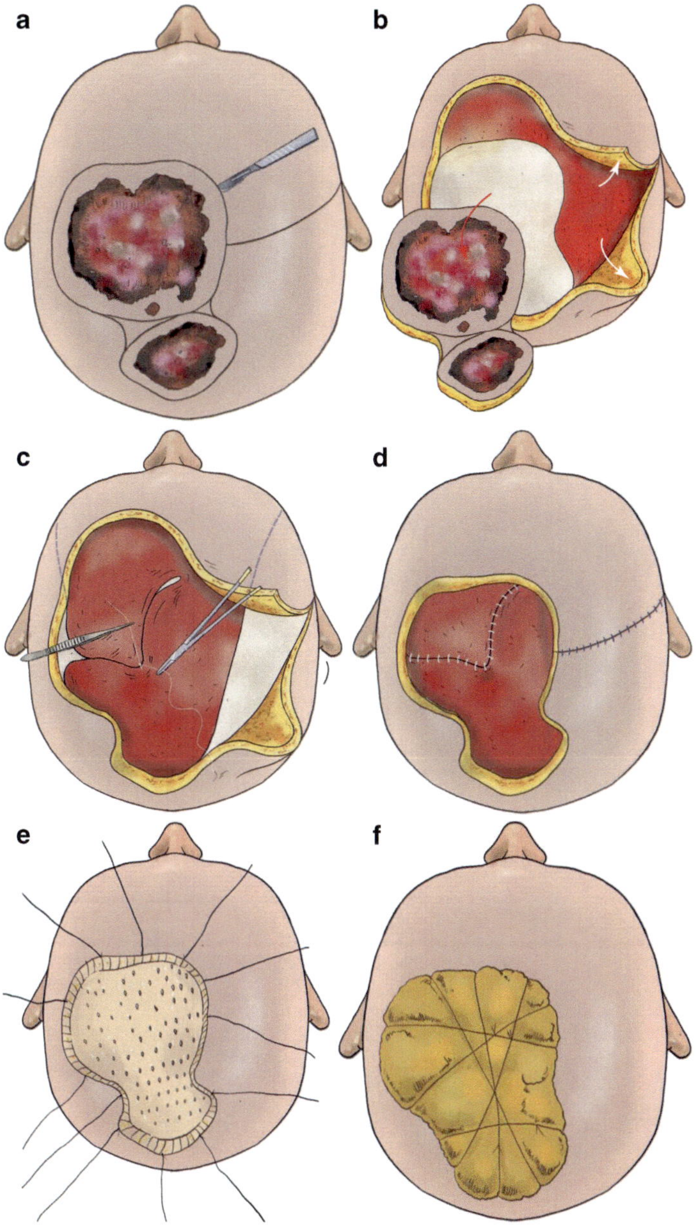

Fig. 5.14 Pericranial flap and skin grafting. (**a**) Markings for excision and scalp flaps, (**b**) "Bare" bone defect following excision and scalp flaps raised in sub galeal plane, (**c**) Pericranial flaps raised and transposed into defect, (**d**) Sutured pericranium covering "bare bone" defect and closure of scalp flaps, (**e**) Split skin graft sutured into defect, (**f**) Tie over bolus dressing in situ, (**g**) Markings for excision and scalp flap, (**h**) Excision defect down to bone, (**i**) Superior scalp flap raised, (**j**) Inferior scalp flap raised and marking for anteriorily based pericranial flap, (**k**) Raised pericranial flap, (**l**) Pericranial flap transposed into defect, (**m**) Scalp flap sutured in place, (**n**) Split skin graft laid over pericranial flap and sutured, (**o**) Tie over bolus dressing in situ

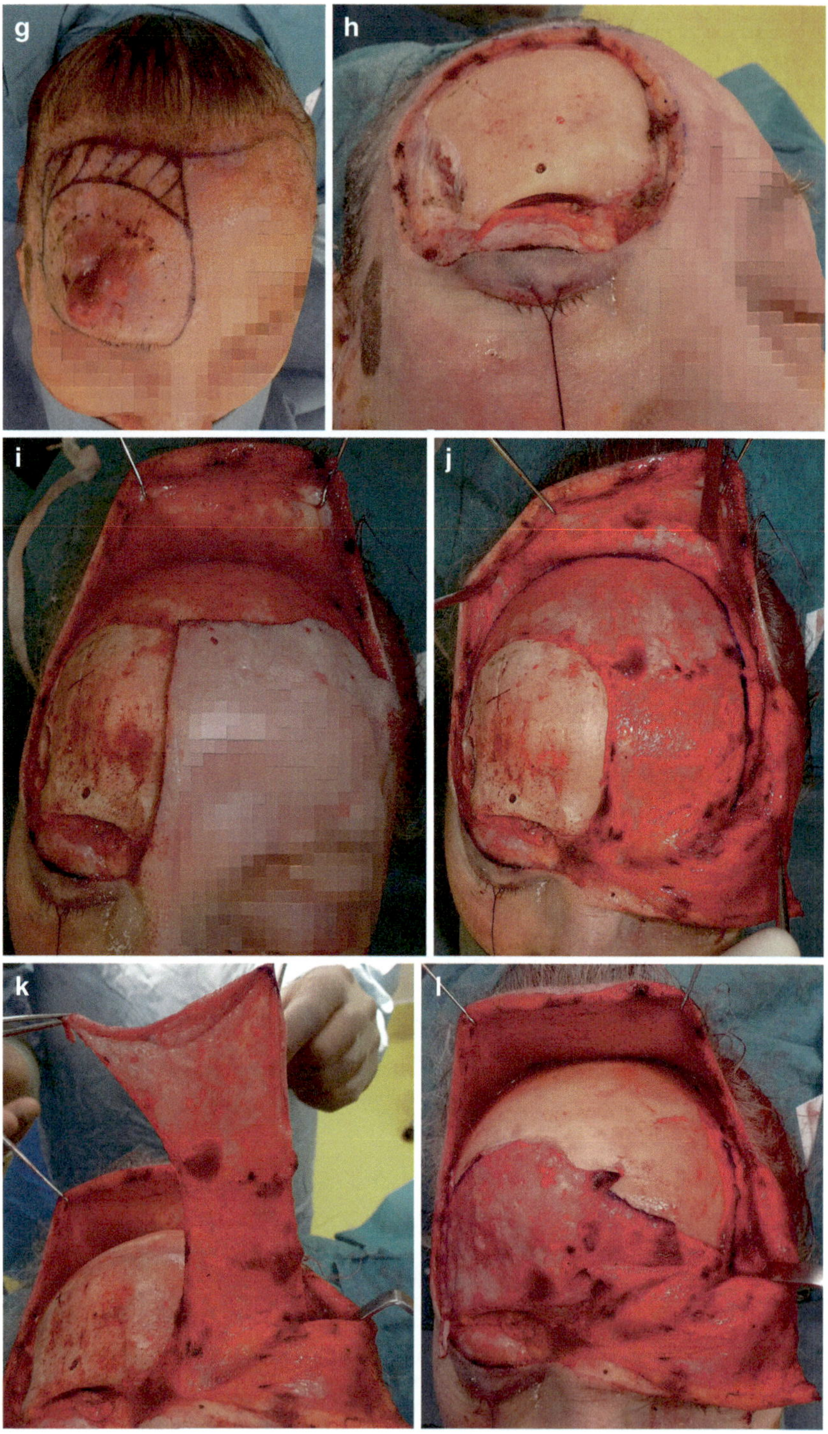

Fig. 5.14 (continued)

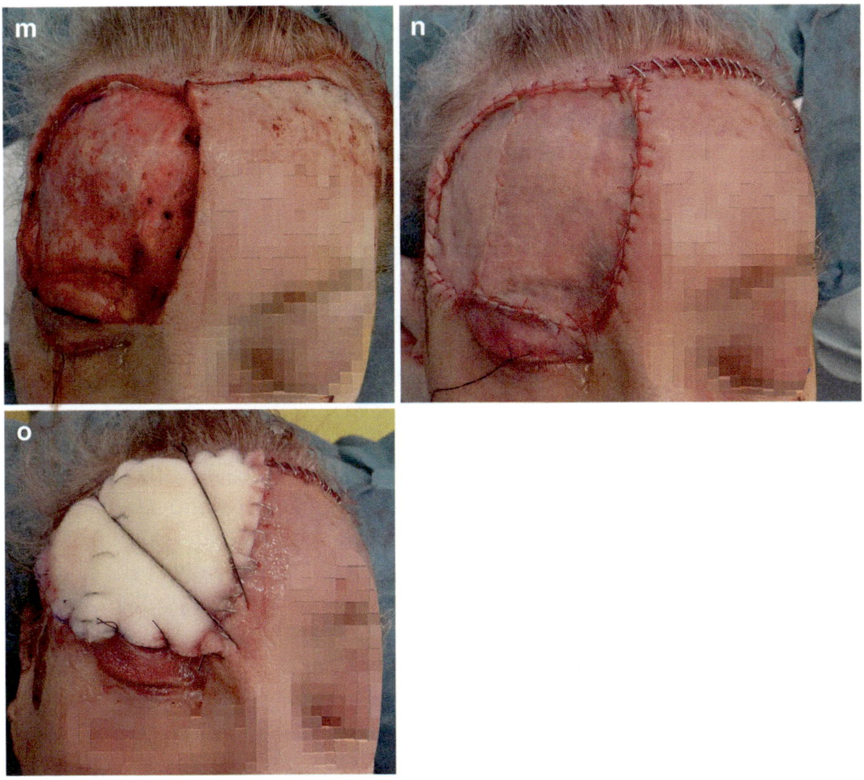

Fig. 5.14 (continued)

Transposition Flap/Skin Grafting of Secondary Defect.

Indications: Medium and large defects (vertex/lateral), defects with exposed bone.

Technique: Transposition flaps can be used to reconstruct defects of various shapes. The principal movement is lateral, and the flap recruits tissue immediately adjacent to or distant to the defect. One of the margins of the defect will form one of the margins of the flap. This could be along most of the length of the flap or just the base, depending on whether the tissue is recruited immediately adjacent or distant (with intervening tissue) to the defect.

Unlike rotation and bilobed flaps, transposition flaps have a linear configuration, and the lateral transposition leads to a decrease in the effective length of the flap. This will have to be considered, when designing the flap. Similarly, the greater the arc of movement the greater the size of the dog ear.

In the case of the standard transposition flap, two parallel incisions are made along the proximal edge of the defect, the width of which is equal to the width of the defect. The length of the flap should be longer than the defect, to account for the decrease in effective length and the flap is often raised in the sub-galeal plane and mobilised into the defect. A 3:1 length to width ratio should usually not be exceeded when designed as a "random" flap. In case of large defects, the flaps are best designed along named vessels as an axial pattern flap. The "secondary" is closed with a skin graft, as it is often not possible to close this primarily. The site and dimensions of the defect (primary and secondary) will principally determine the area of harvest of the flap (Anteriorly based Fig. 5.15a–i, posteriorly based Fig. 5.15j–q). The resultant dog ear is left in-situ and often flattens spontaneously. If persistent, this can be addressed at a later date.

Tips: It is best not the exceed a 3:1 length to width ratio, if designed as a random pattern flap. It is essential that a trial transfer is carried out with a piece of "gauze" to confirm the dimensions and orientation of the flap. The increased dimensions required to compensate for the "convexity" of the skull will also have to be considered. For large defects, the flap is best based on known vessels. The most appropriate patient position during the operation for both excision of the tumour and flap harvest is best trialled in the ward, prior to transfer to the operating table. Galeal scoring can be "carefully" considered to increase the dimensions of the flap, and excessive tension should be avoided at all costs.

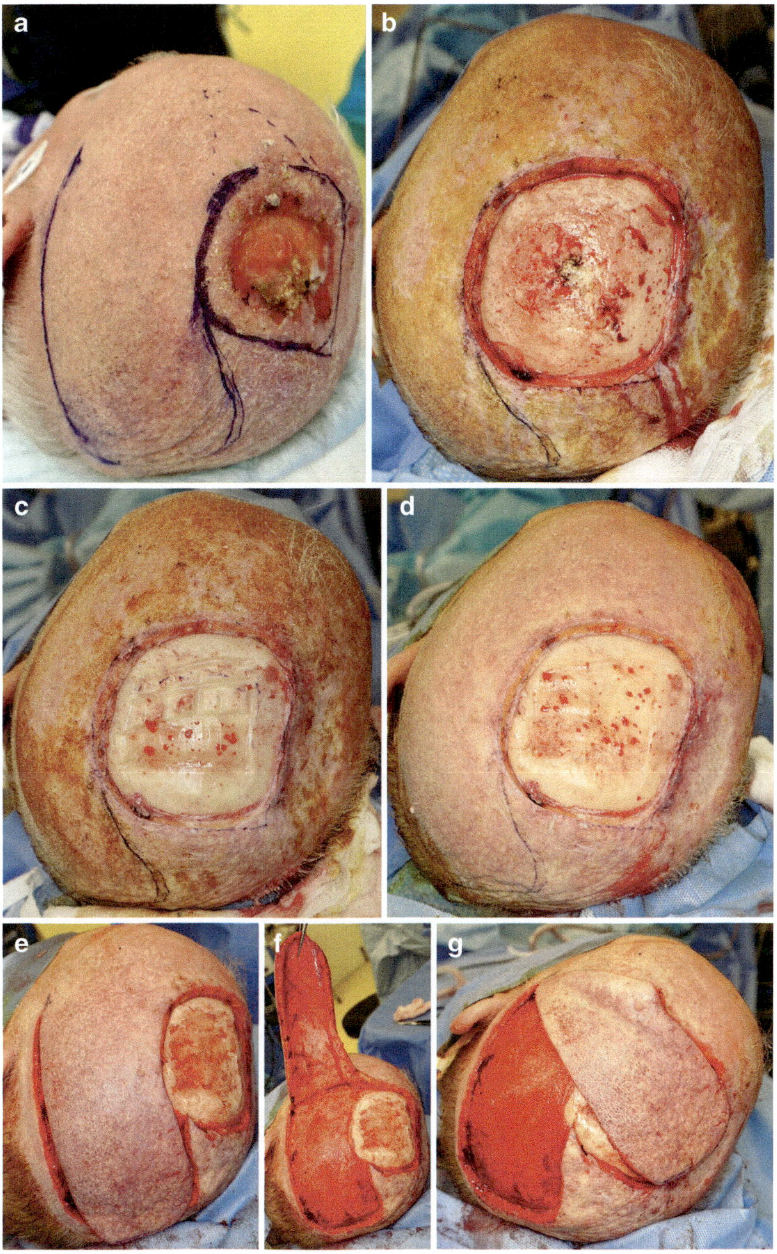

Fig. 5.15 Transposition flaps ((**a**–**i**) anteriorily based; (**j**–**q**) posteriorily based). (**a**) Markings for excision and anteriorly based flap, (**b**) Excision defect down to bare bone, (**c**) Depth orientation grooves for removal of outer cortex, (**d**) Defect follwoing removal of outer cortex, (**e**) Incisions for scalp flap, (**f**) Scalp flap raised in sub galeal plane, (**g**) Falp transposed into defect, (**h**) Split skin graft and flap sutured in place, (**i**) Pressure dressing stapled in situ, (**j**) Markings for excision, (**k**) Defect following excision, (**l**) Markings for a posteriorily based flap, (**m**) Flap raised, (**n**) Flap sutured into defect with dog ear in situ, (**o**) Secondary defect with pericranium in the base, (**p**) Split skin graft held in place with stapled pressure dressing, (**q**) Early post operative result at suture removal

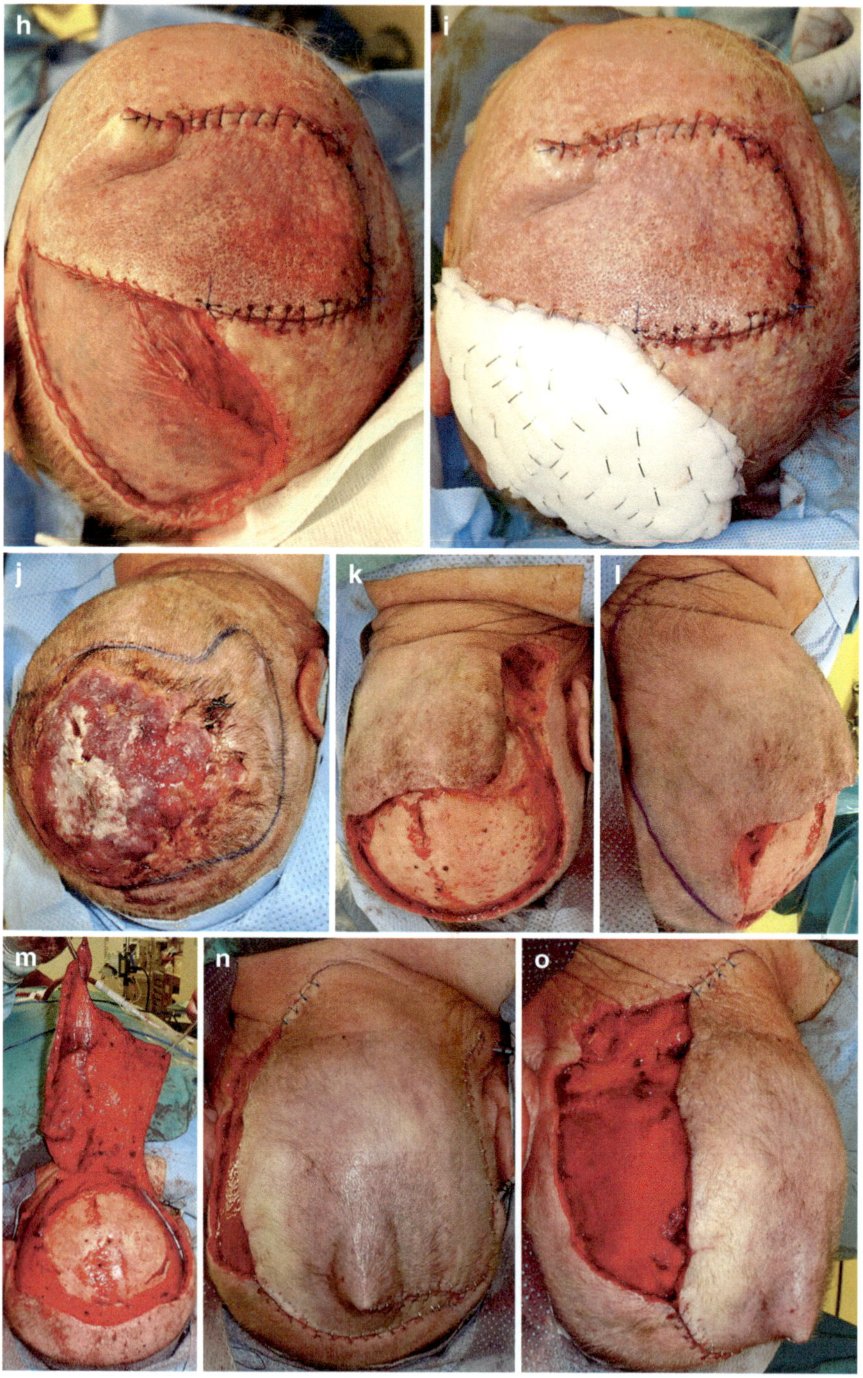

Fig. 5.15 (continued)

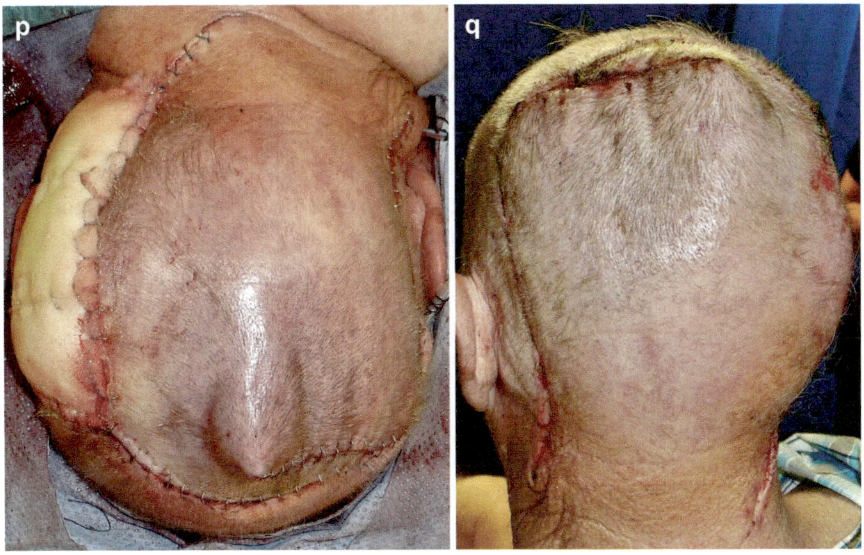

Fig. 5.15 (continued)

Recell

Indications: Medium and large defect with exposed bone.

Technique:

Recell® System (Avita Medical) is an autologous cell harvesting device which allows clinicians to harvest non-cultured skin cells from patients' own skin.

The device consists of a processing unit with a built-in heating mechanism.

The exposed bony defects are debrided with a surgical bur, and multiple bur holes can made within the outer calvarium. A full-thickness or split thickness skin graft is then harvested.

As per manufacturer's guideline, the skin graft is placed in trypsin solution for 15 mins at 37 °C to facilitate intercellular detachment. A scalpel is then used to scrape off the epidermal cells from the dermis for full-thickness skin grafts. Lactate solution was placed over the cells and aspirated with a syringe. The amount of compound sodium lactate solution used is dependent on the size of the skin graft. The aspirated solution is then filtered. The final suspension was sprayed onto the defect via a nozzle.

A non-absorbent dressing Telfa clear (Covidien®) and Tegaderm is then applied and left in place for 1 week. Granulation tissues can be observed in 2-month post-treatment. Complete skin epithelisation was observed 5 months post-operatively (Fig. 5.16a–f).

Tips: A split thickness skin graft will provide a larger volume of epidermal cells. Weekly review of the wound would be helpful to arrest any complications.. Initially, it is important to ensure that the dressings used are clear film dressings which are provided with the Recell® system and work by retaining cell suspension.

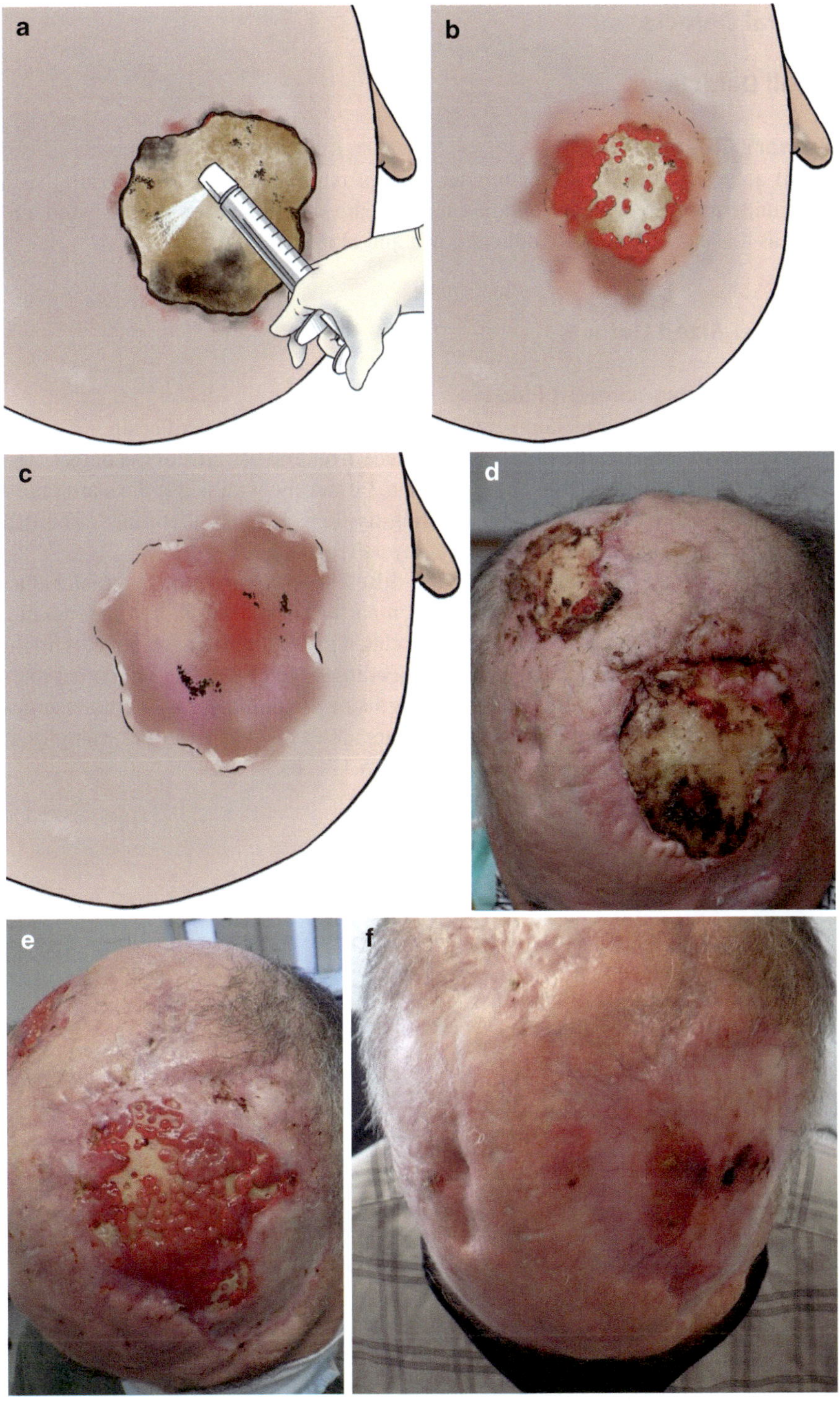

Fig. 5.16 Recell. (**a**) Suspended skin cells sprayed into defect, (**b**) Appearance of granulation tissue, (**c**) Epithelialisation of the defect, (**d**) Defect sprayed with suspended cells, (**e**) Appearance of granulation tissue, (**f**) Appearance follwing epithelialisation of the defect

Lateral Defects

Small Defects

Primary Closure

Small defects in the lateral region can be approximated by primary closure, with wide undermining of the surrounding tissue. Care should be exercised to avoid tension, as this can lead to wound breakdown and alopecia.

Medium-Sized Defects

Unilateral Advancement Flaps

Indication: Small- and medium-sized defects lateral and vertex of scalp.

Technique: Two parallel incisions are made from the margins of the defect. The length of these flaps are ideally no more than 3 times the width. The flaps are raised in the sub-galeal plane, and the surrounding tissue is widely undermined. The flap is advanced into the defect and closed in layers (Fig. 5.17a–h).

Tips: It is important to appreciate the difference in length (outer greater than inner) and thickness (raised flap thinner than native lateral margins) of the two flap margins and this would have to be accommodated in the suturing technique. It might be easier to place all the sutures along the leading edge of the flap and defect margins, before tying them. If the differing lengths of the flap margins are not accommodated during closure, the resulting dog ears are excised as Burrow's triangles at the base or along the margins of the flap (Fig. 5.17g, h).

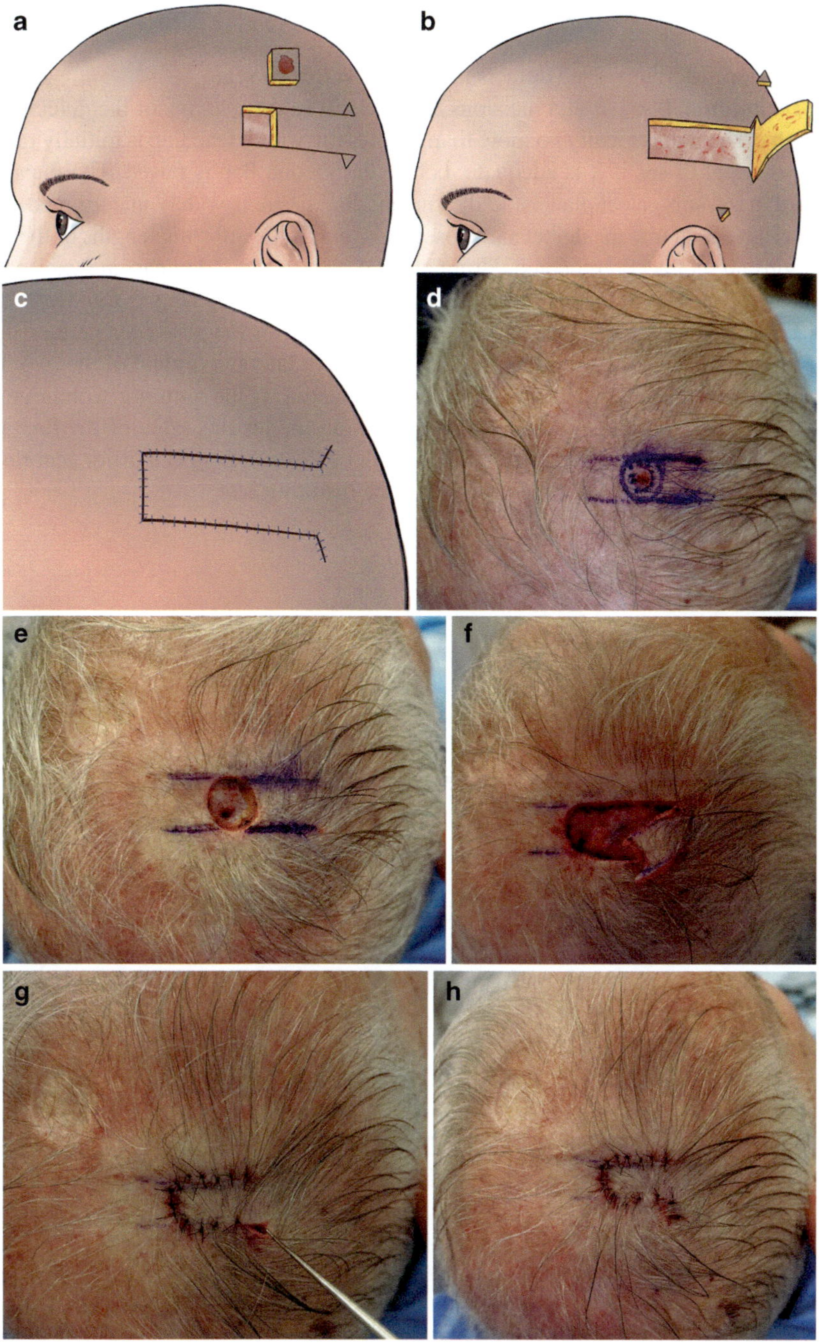

Fig. 5.17 Unilateral advancement flap. (**a**) Defect follwoing excision and flap markings, (**b**) Flap raised in the sub galeal plane, (**c**) Sutured in situ, (**d**) Markings for excision and flap, (**e**) Defect following excision, (**f**) Flap raised in sub galeal plane, (**g**) Flap sutured with dog ear in situ, (**h**) Final closure with correction of dog ear

Bilateral Advancement Flap

Indication: Medium-sized defects lateral and vertex of scalp.

Technique: Two parallel incisions are made from the margins of the defect. The length of the flap is ideally no more than 3 times the width. One flap is initially raised and assessed to see if it is adequate, before the second flap is raised. The flaps are raised in the sub-galeal plane, and the surrounding tissue is widely undermined. The flap is advanced into the defect and closed in layers. If the differing lengths of the flap margins are not accommodated during closure, the resulting dog ears are excised as Burrow's triangles at the base or along the margins of the flap (Fig. 5.18a–f).

Tips: It is important to appreciate the difference in length (outer greater than inner) and thickness (raised flap thinner than native lateral margins) of the two flap margins, and this would have to be accommodated in the suturing technique. It might be easier to place the all the sutures along the leading edge of the flap and defect margins, before tying them. The length of the two flaps can differ according to the relative tissue laxity and position of the resulting scar.

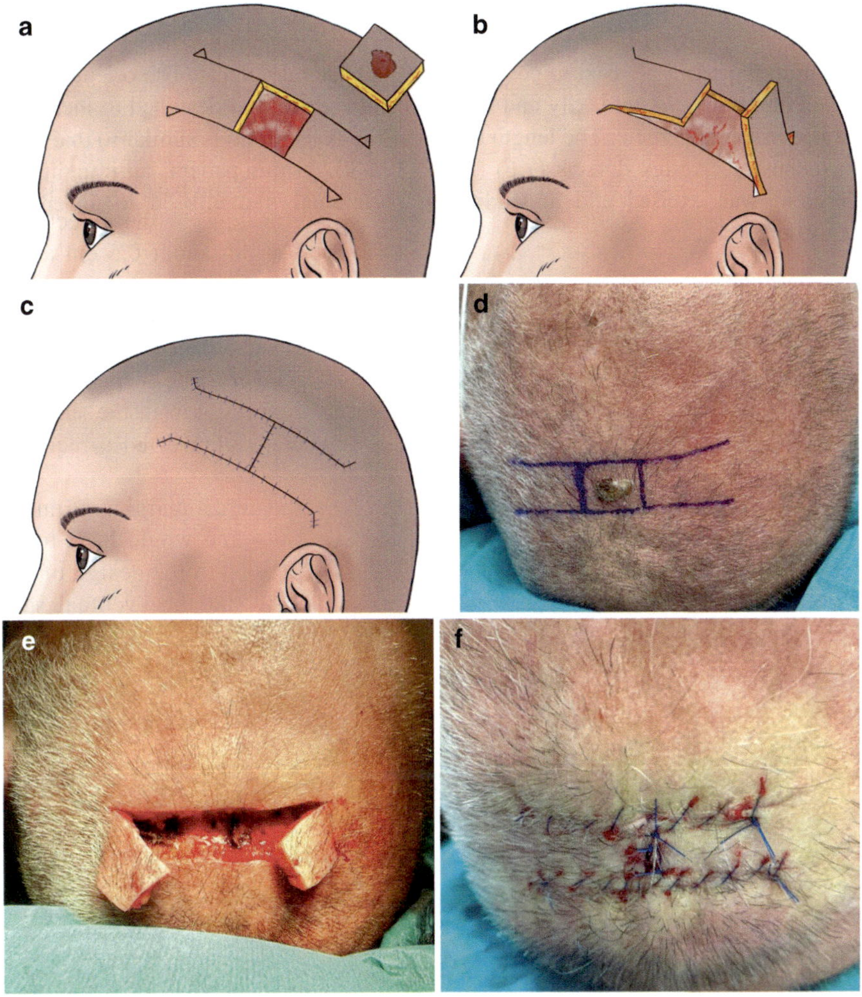

Fig. 5.18 Bilateral advancement flaps. (**a**) Defect following excision and flap markings, (**b**) Flaps raised in sub galeal plane, (**c**) Final closure, (**d**) Markings for excision and flaps, (**e**) Defect following excision and flaps raised, (**f**) Final closure

Rotation/Transposition Flaps

Rotation flaps can be used to cover a variety of lateral defects. The orientation is based on relative tissue laxity and large flaps, these are best designed to include a named vascular pedicle. The length to size of the defect ratio is similar to that used to reconstruct vertex defects (1:6) (Fig. 5.19a–k). In this patient, an intradiploic dermoid was excised and an additional pericranial flap utilised to cover the bony defect.

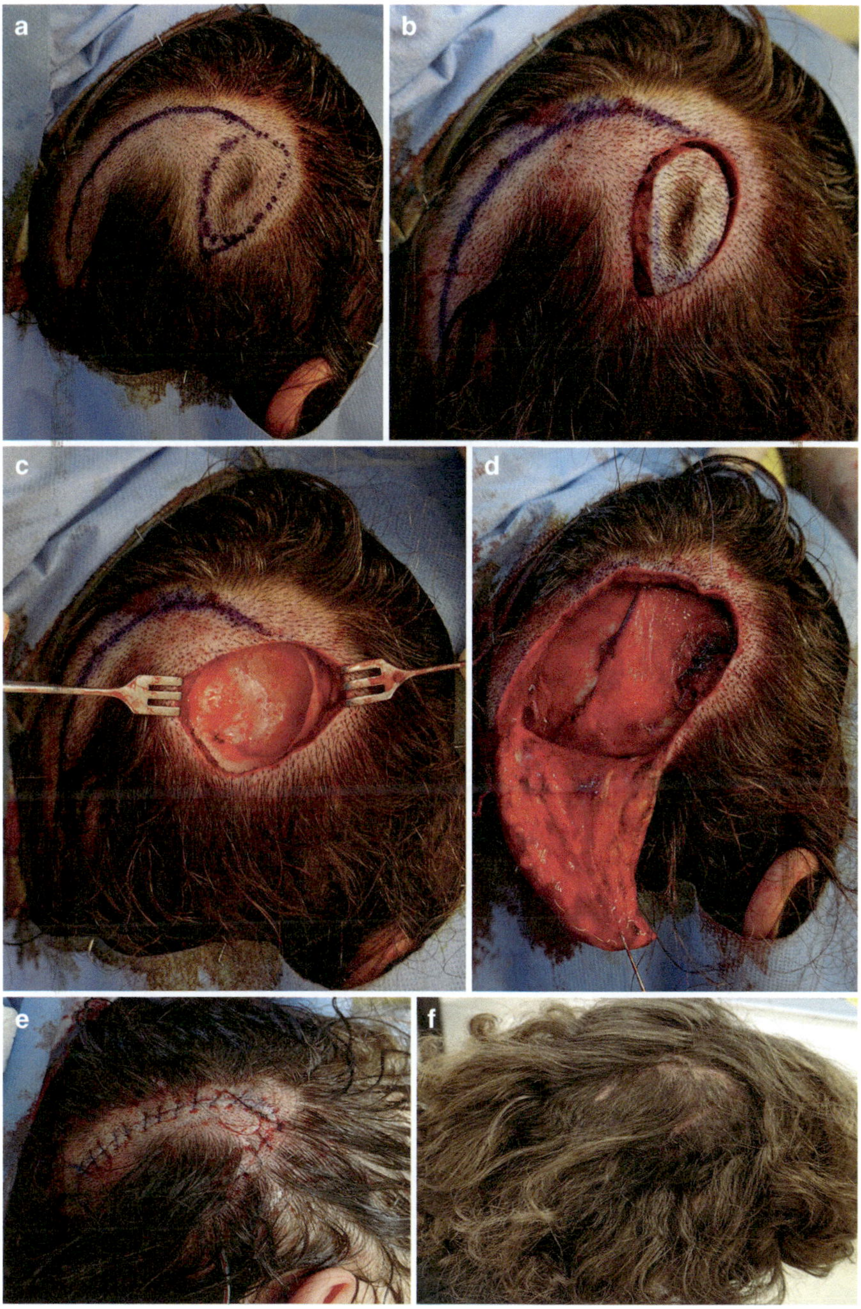

Fig. 5.19 Rotation/transposition flap. (**a**) Markings for excision and flap, (**b**) Excision of lesion, (**c**) Defect following excision, (**d**) Flap raised in sub galeal palne with wide underming of surrounding tissues. Pericranial flap to cover the bone defect, (**e**) Transposition flap sutured in situ, (**f**) Early post operaive result, (**g**) Markings for excision and flap, (**h**) Excision defect, (**i**) Flap raised, (**j**) Flap mobilised into defect, (**k**) Final closure

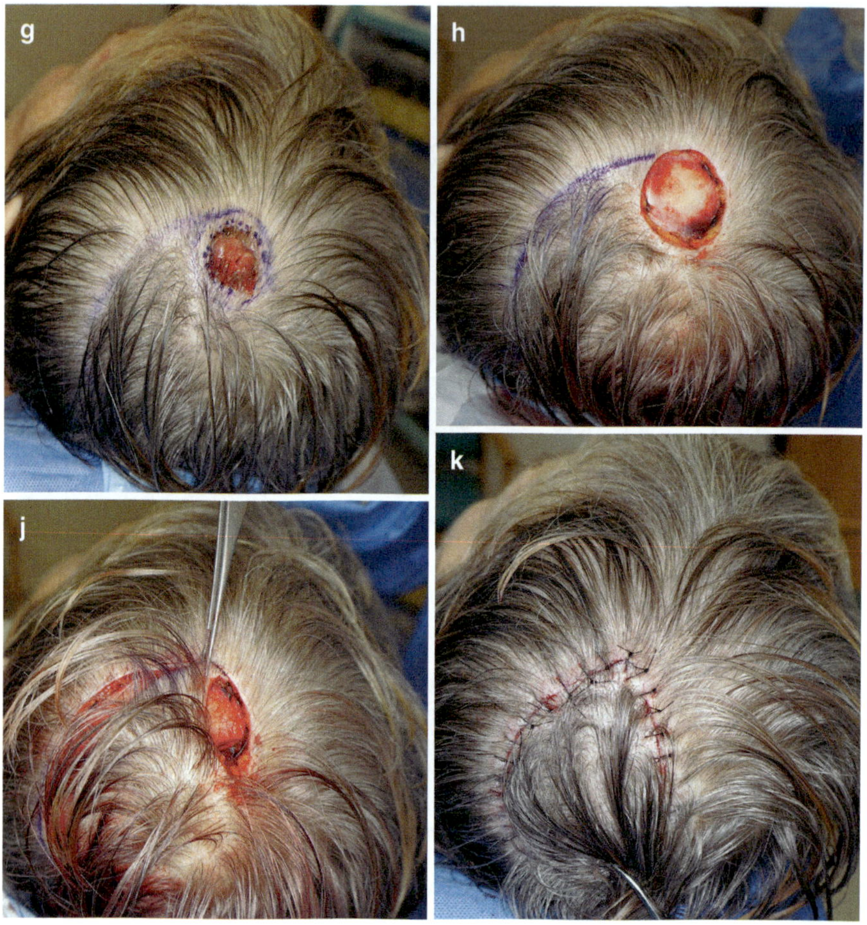

Fig. 5.19 (continued)

Suggested Algorithm

Central (Vertex) Defects

Small

1. Primary closure.
2. Healing by secondary intention.

Medium

1. Rotation/transposition flap.
2. O-Z closure.
3. Unilateral/bilateral advancement flap.
4. Multiple rotation (pin wheel) flap.
5. Multiple Limberg flap.
6. Skin graft.
7. ReCell®.

Large

1. Skin graft.
2. Skin graft with Integra®.
3. Skin graft with pericranial flap.
4. Multiple rotation flap.
5. Rotation/transposition flap with skin graft to secondary defect.

Lateral Defects

Small

1. Primary closure.

Medium

1. Unilateral/bilateral advancement flap.
2. Rotation/transposition flap.
3. O-Z closure.
4. Skin graft.

Large

1. Rotation/transposition flap with skin graft to secondary defect.
2. Skin graft.
3. Skin graft with Integra®.

Forehead Reconstruction 6

Subunits and Anatomical Considerations

The forehead can be divided into central, paramedian and lateral (temple) subunits (Fig. 6.1). In addition, the subunits can be further divided into upper and lower segments for the purposes of reconstruction.

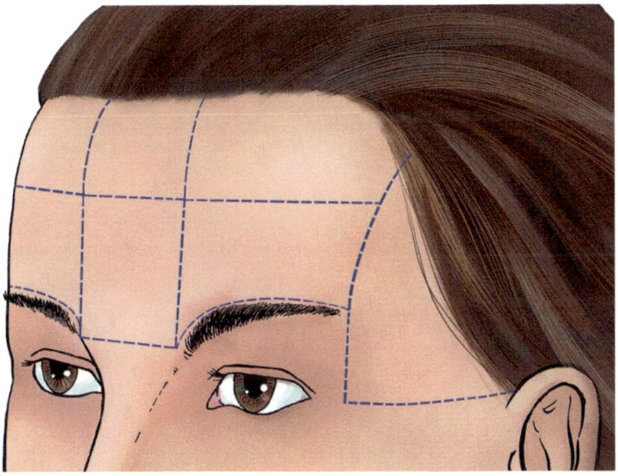

Fig. 6.1 Forehead: Subunits

V. Ilankovan et al., *Local Flaps in Facial Reconstruction*,
https://doi.org/10.1007/978-3-031-49464-2_6

The supra-orbital and supra-trochlear nerves traverse the bony orbital margins, pierce the overlying muscles and run in the subcutaneous plane, just above the frontalis/galea up to the vertex (Fig. 6.2). If attempting to preserve the sensation of the forehead, horizontal incisions and undermining should be limited to the subcutaneous plane. In case of central vertical incisions, undermining can be undertaken in the plane deep to frontalis/galea.

In the central forehead, the frontalis muscle is often separated in the lower part before they join together to form a raphae. This along with the creases created by the "corrugator supercilli" offer the possibility of utilising vertical scars in this area. In the para median and lateral subunits, the RSTLs lie horizontally and offer good camouflage to scars (Fig. 6.3).

The temporal branch of the facial nerve runs on the deep surface of the frontalis/galea and therefore incisions and dissections should be above this plane. It is also important that any transection of the frontalis is repaired to restore continuity of the muscle, so as to avoid drooping of the eyebrow.

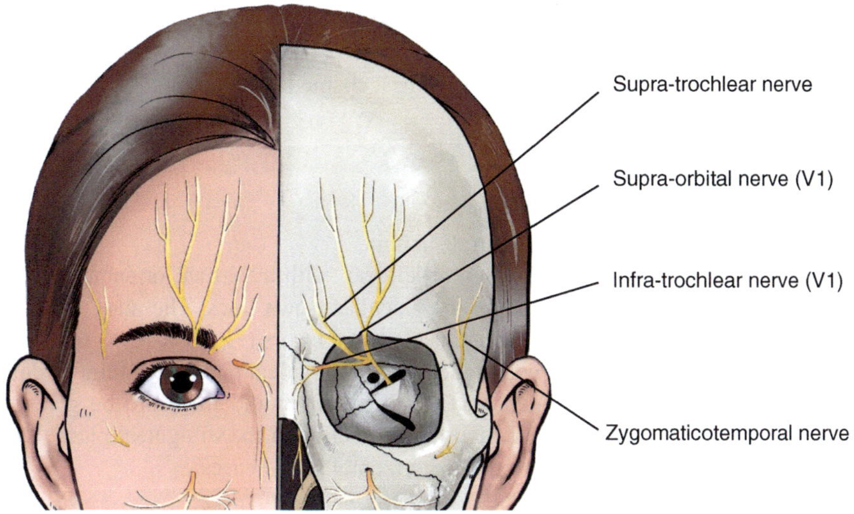

Fig. 6.2 Nerve supply of forehead

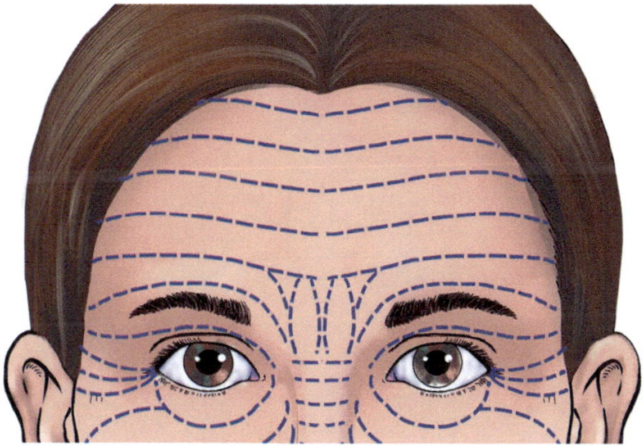

Fig. 6.3 Orientation of RSTL's in the forehead

Central Defects (Between the Medial End of the Eyebrows)

Vertical orientation of the scars offers the best cosmetic outcome.

Elliptical Excision

Indication: Small lesion in the central subunit.

Technique: The lesion is excised an ellipse, with a vertical orientation. This enables placement of the scar along the glabellar frown lines. The margins of the defect are undermined, and the wound is closed in layers (Fig. 6.4a–c).

Tips: Undermining is best undertaken in the sub-galeal plane, to minimise damage to the adjacent sensory nerves. Consideration should therefore be given to remove additional deep tissue, to facilitate dissection in the sub-galeal plane. Care should be taken to accurately orient the horizontal skin creases.

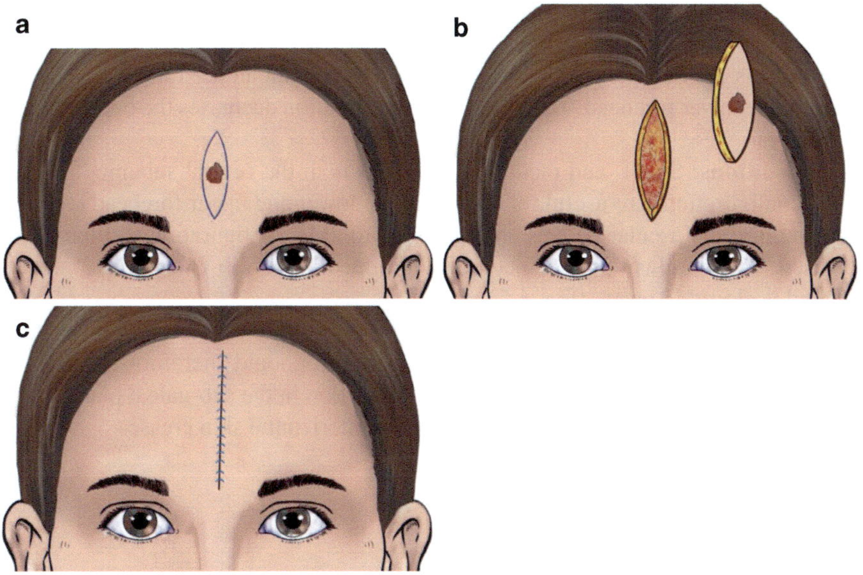

Fig. 6.4 Vertical elliptical excision and primary closure. (**a**) Marking for excision, (**b**) Excision defect, (**c**) Final closure

M & W Flaps

The defects are best closed as "M" flaps if present in the upper forehead and "W" flaps in the lower forehead. The "M & W" configuration decreases the overall length of the scar.

Indications: Small- and medium-sized defects in the central subunit. "M" and "W" configurations are useful for defects in the lower and upper forehead regions.

Technique: Circular defects are converted to "M" configuration and the lesion excised. The margins of the defect are undermined in the sub-galeal plane, and the wound is closed in layers (Fig. 6.5a–g).

Tips: Undermining is best undertaken in the sub-galeal plane, to minimise damage to the adjacent sensory nerves. Consideration should therefore be given to remove additional deep tissue, to facilitate dissection in the sub-galeal plane.

Care should be taken to accurately orient the horizontal skin creases.

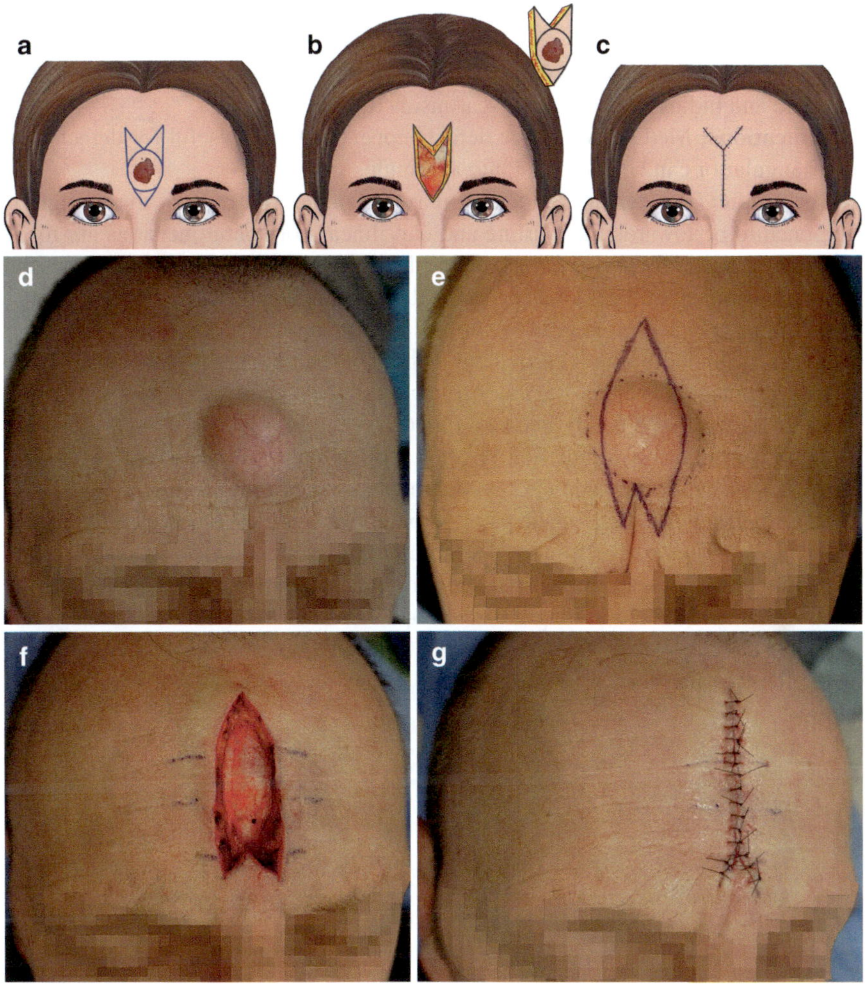

Fig. 6.5 W and M excision and closure. (**a**) M excision markings, (**b**) Defect following excision, (**c**) Final closure, (**d**) Lesion central forehead, (**e**) W excision markings, (**f**) Defect following excision, (**g**) Final closure maintaing horizontal skin creases

Upper Forehead

V-T flap: A "V-T" flap offers the advantage of utilising a vertical scar in the central forehead and hiding the horizontal scar inside the hairline.

Indications: Medium and large defects upper forehead. Useful for defects that are triangular or can be converted into a triangle.

Technique: The defect is modified into a triangle. The base of the triangle is fashioned to be towards the hairline and curvilinear horizontal incisions are made laterally from the base of the defect, inside the hairline. The horizontal incisions and any undermining are best carried out in the subcutaneous plane if an attempt is made to preserve sensation to the scalp and avoid transecting the frontalis. In other instances the undermining is carried out in the sub galeal/frontalis plane. The wound is sutured in layers and any Burrow's triangles are best positioned superiorly at the lateral margins (Fig. 6.6a–d). See also Fig. 6.14.

Tips: Subcutaneous dissection is often tedious and is best carried out with a blade. It is essential to avoid buttonholing the flap and compromising the blood supply. The hairline incision is made parallel to the hair follicles to decrease the risk of alopecia. Sub-galeal dissection results in a more robust flap, which is easier to raise, but will result in transection of the supra-orbital and supra-trochlear nerve at the hairline. The difference in length of the flaps can often be accommodated by differential suturing, but if dog ears are to be excised, these are best done superiorly inside the hairline. Care should be taken to accurately orient the horizontal skin creases.

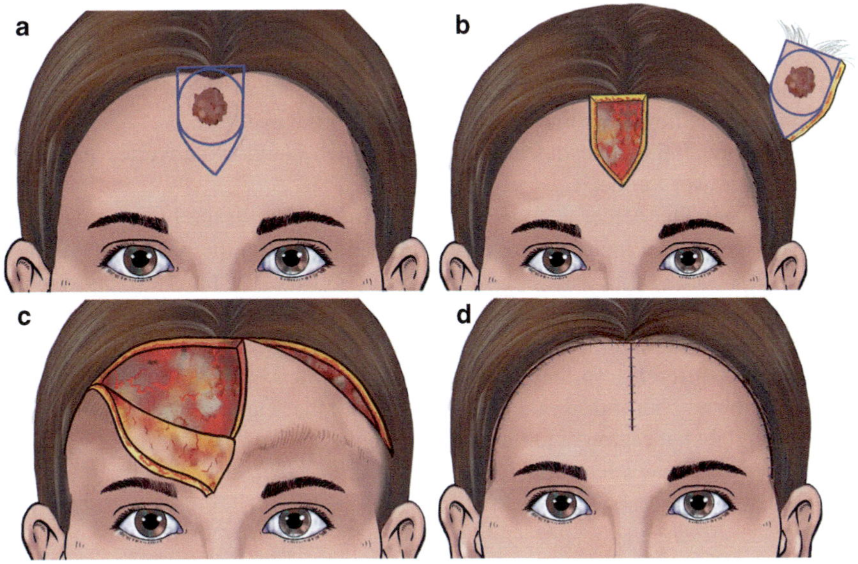

Fig. 6.6 V-T flap. (**a**) Markings of excision and flap, (**b**) Excision defect, (**c**) Flaps raised the appropriate plane, (**d**) Final closure

Lower Forehead

A-T flap: The "A-T" flap offers the advantage of utilising a vertical scar in the forehead and positioning the horizontal incisions along the eyebrow.

Indications: Triangular defects or defects which could be converted into a triangle in the lower forehead.

Technique: The defect is converted into a triangle, with the base in the lower forehead. Horizontal incisions are extended laterally, from the base of the defect, along the forehead skin creases just above the eyebrows. The flaps are raised in the subcutaneous plane if an attempt is made to preserve sensation to the scalp and avoid transecting the frontalis. The wound is sutured in layers (Fig. 6.7a–c).

Tips: The difference in length of the flaps can often be accommodated by differential suturing, but if dog ears are to be excised, these are best positioned inferiorly in the glabellar region or at the lateral extremity to hide the scar in the glabellar frown lines and crow's feet, respectively. Care should be taken to accurately orient the horizontal skin creases.

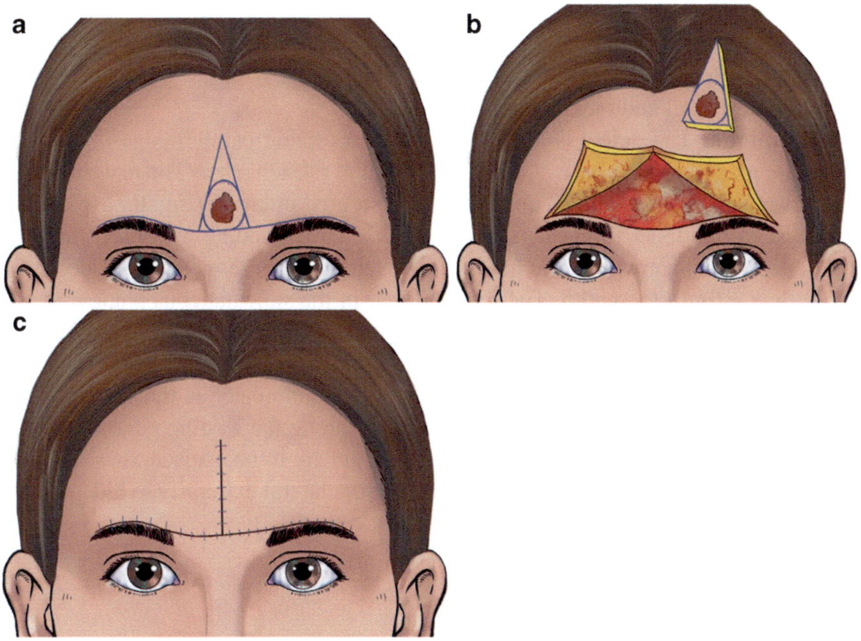

Fig. 6.7 A-T flap. (**a**) Markings for excision and flap, (**b**) Excision defect and flaps raised, (**c**) Final closure

Upper and Lower Forehead

Unilateral Advancement Flaps

Indication: Small and medium defects.

Technique: The defect is ideally converted to obtain parallel edges. Two incisions are made from the base of the defect, parallel to each other. The margins of the defect are widely undermined and the wound sutured in layers (Fig. 6.8a–c).

Tips: In the upper forehead, one could consider expanding the defect, to place the superior incision within the hairline. The length of these incisions is ideally no more than 3 times the width. The flap is raised in the subcutaneous plane if sensation is to be preserved. It is important to appreciate the difference in length (outer greater than inner) and thickness (raised flap thinner than native lateral margins) of the two flap margins and this would have to be accommodated in the suturing technique. It might be easier to place all the sutures along the leading edge of the flap and defect margins, before tying them. If dog ears are to be excised, these are best positioned medially in the glabella region or at the lateral extremity to hide the scar in the glabella frown lines and crow's feet, respectively.

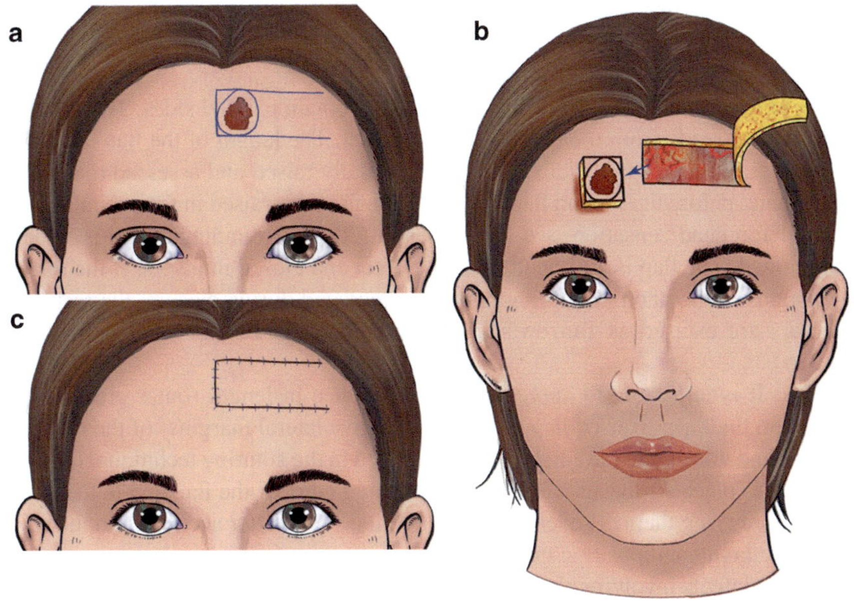

Fig. 6.8 Unilateral advancement flap. (**a**) Markings for excision and flap, (**b**) Excision defect and flap raised, (**c**) Final closure

Bilateral Advancement Flap

Indications: Medium defects in the forehead.

Technique: The defect is ideally converted to obtain parallel sides. Two parallel incisions are made from the margins of the defect. The length of the flap is ideally no more than 3 times the width. One flap is initially raised and assessed to see if it is adequate, before the second flap is raised. The flaps are raised in the subcutaneous plane if forehead sensation is to be preserved. The surrounding tissue is widely undermined. The flap is advanced into the defect and closed in layers. If the differing lengths of the flap margins are not accommodated during closure, the resulting dog ears are excised as Burrow's triangles at the base or along the margins of the flap.

Tips: It is important to appreciate the difference in length (outer greater than inner) and thickness (raised flap thinner than native lateral margins) of the two flap margins and this would have to be accommodated in the suturing technique. It might be easier to place all the sutures along the leading edge of the flap and defect margins, before tying them. The length of the two flaps can differ according to the relative tissue laxity and position of the resulting scar (Fig. 6.9a–g).

Larger defects involving the upper and lower forehead can be closed with bilateral advancement flaps, with the superior horizontal incision placed just within the hairline and the inferior, just above the eye brow. In these instances, large flaps are raised, the incision is made down to the periosteum and the flaps raised in the subgaleal plane to avoid compromising its vascularity by preserving the anterior branch of the superficial temporal vessels. The position of the eyebrow is maintained by anchoring it to the periosteum at the desired level.

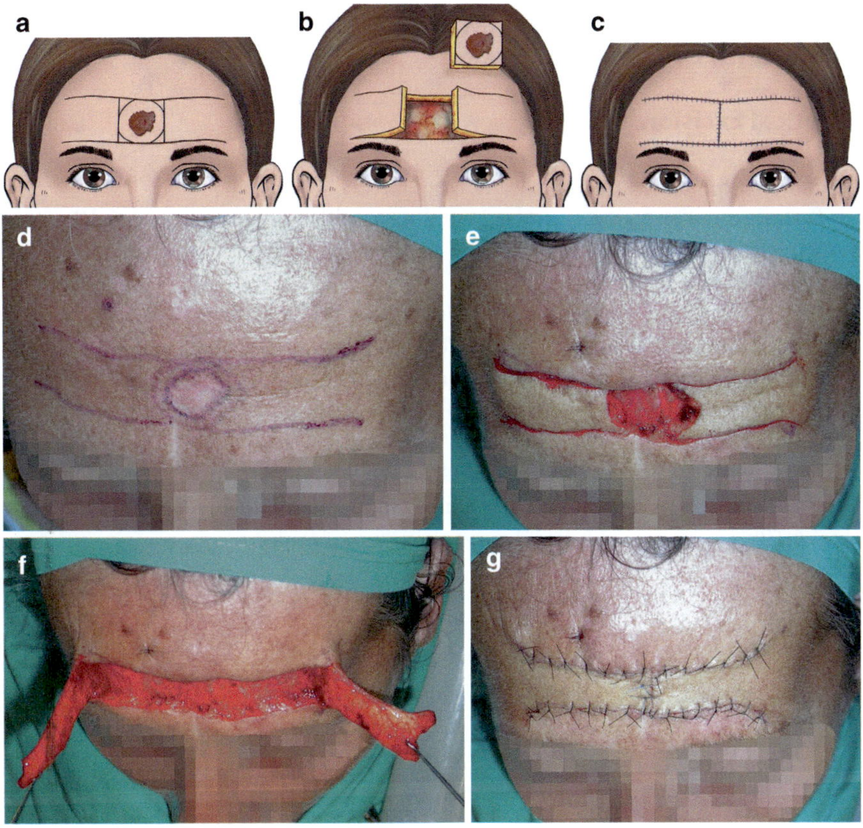

Fig. 6.9 Bilateral advancement flap. (**a**) Markings for excision and flaps, (**b**) Excision defect and flaps raised, (**c**) Final closure, (**d**) Markings for excision and flaps, (**e**) Excision defect and flap incisions, (**f**) Flaps raised, (**g**) Final closure

Paramedian Defects (Between Medial End of the Eyebrow and Lateral Orbital Rim)

Elliptical Excision

Indication: Small central and paramedian defects.

Technique: The lesion is excised an ellipse, with a horizontal (Fig. 6.10a–d) or vertical (Fig. 6.10e–g) orientation. The margins of the defect are undermined and the wound closed in layers.

Tips: Undermining is best undertaken in the sub-galeal plane, to minimise damage to the adjacent sensory nerves. Consideration should therefore be given to remove additional deep tissue, to facilitate dissection in the sub-galeal plane. Care should be taken to accurately orient the horizontal skin creases and prevent distortion of the eyebrows.

To decrease the overall length of the scar, the lateral margins of the defect can be converted to a "W," with the scar still lying parallel to the forehead furrows (Fig. 6.10h–j).

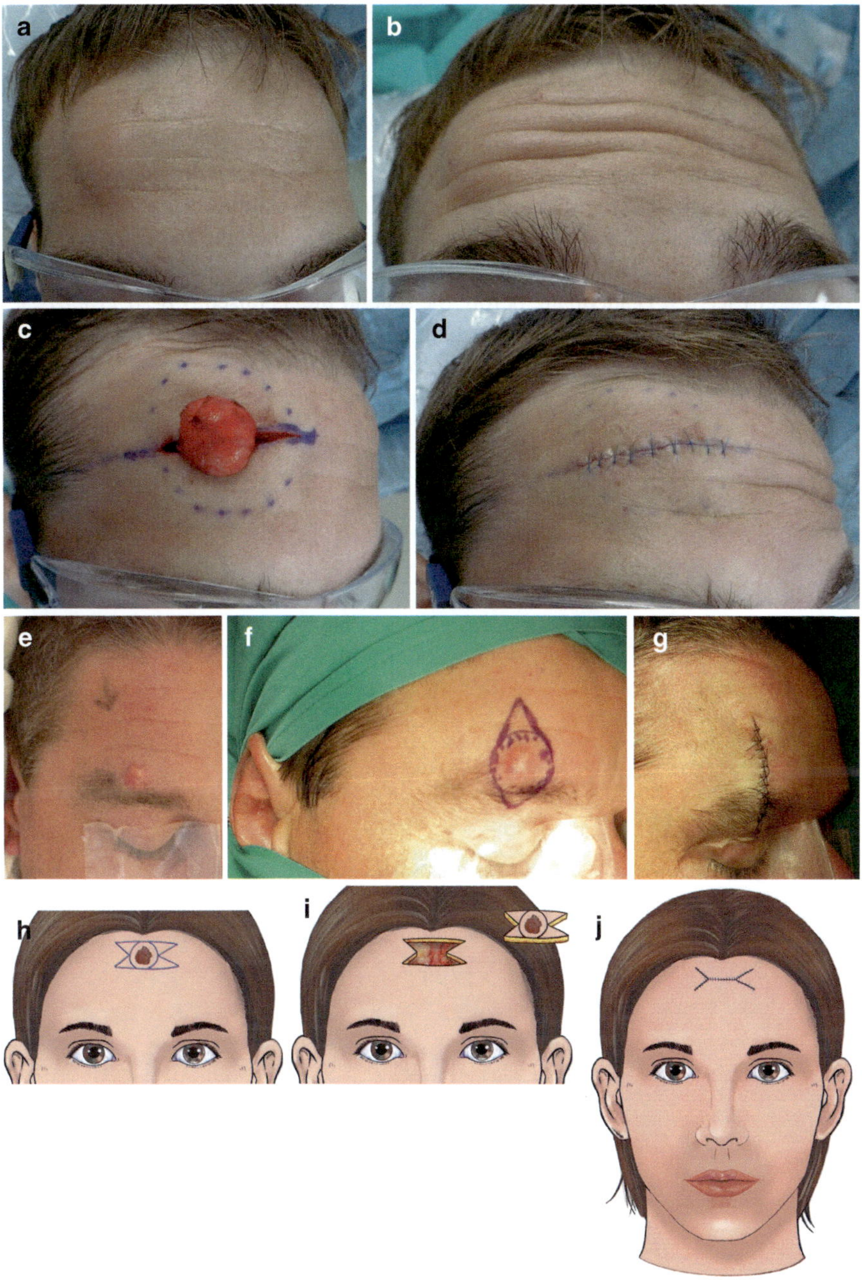

Fig. 6.10 Horizontal and Vertical excision and primary closure. (**a**) Lesion lateral forehead, (**b**) Orientation of horizontal skin creases, (**c**) Horizontal excision of lesion, (**d**) Final closure, (**e**) Lesion lateral forehead/eyebrow, (**f**) Markings for vertical excision of lesion, (**g**) Final closure, (**h**) Markings for lying "W" excision, (**i**) Excision defect, (**j**) Final closure

Unilateral/Bilateral Advancement Flaps

Indications: Small, medium defects. Advantage of placing the incisions along the forehead skin creases.

Technique: The defect is ideally converted to have parallel sides. Horizontal incisions are made from the base of the defect and extend laterally and/or medially, parallel to the frown lines. The incisions and any undermining are best carried out in the subcutaneous plane in an attempt to preserve sensation to the scalp and avoid transecting the frontalis. In the case of bilateral flaps, one flap is initially raised and assessed to see if it is adequate, before the second flap is raised (Fig. 6.11a, b).

Tips: Due to the difference in the lengths of the flap adjacent to the horizontal incisions, Burrow's triangles will have to be excised and are best positioned medially in the glabellar region or laterally in the crow's foot region.

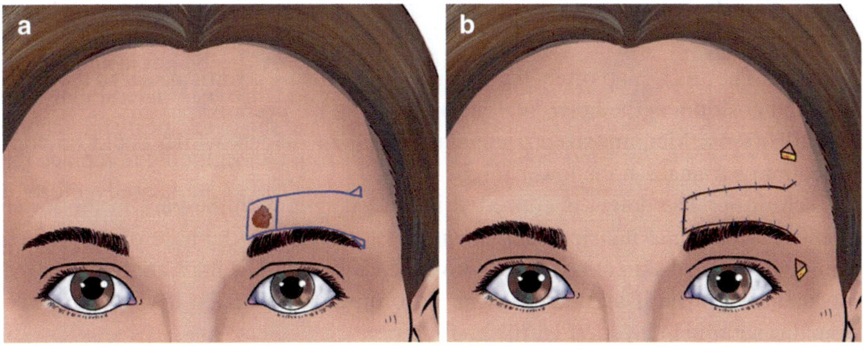

Fig. 6.11 Unilateral advancement flap. (**a**) Markings for excision and flap, (**b**) Final closure with excision of dog ears

Lower Forehead

A-T flap: The "A-T" flap offers the advantage of utilising a vertical scar in the forehead and positioning the horizontal incisions along the eyebrow.

Indications: Medium-sized triangular defects or defects which could be converted into a triangle in the lower forehead.

Technique: The defect is converted into a triangle, with the base in the lower forehead. Horizontal incisions are extended laterally, from the base of the defect, along the forehead skin creases/just above the eyebrows. The flaps are raised in the subcutaneous plane if an attempt is made to preserve sensation to the scalp. The wound is sutured in layers (Fig. 6.12a–f).

Tips: The difference in length of the flaps can often be accommodated by differential suturing, but if dog ears are to be excised, these are best positioned inferiorly in the glabellar region or at the lateral extremity to hide the scar in the glabellar frown lines and crow's feet respectively. Care should be taken to accurately orient the horizontal skin creases. It is often necessary to excise additional deep tissue to prevent "bunching" of the tissues and these can be made away from the nerves.

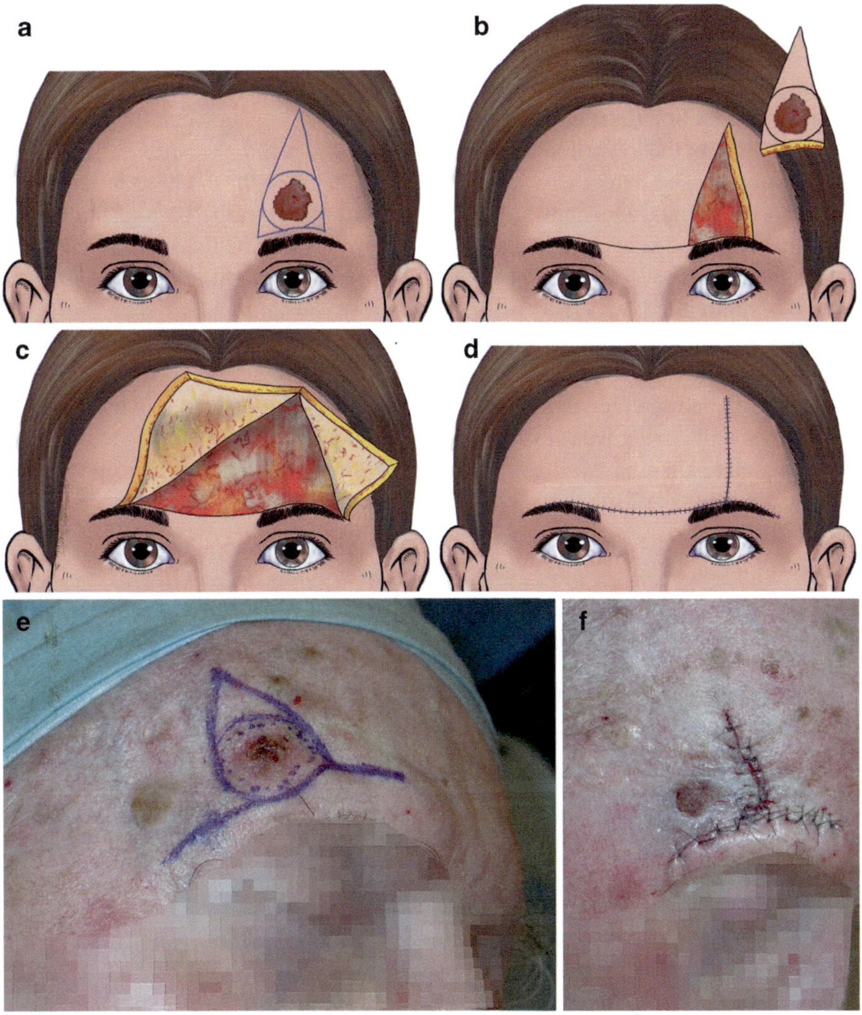

Fig. 6.12 A-T flap. (**a**) Markings for excision, (**b**) Excision defect and markings for flap, (**c**) Flaps raised in an appropriate plane, (**d**) Final closure, (**e**) Markings for excision and flap, (**f**) Final closure

V-T Flap

The "V - T" flap offers the advantage of utilising a horizontal scar in the forehead and positioning the vertical incision in the eyebrow.

Indications: Small-sized triangular defects or defects which could be converted into a triangle in the lower forehead.

Technique: The defect is converted into a triangle, with the base in the upper forehead. Horizontal incisions are extended laterally, from the base of the defect, along the forehead skin creases/just above the eyebrows. The flaps are raised in the subcutaneous plane if an attempt is made to preserve sensation to the scalp. The wound is sutured in layers (Fig. 6.13a–c).

Tips: The difference in length of the flaps can often be accommodated by differential suturing, but if dog ears are to be excised, these are best positioned inferiorly in the glabellar region or at the lateral extremity to hide the scar in the glabellar frown lines and crow's feet, respectively. Care should be taken to accurately orient the horizontal skin creases. It is often necessary to excise additional deep tissue to prevent "bunching" of the tissues and these can be made away from the nerves.

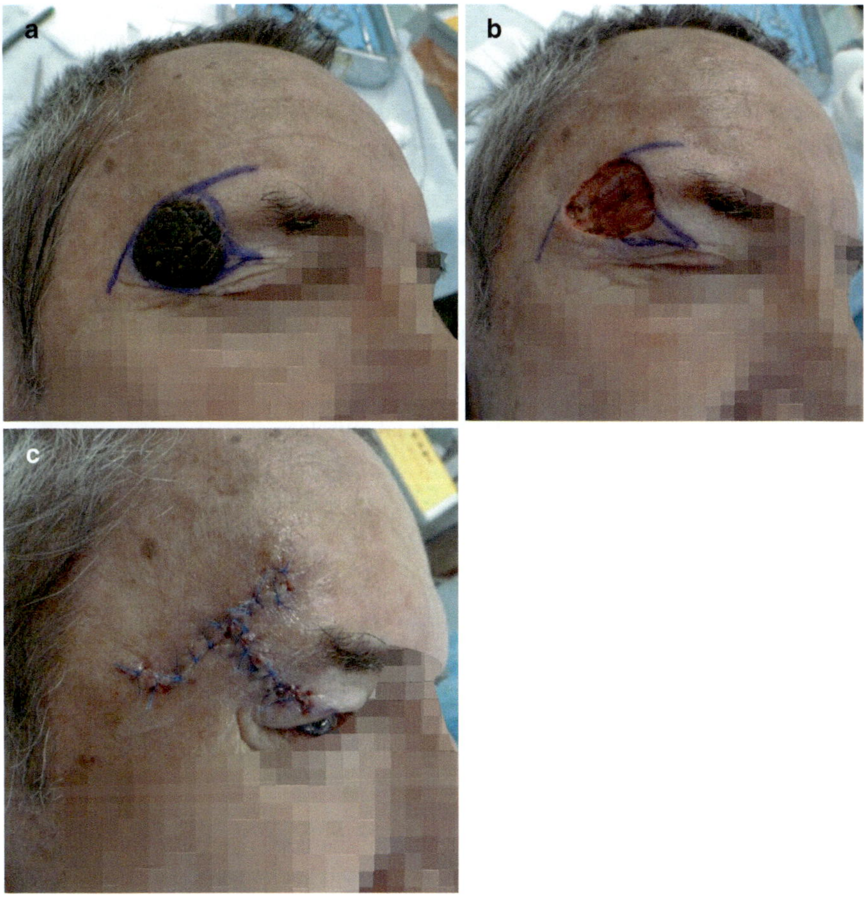

Fig. 6.13 V-T flap. (**a**) Markings for excision and flap, (**b**) Excision defect, (**c**) Final closure

Upper Forehead

V-T flap: Medium and large defects. See medial defects (Figs. 6.6a–d and 6.14).

Tips: In addition, the lateral flap is raised in the subcutaneous plane to avoid damage to the frontal branch of the facial nerve.

Lateral Forehead/Temple (Between the Lateral Orbital Rim and Zygomatic Arch)

Elliptical excision: Small defects can be converted into an ellipse, oriented to lie parallel to the crow's foot. The incisions and any undermining are best carried out in the subcutaneous plane in an attempt to avoid damage to the temporal branch of the facial nerves, which runs deep to the facial muscles.

V-T Flap

Indication: For defects that are triangular or can be converted into a triangle. The "V-T" flap offers the advantage of utilising a vertical scar in crow's foot and hiding the horizontal scar inside the hairline.

Technique: The base of the triangle is fashioned to be towards the hairline, with horizontal incisions extending laterally from the margins of the basal defect, inside the hairline. The horizontal incisions and any undermining are best carried out in the subcutaneous plane in an attempt to avoid damage to the temporal branch of the facial nerve (Fig. 6.14a–j).

Tips: Due to the difference in the lengths of the flap adjacent to the horizontal incisions, Burrow's triangles will have to be excised and are best positioned superiorly, within the hairline.

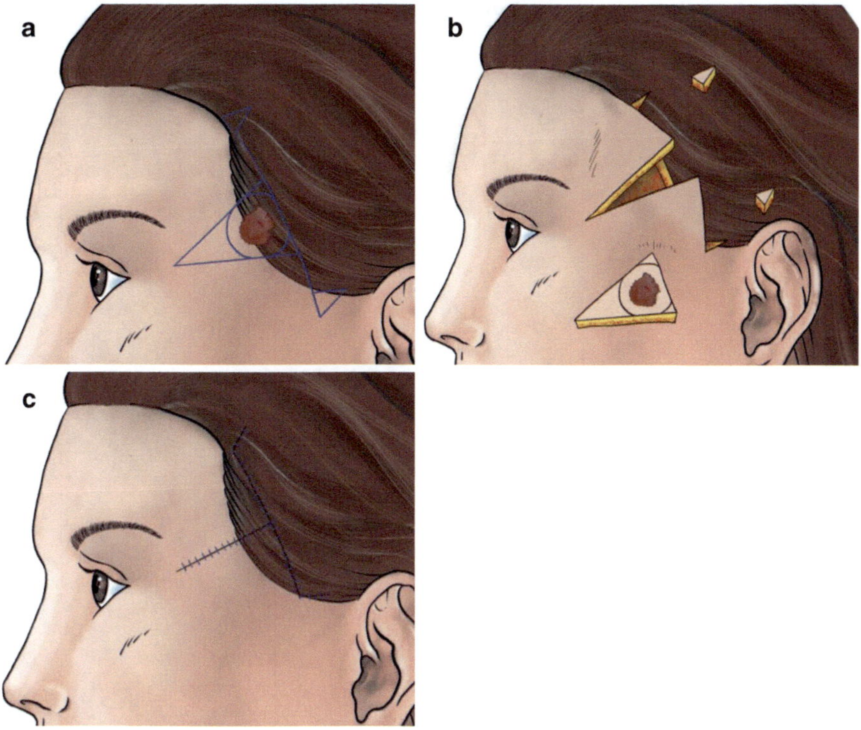

Fig. 6.14 V-T flap. (**a**) Markings for excision and flap, (**b**) Excision defect, flaps raised and dog eras excised, (**c**) Final closure, (**d**) Markings for excision and flap, (**e**) Excision defect, (**f**) Incisions for flap, (**g**) Flaps raised and undermined, (**h**) Trial transposition, (**i**) Closure with delineation of dog ears, (**j**) Final closure

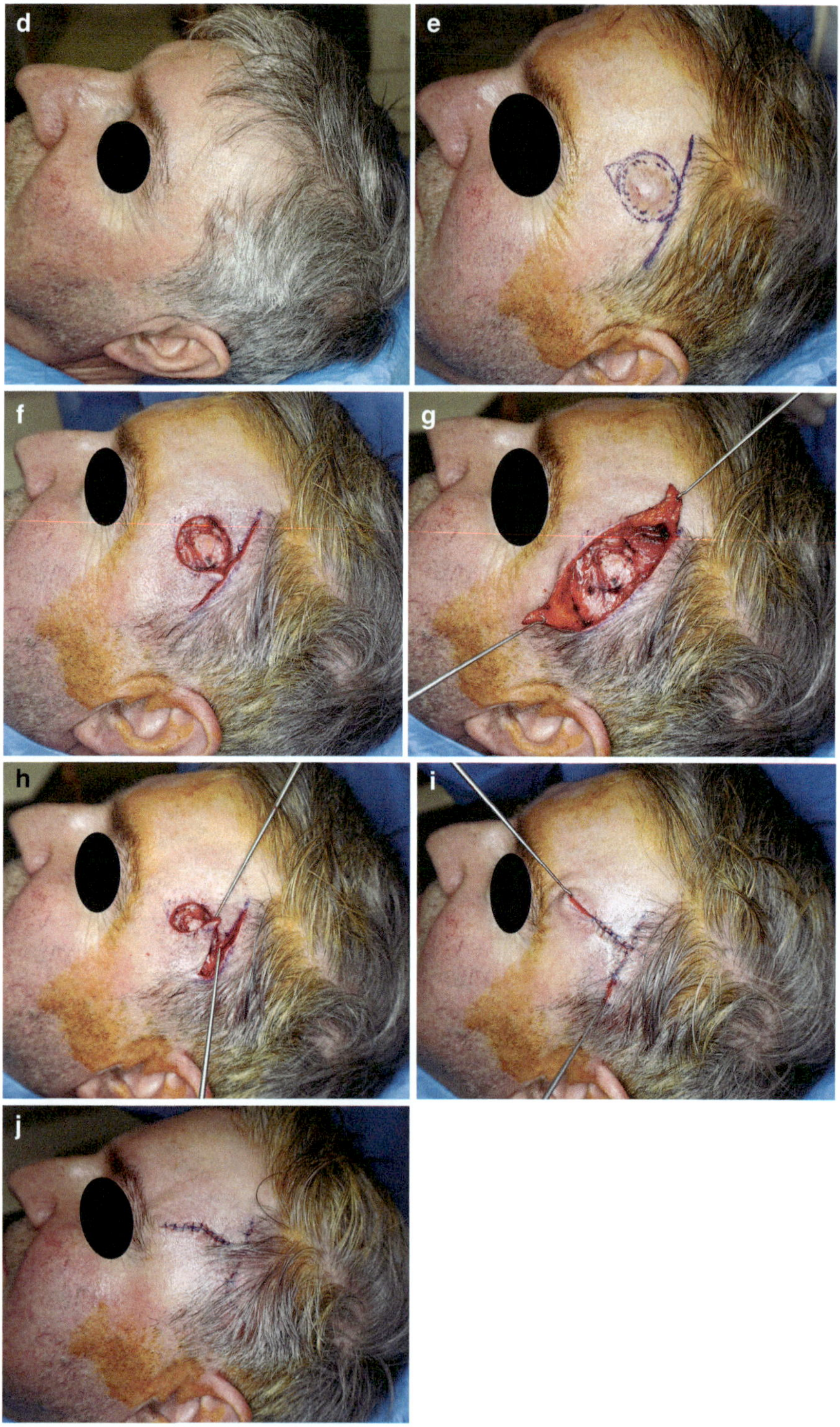

Fig. 6.14 (continued)

Rotation/Transposition Flap

Indications: Medium defects. For defects that are triangular or can be converted into a triangle, a rotation/transposition flap offers the advantage of utilising a vertical scar in crow's foot and hiding the curvilinear scar inside the hairline.

Technique: The base of the triangle is fashioned to be towards the hairline, with the curvilinear incision extending laterally from the margin of the basal defect, inside the hairline, towards the pre-auricular skin crease. The tissue laxity in the temporal/pre-auricular region is utilised to close the defect (Fig. 6.15a–c).

Tips: Due to the difference in the lengths of the flap adjacent to the curvilinear incision, Burrow's triangles will have to be excised and are best positioned superiorly, within the hairline.

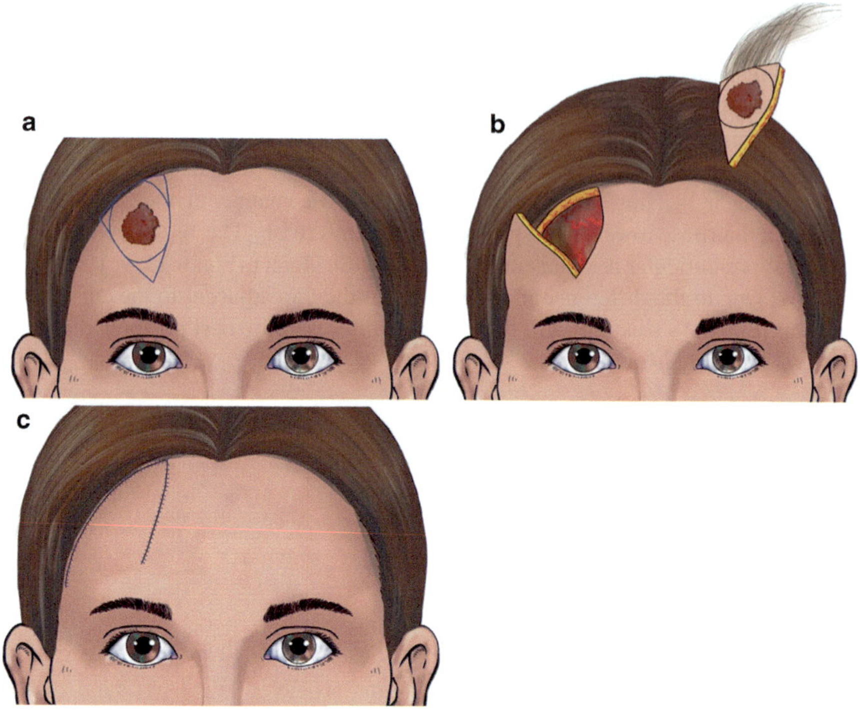

Fig. 6.15 Rotation/transposition flap. (**a**) Markings for excision and flap, (**b**) Defect folllowing excision and flap raised, (**c**) Final closure

Rhombic Flap (Limberg Flap)

Indications: Medium defects. For defects that are rhomboid or can be converted into a rhombus, the Limberg flap offers the advantage of utilising the skin laxity adjacent to the lateral canthus.

Technique: Technically, four flaps can be raised for any given defect, and the final decision is based on tissue laxity and the orientation of the eventual scars. An incision is made by extending the short diagonal by a length equal to one side of the defect and a further incision is made from its extremity parallel to the adjacent side of the defect, again of equal length. The incision and any undermining are best carried out in the subcutaneous plane in an attempt to avoid damage to the temporal branch of the facial nerve. The wound is closed in layers (Fig. 6.16a–h).

Tips: The amount of skin available in the adjacent area can be assessed using the "pinch test." With a rhomboid flap, some but not all the scars can be placed along the skin creases. It is often easier to close the secondary defect first followed by the primary defect. In the case of circular defects, it is not always necessary to remove additional tissue to convert the defect into a rhomboid.

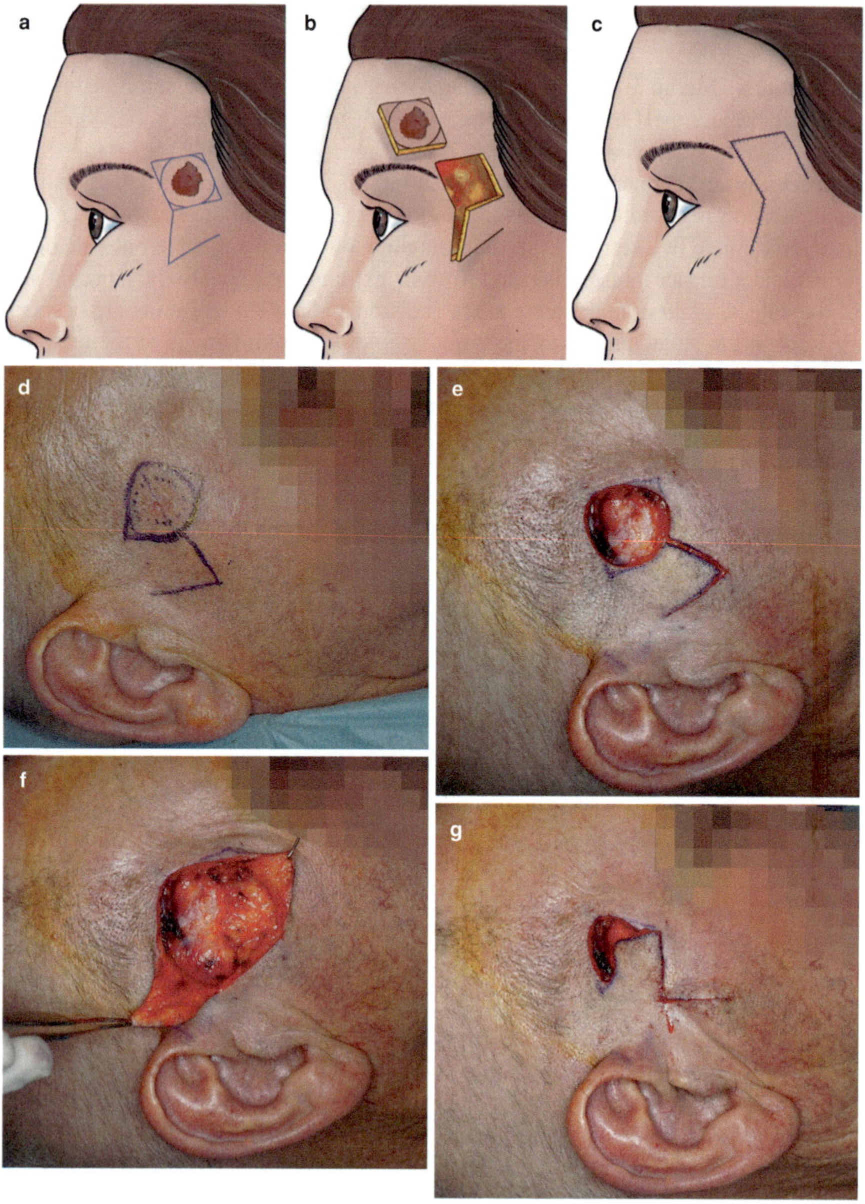

Fig. 6.16 Rhombic flap. (**a**) Markings for excision and flap, (**b**) Excision defect and flaps raised, (**c**) Final closure (**d**) Markings for excision and flap, (**e**) Excision defect and flap incisions, (**f**) flap raised and undermining of margins, (**g**) closure of secondary defect, (**h**) Final closure

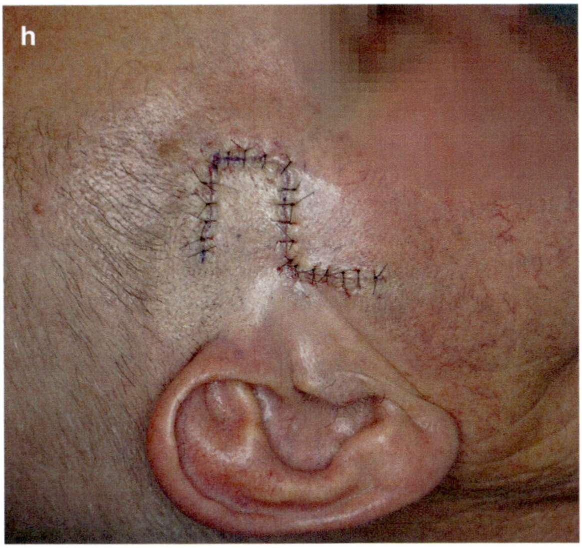

Fig. 6.16 (continued)

Unilateral/Bilateral Advancement Flaps

Indications: Small, medium defects.

Technique: The defect is ideally converted to have parallel sides. Parallel curvilinear incisions are made from the base of the defect and extend laterally and/or medially, parallel to the frown lines. The incisions and any undermining are best carried out in the subcutaneous plane in an attempt to avoid damage to the frontal branch of the facial nerve. In the case of bilateral flaps, one flap is initially raised and assessed to see if it adequate, before the second flap is raised (Fig. 6.17a–e).

Tips: Due to the difference in the lengths of the flap adjacent to the horizontal incisions, Burrow's triangles will have to be excised and are best positioned medially in the glabellar region or laterally in the crow's foot region.

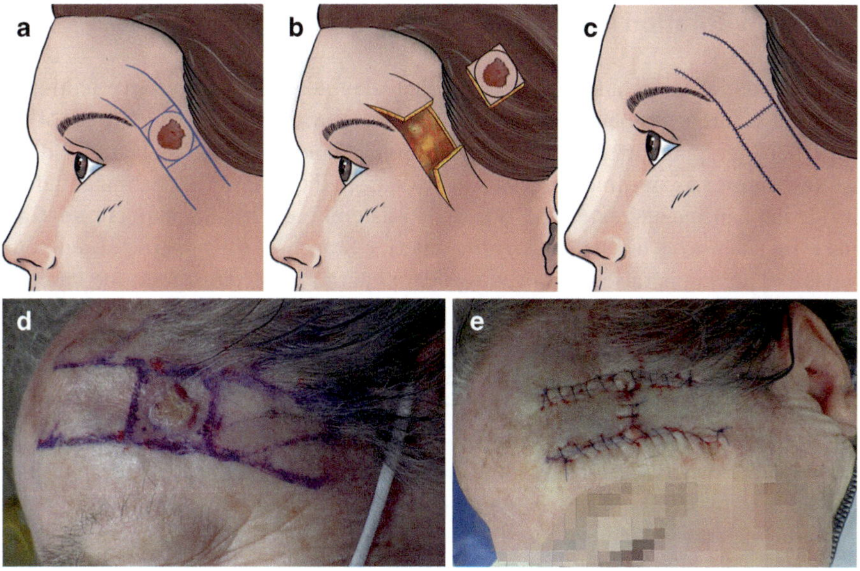

Fig. 6.17 Bilateral advancement flaps. (**a**) Markings for excision and flaps, (**b**) Excision defect and flaps raised, (**c**) Final closure, (**d**) Markings for excision and flaps, (**e**) Final closure

Forehead Rotation Flap

Indications: Medium and large defects that triangular on can be converted into a triangle. A forehead rotation flap based on the contralateral anterior branch of the superficial temporal artery, supra-orbital/supra-trochlear vessels can be utilised.

Technique: A curvilinear incision is made from the base of the triangular defect, inside the hairline and extended to the contralateral pre-auricular skin crease. Care must be taken to avoid damage to the anterior branch of the superficial temporal vessels. The flap is raised in the sub-galeal plane to avoid damage to the vascular supply and beneath the superficial layer of the deep temporal fascia to avoid damage to the temporal branch of the facial nerve. The wound is closed in layers and a pressure dressing/drain utilised as appropriate (Fig. 6.18a–c).

Tips: Due to the difference in the lengths of the wound margins adjacent to the curvilinear incision, Burrow's triangles often have to be excised and are best positioned superiorly/posteriorly, within the hairline. The placement of the incisions should take into account any potential changes to the hairline. Any dog ear is the supra-orbital area which is revised to lie within the glabellar frown lines. The revision is best undertaken at a later date, to avoid vascular compromise.

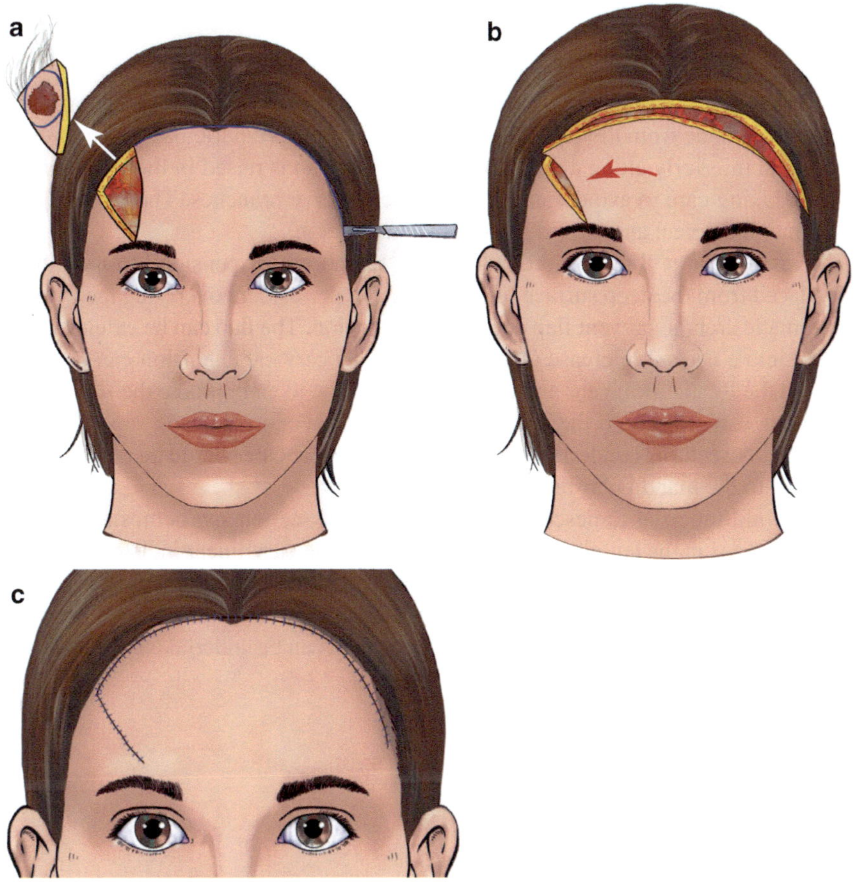

Fig. 6.18 Forehead rotation/transposition flap. (**a**) Excision defect and flap markings, (**b**) Flap raised and rotated into defect, (**c**) Final closure

Cervical/Cheek Rotation Flap

Indications: Medium/Large defects.

Technique: The defect is converted into a triangle, with the base laterally. The incision is made from the base of the defect, along the pre-auricular skin crease and extended inferiorly along a neck skin crease. The flap is raised in the subcutaneous plane, taking care to avoid damage to the facial nerve branches. The flap is mobilised into the defect and closed in layers (Fig. 6.19a–h).

Tips: If a large flap is raised, additional "anchoring/suspension" sutures should be placed from the deep surface of the flap to the periosteum overlying the zygoma/zygomatic arch, to prevent flap decent and ectropion. The flap can be extended inferiorly into a neck skin crease (cervicofacial). The cervical extension can be placed behind the lobule of the ear and close to the hairline to camouflage the scars.

When extending into the neck, the plane of dissection is in the supraplatysmal plane. If dissection is undertaken deep to the platysma, care should be taken to avoid damage to the mandibular branch of the facial nerve.

The infiltration of tumescent solution can aid dissection and hemostasis. Due to the difference in the lengths of the flap adjacent to the curvilinear incision, Burrow's triangles will have to be excised and are best positioned superiorly/posteriorly, within the hairline and behind the ear lobe. The dog ear is the lateral canthus which is revised to lie within the crow's feet. The revision can be undertaken at a later date, to avoid vascular compromise.

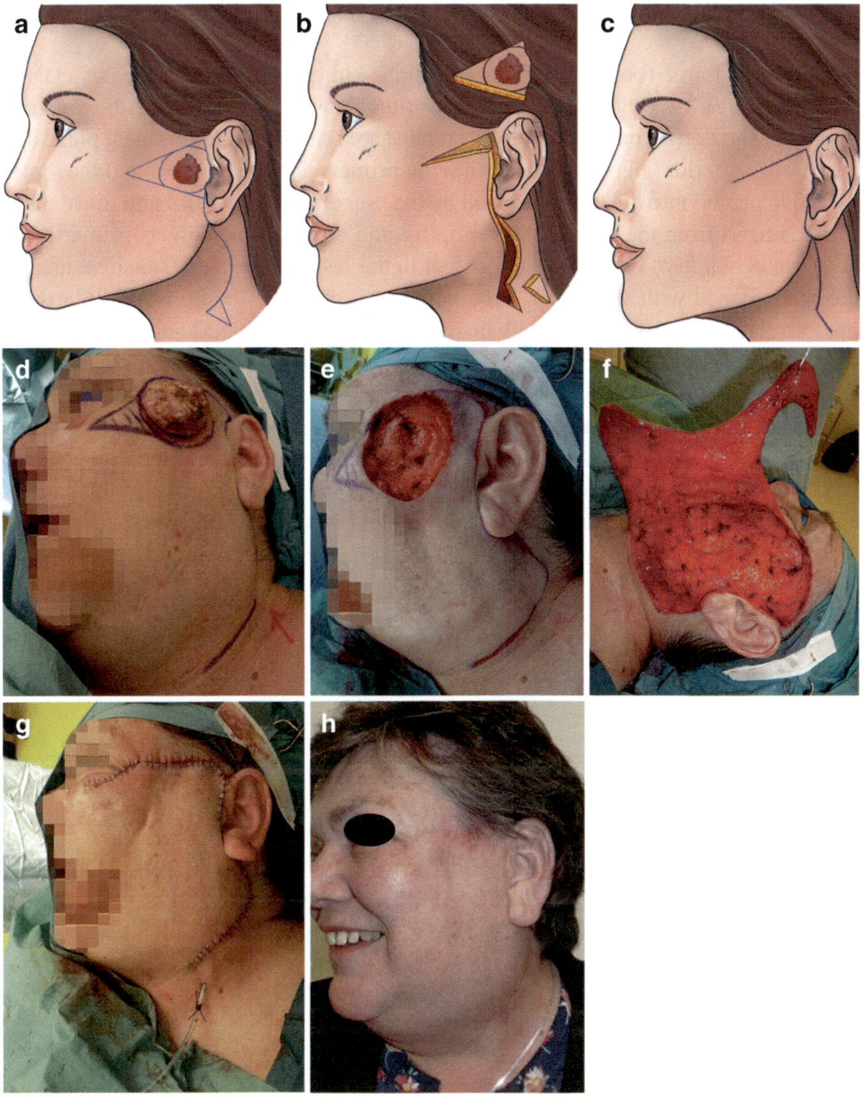

Fig. 6.19 Cervical/Cheek rotation flap. (**a**) Markings for excision and flap, (**b**) Excision defect and flap raised, (**c**) Final closure, (**d**) Markings for excision and flap, (**e**) Excision defect and flap incisions, (**f**) Flap raised, (**g**) Final closure, (**h**) Early post operative result

Multiple Transposition Flaps ± Skin Grafts

Indications: Large forehead defects, avoiding skin graft at the primary defect.

Technique: Two overlapping transposition flaps are raised from the superior margin of the defect, based laterally. The flaps are raised in the sub-galeal plane and the more "superior" flap transposed into the primary forehead defect and the "inferior" flap placed into the defect created by the "superior" flap. Third and fourth flaps can be raised from the posterior scalp to try and close all the defects primarily (al la - Orticochea flap) or the residual defect in the less aesthetically sensitive area of the scalp closed with skin grafts. The dog ears created by the transposed flaps are not corrected initially and are left in situ to preserve the blood supply. The often flatten out spontaneously or can be corrected later (after 6 weeks) (Fig. 6.20a–i).

Tips: Meticulous planning is necessary to get the orientation of the flaps correct and trial movements with a piece of towel is helpful. Do not be tempted to correct the dog ears at the initial stage. The position of the eyebrows and the dog ears can be corrected as a second-stage procedure. Depending on the hairline of the patient, hair is likely to be transferred to the forehead and would have to be addressed.

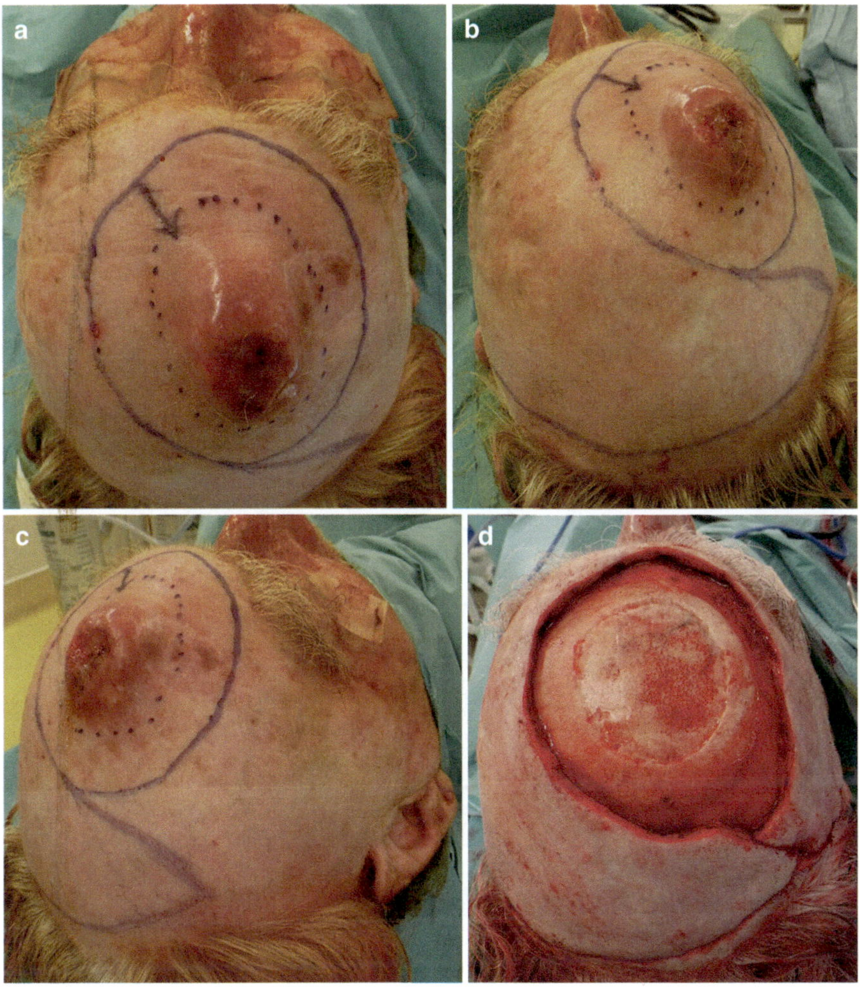

Fig. 6.20 Multiple transposition flaps. (**a**) Markings for excision - anterior view, (**b**) Markings for excision - poster view, (**c**) Markings for excision - lateral view, (**d**) Excision deefect and flap incisions, (**e**) Flaps raised, (**f**) Posterior flap transposed into anterior defect, (**g**) Anterior flap transposed into posterior defect, (**h**) Final closure with skin grafting of tertiary defect, (**i**) Ealy post operative result with dog ear in situ

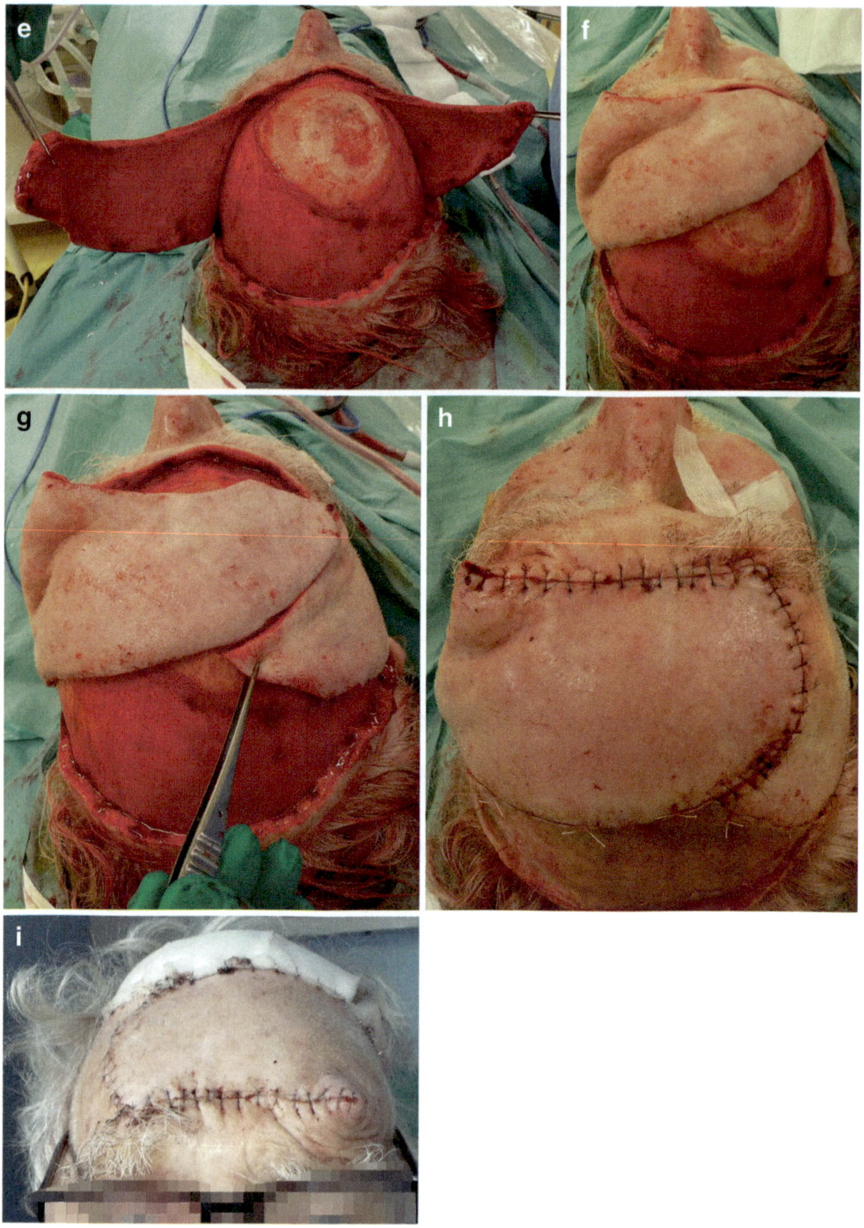

Fig. 6.20 (continued)

Skin Graft

Indications: Medium and large defects can be reconstructed with a full or partial thickness skin graft.

Technique: A suitable template is made of the defect, which is transferred to the donar site to harvest the graft. The graft is sutured to the defect, with additional "long" sutures that can be used for "tying" over the bolus. If possible, the graft can be "quilted" to the base, to decrease the risk of haematoma and dead space. A non-adherent dressing is laid over the sutured graft, over which a cotton wool ball/sponge soaked in proflavin or a suitable antibiotic ointment is placed. The tie-over bolus sutures are now used to hold the dressing in place. Alternatively the dressing could be held in place with skin staples (Fig. 6.21a–d).

Tips: The cosmetic outcome is acceptable in the upper and lateral forehead, where it can be "hidden" by alterations to the hair style.

In addition, very large defects involving most of the forehead can be satisfactorily reconstructed with a skin graft, provided care is taken to place the margins along the eyebrows, bridge of nose and hairline. The "take" of the skin graft is significantly improved, when placed on a well-vascularised bed. The "take" on exposed bone can be improved by utilising Ingetra® or a pericranial transposition flap (see Chap. 5—Figs. 5.13 and 5.14).

Tissue expansion: This can be considered for large forehead defects when staged reconstruction is planned for closure of the primary or secondary defect. It can also be considered, when adequate time and tissue are available to carry out the required expansion, prior to excision of the index pathology.

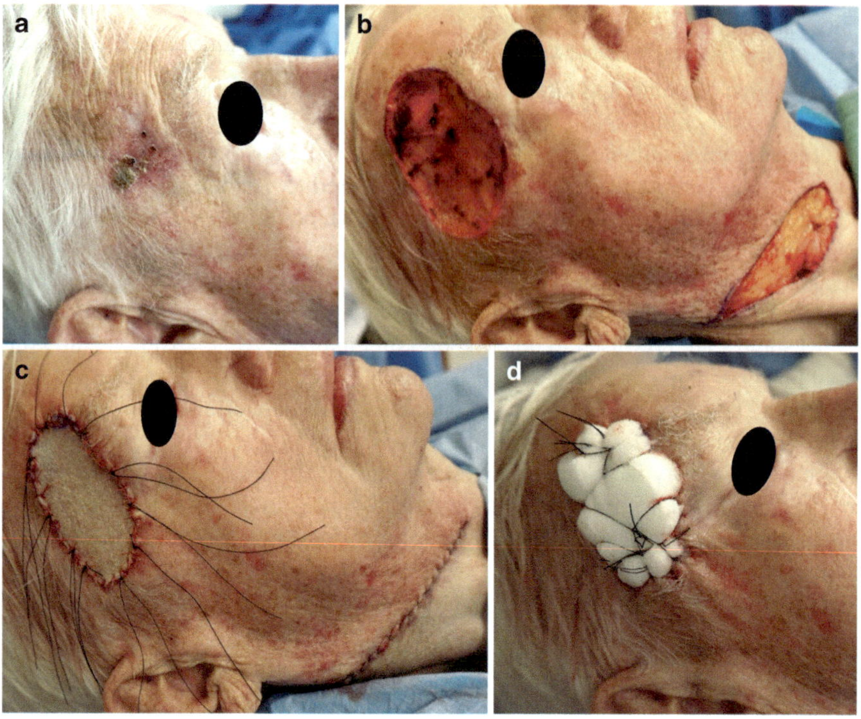

Fig. 6.21 Skin grafting. (**a**) Lesion temple, (**b**) Excision defect and skin graft harvest site, (**c**) Graft sutured in place with tie over sutures. Donar site sutured, (**d**) Tie over bolus dressing

Suggested Algorithm

Forehead

Central Defects

Small
1. Primary closure (vertical).
2. "M" excision (Superior)
3. "W" excision (Inferior)

Medium
Upper
1. V-T flap.
2. Unilateral/bilateral advancement flap.

Lower
1. A-T flap.
2. Unilateral/bilateral advancement flap.

Paramedian

Small
1. Primary closure (Vertical/horizontal).

Medium
Upper
1. V-T flap.
2. Unilateral/bilateral advancement flap.
3. Rotation/transposition flap.

Lower
1. A-T, V-T flap.
2. Unilateral/bilateral advancement flap.

Temple/Lateral Forehead

Small
1. Primary closure (along crow's feet).

Medium

1. V-T flap.
2. Rotation/transposition flap.
3. Unilateral/bilateral advancement flap.
4. Rhomboid flap.
5. Skin graft.

Large Defects

1. Multiple transposition flaps.
2. Rotation/transposition flap with skin grafting of secondary defect.
3. Skin graft.
4. Skin graft with Integra®.
5. Tissue expansion.

Nose

7

Subunits and Anatomical Considerations

The nose is a complex structure and lends itself to being further divided into subunits, separated by less discrete borders. It is typically divided into nine subunits; columella, tip, dorsum and paired sidewalls, ala and nasal facets (Fig. 7.1).

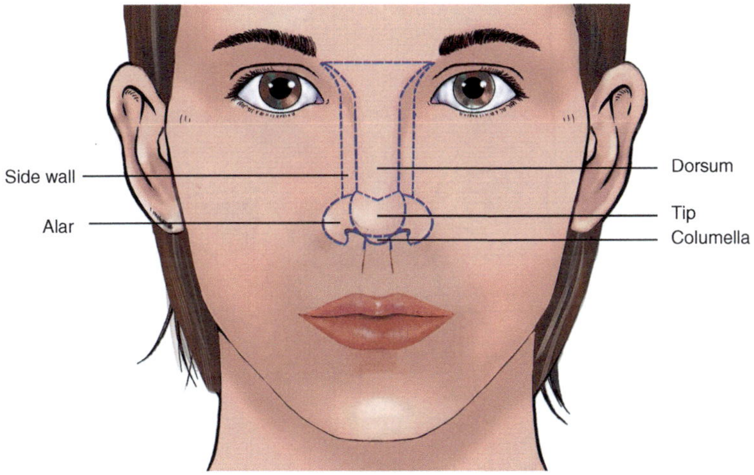

Fig. 7.1 Nasal subunits

V. Ilankovan et al., *Local Flaps in Facial Reconstruction*,
https://doi.org/10.1007/978-3-031-49464-2_7

The complex three-dimensional shape is supported by a bony and cartilaginous framework. The overlying skin is of varying thickness and mobility, and the deep surface is lined by mucous membrane. It is thick and less mobile caudally around the tip and ala and thinner and more mobile in the cephalic region along the dorsum and sidewalls. The nasal bones, upper lateral and septal cartilage provided support to the dorsum and sidewalls and the lower lateral cartilage to the ala. The tip and columella are supported by the septal and lower lateral cartilages (Fig. 7.2).

The concept of "sub-unit" reconstruction was initially popularised for the nose and often involves altering the size and shape of the defect to reconstruct a full subunit, if the defect involves more than half the subunit, so that the scars lie in the most advantageous positions and deceive the eye. Adequate cartilage and skeletal support should be provided to support the reconstruction. The ala contains the lower lateral cartilage in its medial/superior aspect and only fibrofatty tissue in its lateral/inferior aspect. Cartilage support may be required for reconstruction of the ala subunit to prevent collapse, even if the defect only involves the lateral aspect.

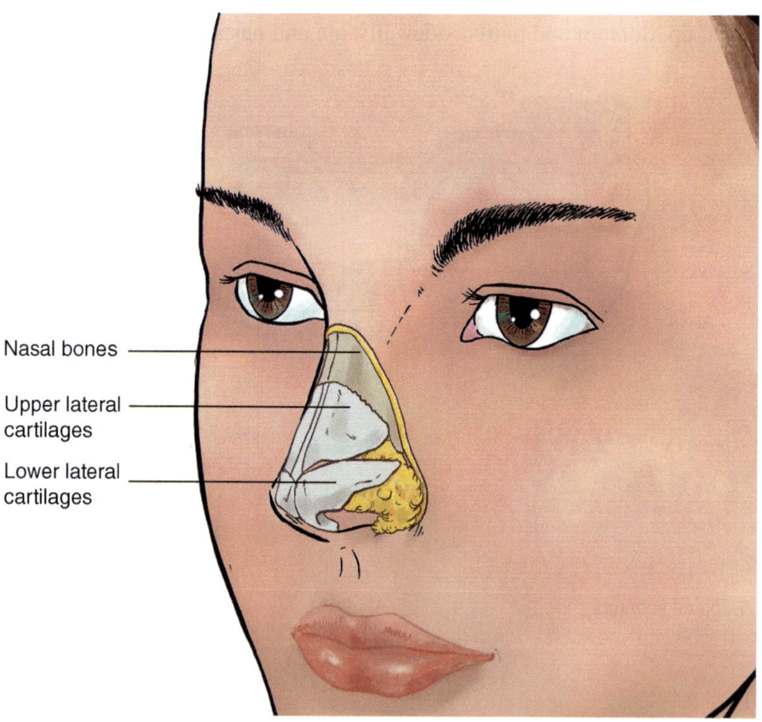

Fig. 7.2 Nasal bone, cartilage abd fibrofatty tissue

Nasal Dorsum Defects

Primary Closure (Vertical)

Indication: Small defect.

Technique: The defect is converted into an ellipse to lie along the vertical glabella RSTLs. The wound margins are undermined in the subcutaneous plane superiorly and in the sub-muscular plane in the mid/lower dorsum. The wound edges are mobilised and closed in layers (Fig. 7.3a–f).

Tips: Determine tissue laxity prior to procedure, if considering closure of mid/lower dorsum defects. Closure of larger upper defects can "medialise" the eyebrows and needs to be taken into account and discussed with the patient.

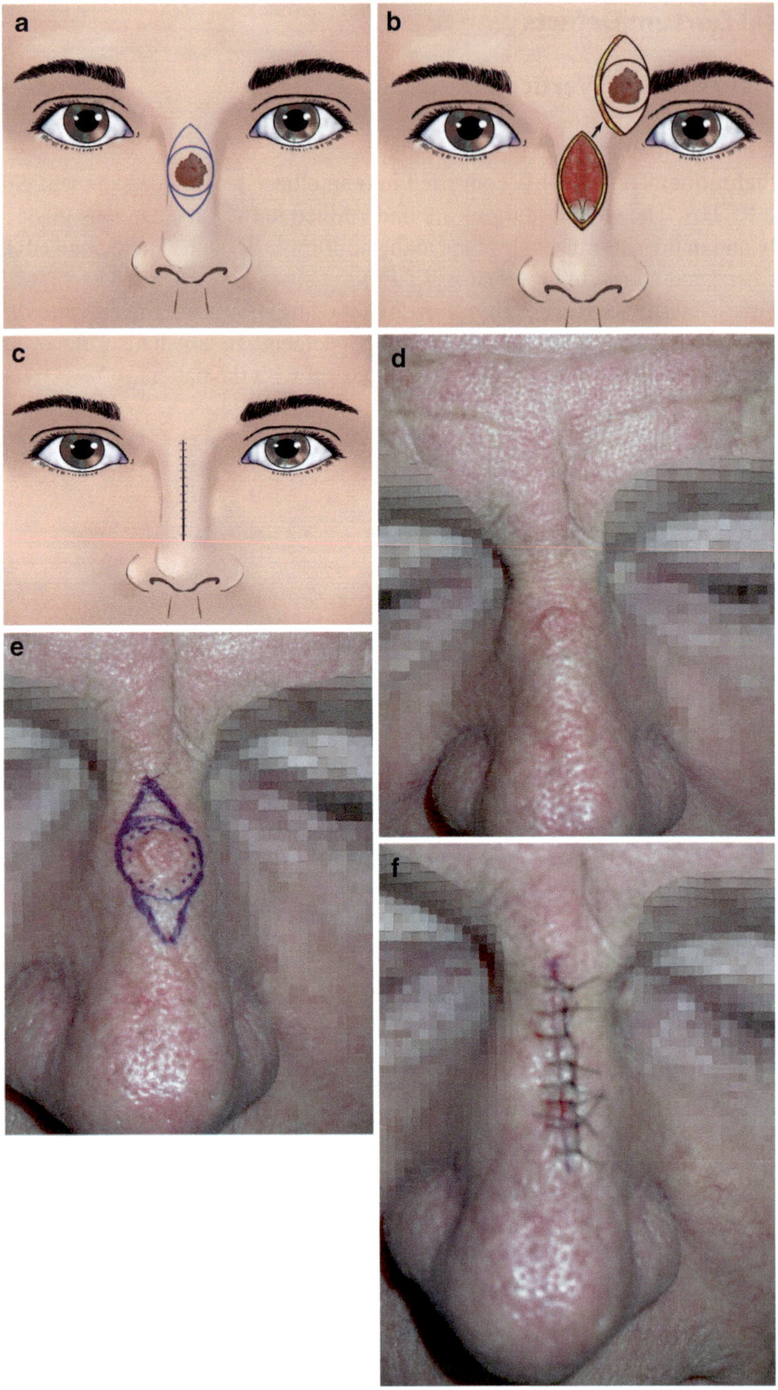

Fig. 7.3 Vertical excision and primary closure. (**a**) Marking for excision, (**b**) Excision defect, (**c**) Final closure, (**d**) Lesion dorsum nose, (**e**) Markings for excision, (**f**) Final closure

Primary Closure (Horizontal)

Indication: Small defect.

Technique: The defect is converted into an ellipse to lie along a horizontal skin crease. The wound margins are undermined in the subcutaneous plane superiorly and in the sub-muscular plane in the mid and lower dorsum. The wound edges are mobilised and closed in layers (Fig. 7.4a–d).

Tips: Determine tissue laxity prior to procedure, if considering closure of mid/lower dorsum defects. Closure of larger defects can alter the position of the nasal tip, which can be advantageous in some circumstances.

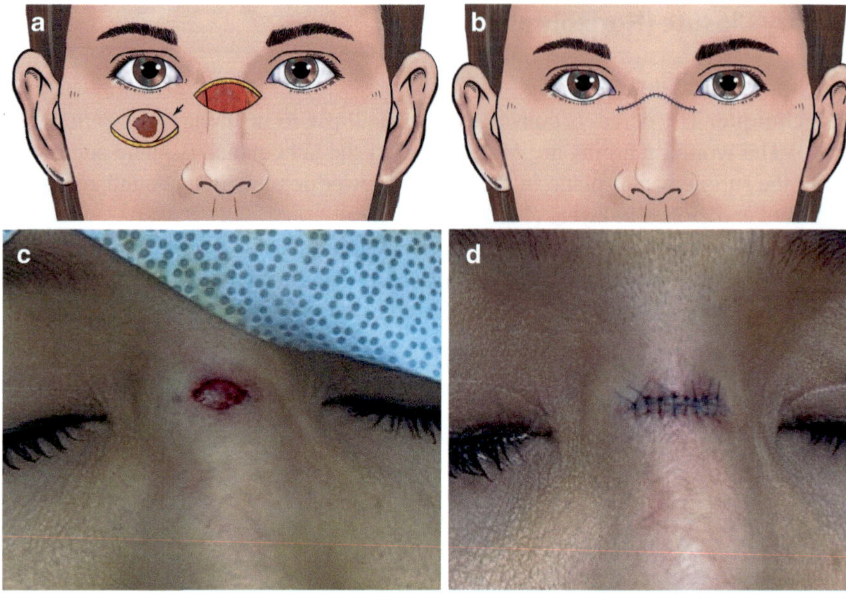

Fig. 7.4 Horizontal excision and primary closure. (**a**) Excision defect, (**b**) Final closure, (**c**) Excision defect, (**d**) Final closure

Glabellar Advancement Flap

Indications: Medium defect, mid/lower dorsum, nasal tip.

Technique: The defect is "squared off" to have parallel edges. Two incisions are made from the superior margins of the defect, along the junction of the dorsum and sidewalls, up to and if necessary just past the glabella. The flap is raised in the submuscular plane. The surrounding wound edges are undermined and closed in layers (Fig. 7.5a–i).

Tips: Skin laxity in the glabella and nasal dorsum should be determined prior to utilising this flap. A flap length of up to 3 times the size of the defect can be raised, but it is mandatory to avoid tension on closure. A flap of inadequate length can lead to an unsatisfactory upturned nasal tip, though in the elderly this might be advantageous.

It is important to anchor the deep surface of the flap to the underlying tissues at the root of the nose to prevent "tenting." The difference in the length of the wound margins can be accommodated by differential suturing and Burrow's triangles are best excised in the glabella skin creases.

Open rhinoplasty techniques can be utilised to address nasal humps (if present), which can also provide additional "length" to the flap and facilitate closure (Fig. 7.5e–g).

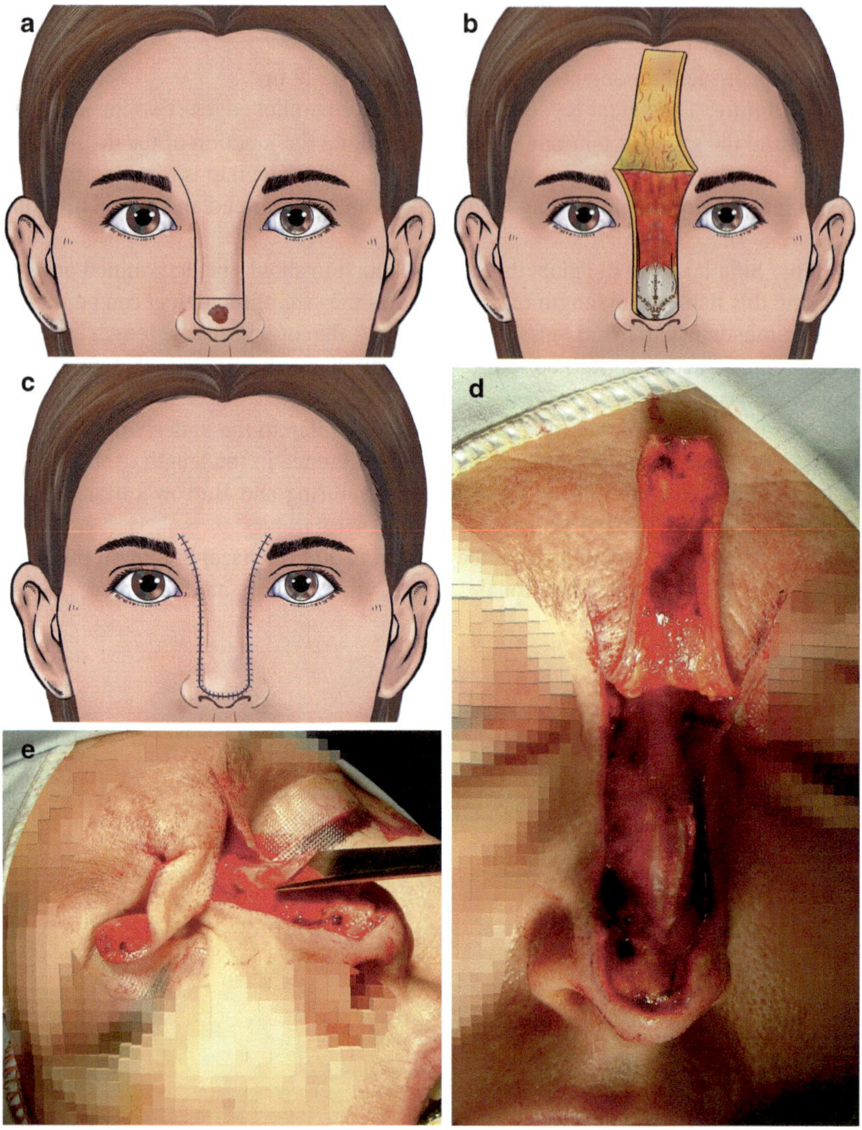

Fig. 7.5 Glabella advancement flap. (**a**) Markings for excision and flap, (**b**) Excision defect and flap raised, (**c**) Final closure, (**d**) Excision defect and flap raised. Dorsal hump, (**e**) Dorsal hump reduction, (**f**) Post hump reduction, (**g**) Medialising upper lateral cartilage, (**h**) Final closure - frontal view, (**i**) Final closure - lateral view

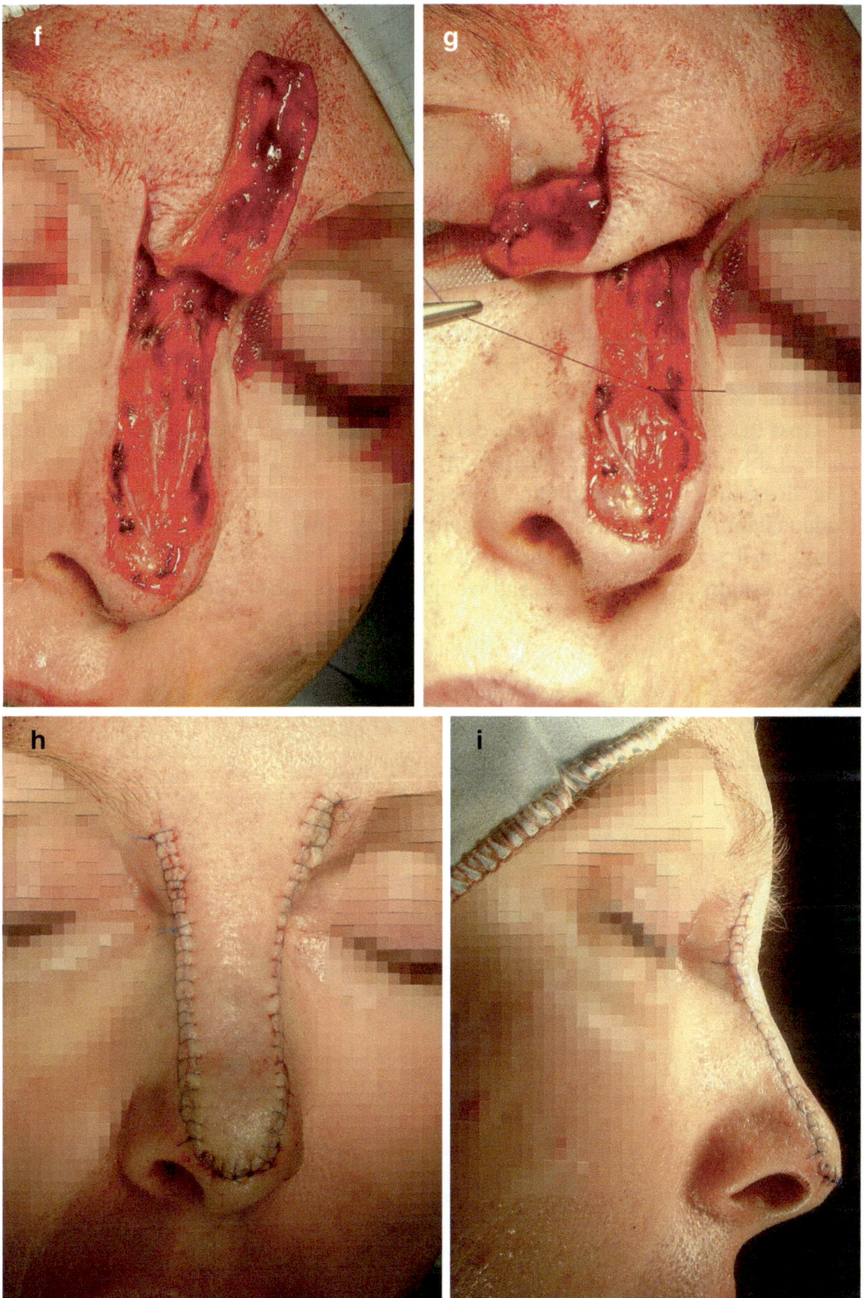

Fig. 7.5 (continued)

Glabella Transposition Flap

Indications: Medium defect mid/lower dorsum/side wall.

Technique: The defect is modified into a triangle with a horizontal long axis. A curvilinear incision is made from the superior edge of the defect, along the junction between the cheek and the nasal sidewall. It is extended superiorly into the glabella skin crease, passing about 0.5 cm away from the medial canthus. A back cut is made from the summit, across to the contralateral medial canthus. The nasal component of the flap is raised in the sub-muscular plane and the glabellar component in the subcutaneous plane. The wound margins are widely undermined and closed in layers. The secondary glabellar/nasal root defect is closed primarily and any excess skin in the superior aspect of the flap discarded. Dog ear at the primary defect is corrected as required (Fig. 7.6a–f).

Tips: In case of smaller/midline defects, the superior curvilinear incision can be made at the junction of the nasal dorsum and side wall. The flap might require thinning along the caudal margin and medial canthus region for better inset. A flap of inadequate mobility can lead to an unsatisfactory upward displacement of nasal tip, though in the elderly this might be advantageous. Primary closure of the glabella defect medialises the eyebrows and would have to be taken into account when considering this flap.

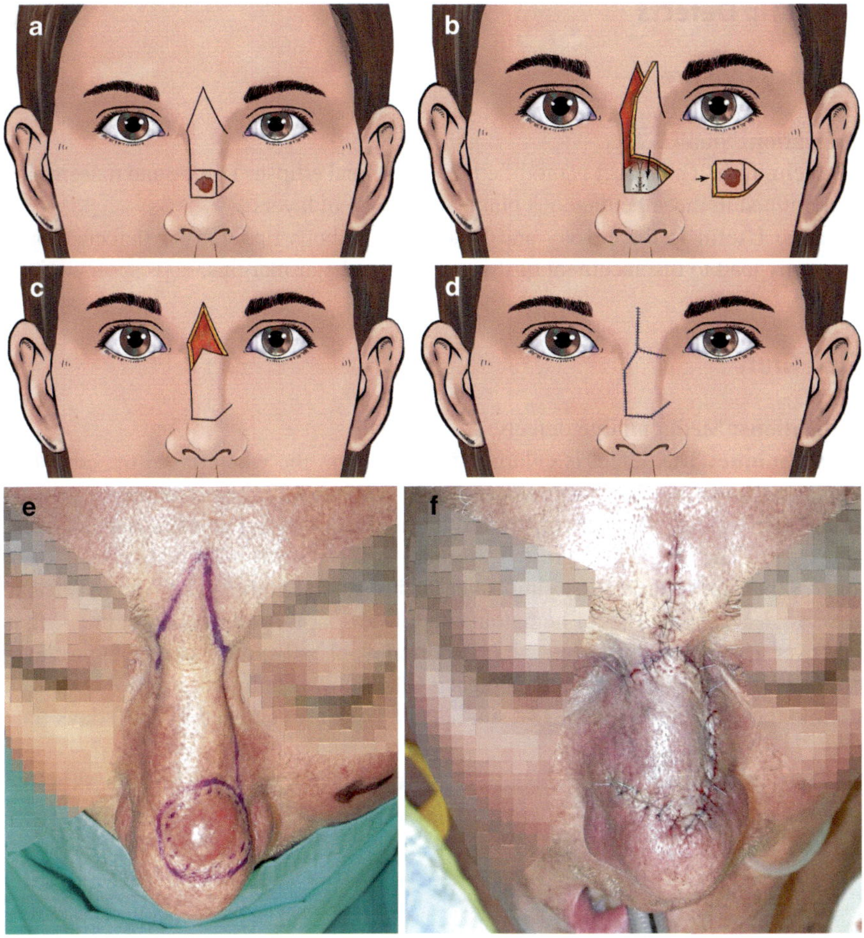

Fig. 7.6 Glabella transposition flap. (**a**) Markings for excision and flap, (**b**) Excision defect and flap raised, (**c**) Flap transposed into defect, (**d**) Final closure, (**e**) Markings for excision and flap, (**f**) Final closure

Nasal Tip Defects

Primary Closure

Indication: Small defect.

Technique: The defect is modified into a vertical ellipse. The wound margins are undermined in the subcutaneous plane and closed in layers.

Tips: Useful in the elderly and those with bulbous tips. Larger defects closed primarily lead to displacement of the nasal tip and alar margins.

Skin Graft

Indications: Medium/large defects.

Technique: The defect is enlarged to encompass the whole nasal tip subunit if the initial defect involves more than half the subunit. An accurate template is made of the final defect, which is transferred to the donar site to harvest a full-thickness skin graft. The "defatted" graft is sutured to the defect, with additional "long" sutures that can be used for "tying" over the bolus. The graft can be "quilted" to the base, to decrease the risk of hematoma and dead space. A non-adherent dressing is laid over the sutured graft, over which a cotton wool ball/sponge soaked in proflavin or a suitable antibiotic ointment is placed. The tie-over bolus sutures are now used to hold the dressing in place. The sutures and pack are removed in 7–10 days time (Fig. 7.7a–d).

Tips: A more acceptable result is obtained in individuals with thin skin and superficial defects.

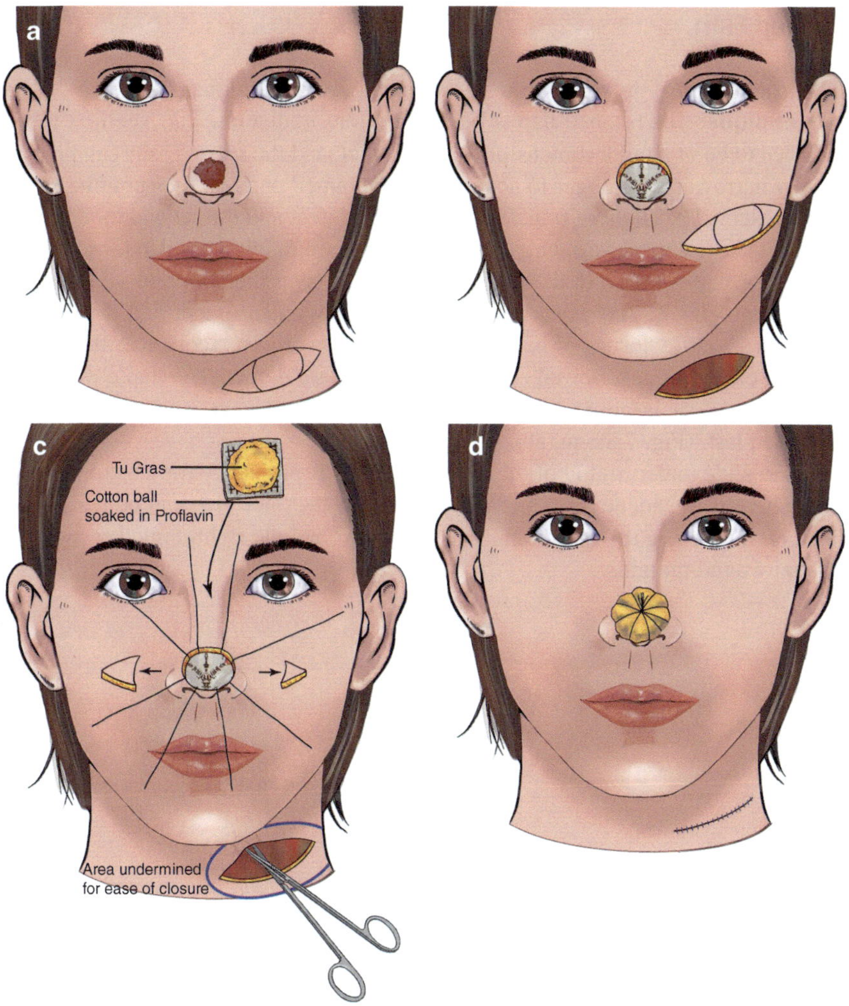

Fig. 7.7 Skin grafting for nasal tip defect. (**a**) Markings for excision, (**b**) Excision defect and skin graft harvest from neck, (**c**) Graft prepared for placement into defect, (**d**) Graft held in place with tie over bolus dressing. Donor site in neck closed

Bilobed Flap

Indications: Nasal tip, lower/mid sidewall, alar (away from margin).

Technique: The bilobed flap is best suited for circular defects. The first lobe is designed to be of similar dimensions to the defect, and the second lobe can be made slightly narrower, but longer to accommodate pointed ends on the summit, for primary closure. The angle of transfer between the defect and the second lobe is based on the site of tissue recruitment, which is often the remaining nasal sidewall/medial cheek. The flap is raised in the sub-muscular plane over the nose and subcutaneous plane in the cheek. The wound margins are widely undermined, and the defect is closed in layers. Closure is best carried out in an orderly sequence; the tertiary defect is closed first, followed closure of the primary defect. The flap covering the secondary defect is appropriately trimmed and closed next, and the dog ear is addressed last. (Fig. 7.8a–m, also see Fig. 3.5).

Tips: Wide undermining of the wound margins is necessary for tension free closure. There is a tendency for "pin cushioning" of the flap. This can be partly mitigated by modifying the defect and flap margin to include right-angled corners and parallel wound margins.

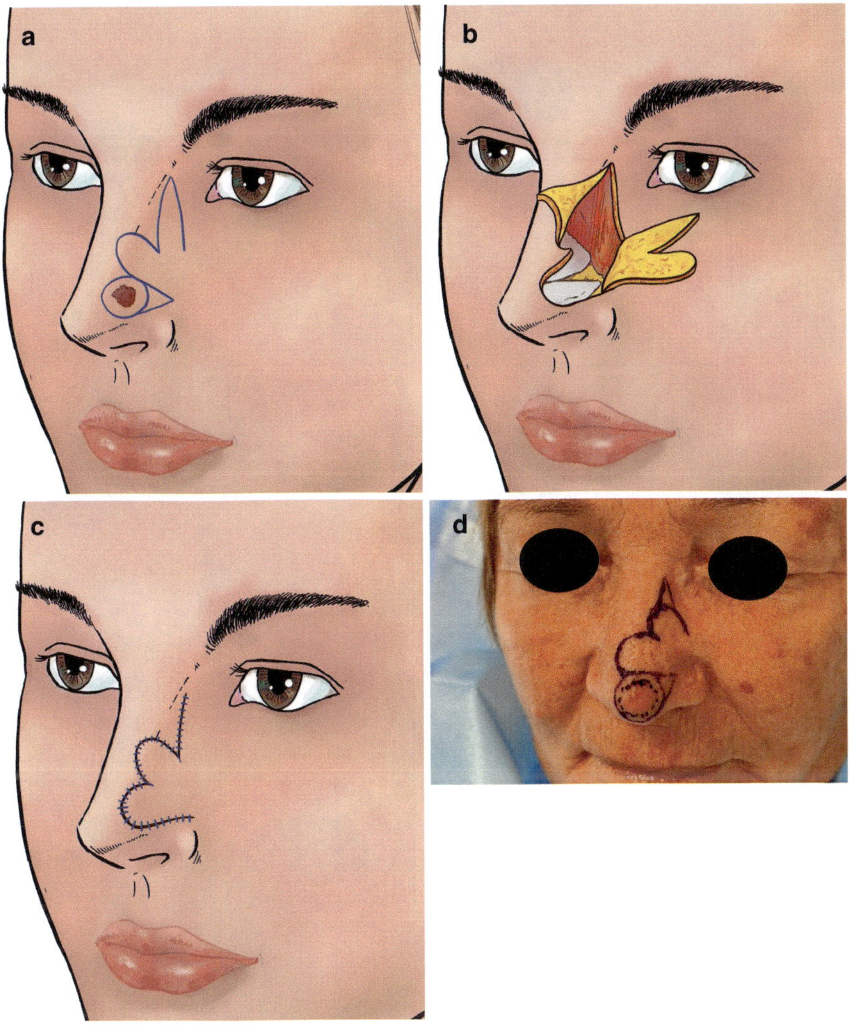

Fig. 7.8 Laterally based bilobed flap. (**a**) Markings for excision and flap, (**b**) Excision defect and flaps raised, (**c**) Final closure, (**d**) Markings for excision and flap, (**e**) Excision defect, (**f**) Flaps raised, (**g**) Wide undermining of surrounding tissues, (**h**) Initial closure of tertiary defect, (**i**) Subsequent closure of primary defect, (**j**) Adjustment and closure of secondary defect, (**k**) Final correction of dog ear, (**l**) Final closure, (**m**) Late result with no further revisions

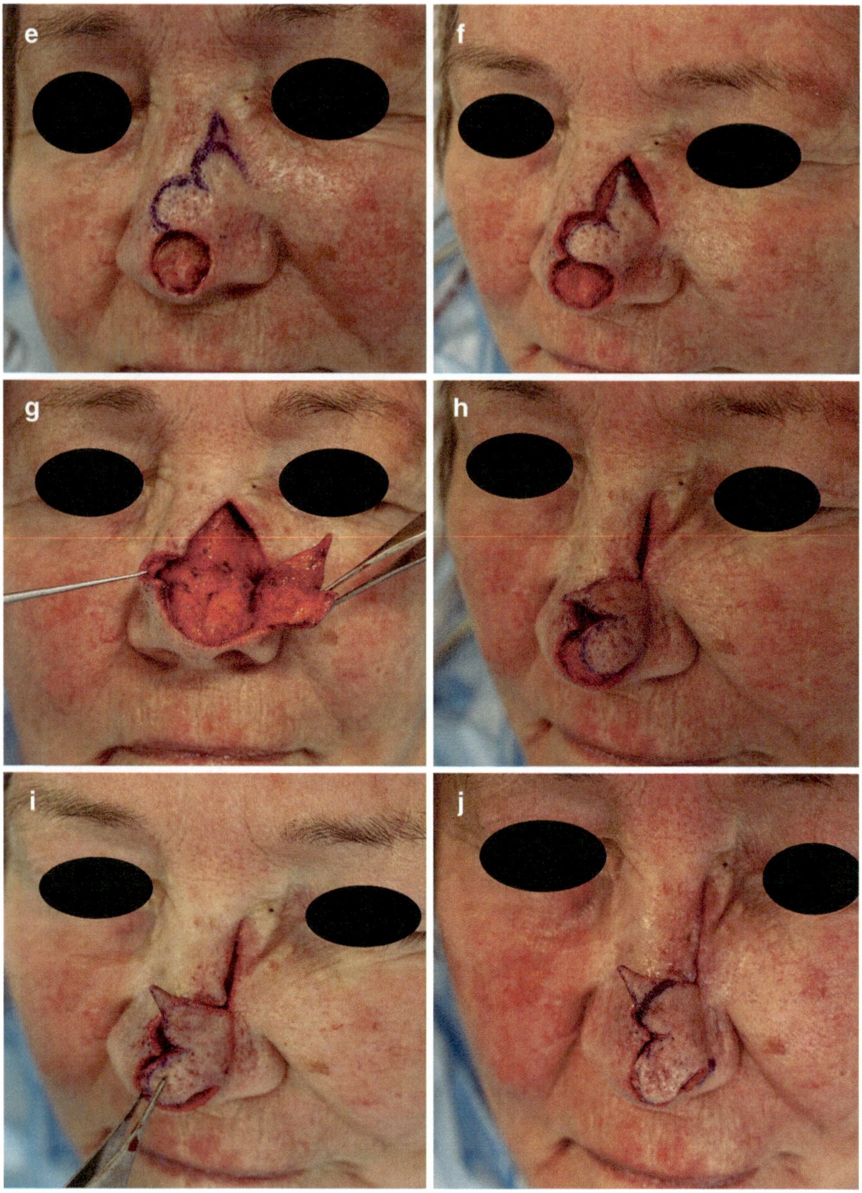

Fig. 7.8 (continued)

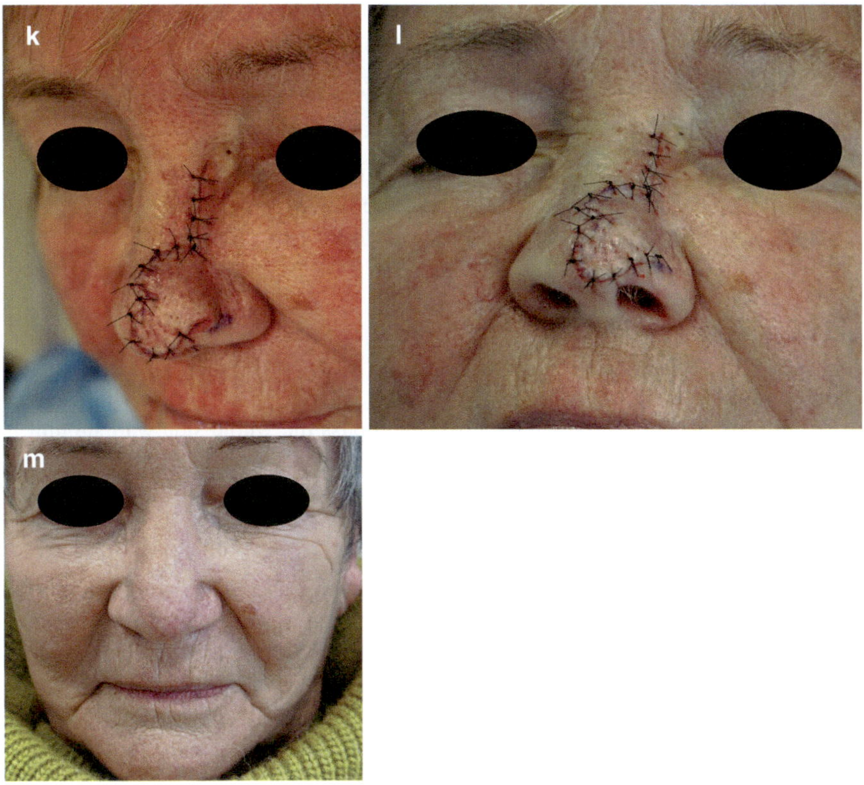

Fig. 7.8 (continued)

Sidewall Defects

Primary Closure

Indication: Small defect.

Technique: The defect is modified into a vertical ellipse. The wound margins are undermined in the subcutaneous plane and closed in layers.

Tips: Tissue laxity should be assessed prior to the procedure.

Skin Grafts

Indications: Medium/large defects.

Technique: The defect is enlarged to encompass the whole side wall subunit if the initial defect involves more than half the subunit. An accurate template is made of the defect, which is transferred to the donar site to harvest a full-thickness skin graft. The "defatted" graft is sutured to the defect, with additional "long" sutures that can be used for "tying" over the bolus. The graft can be "quilted" to the base, to decrease the risk of hematoma and dead space. A non-adherent dressing is laid over the sutured graft, over which a cotton wool ball/sponge soaked in proflavin or a suitable antibiotic ointment is placed. The tie-over bolus sutures are now used to hold the dressing in place. The sutures and pack are removed in 7–10 days time (see Fig. 7.7a–d).

Tips: A more acceptable result is obtained in individuals with thin skin and superficial defects.

Glabella Transposition Flap

Indications: Medium defect, upper and mid sidewall.

Technique: The defect is modified into a triangle with the base placed laterally. A curvilinear incision is made from the superior edge of the defect and extended superiorly into the glabella skin crease, passing about 0.5 cm away from the medial canthus. A back cut is made from the summit, across to the contralateral medial canthus. The nasal component of the flap is raised in the submuscular plane and the glabellar component in the subcutaneous plane. The wound margins are widely undermined and closed in layers. The secondary glabellar/nasal root defect is closed primarily and any excess skin in the superior aspect of the flap discarded. Dog ear at the primary defect is corrected as required (Fig. 7.9a–m).

Tips: The flap often has to be thinned, to match the defect margins. Primary closure of the glabella defect medialises the eyebrows and would have to be taken into account, when considering this flap. Variations to the design of the flap can be utilised to best accommodate the defect and the eventual scar (Fig. 7.9e–m).

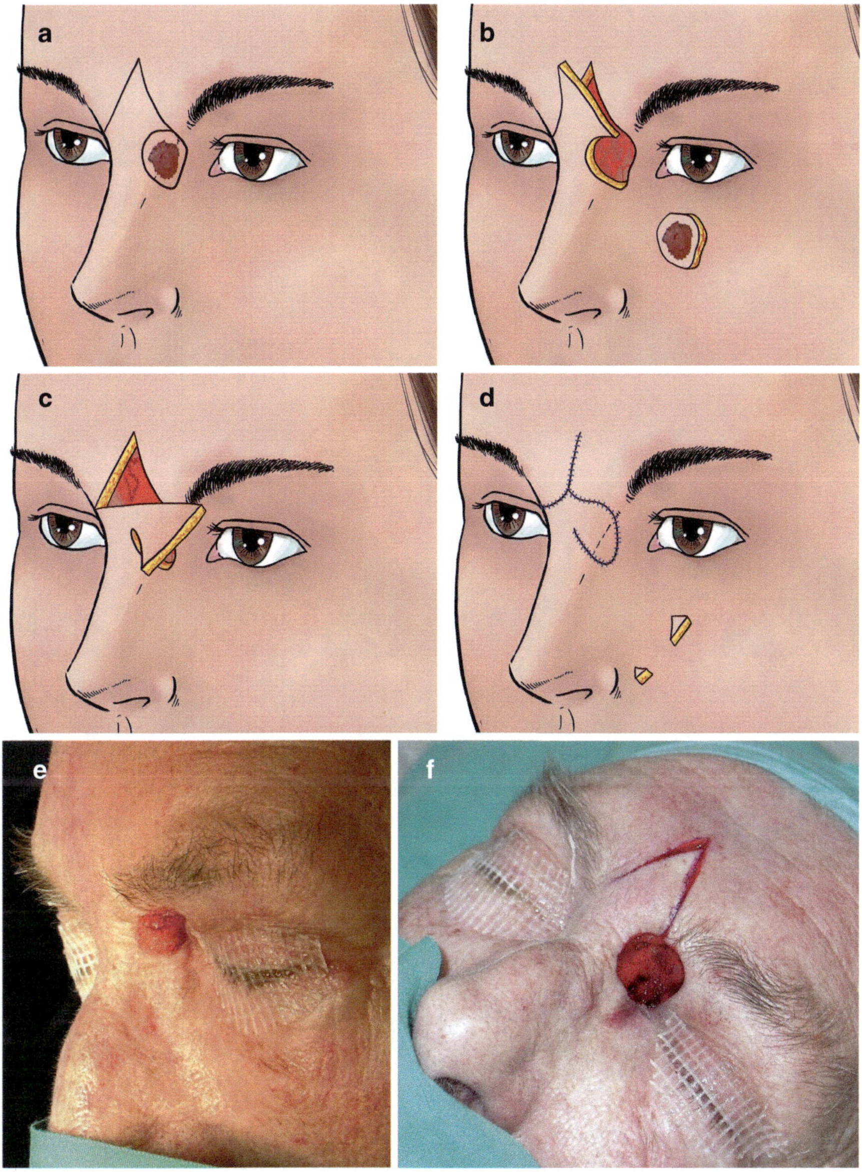

Fig. 7.9 Glabela transposition flap. (**a**) Markings for excision and flap, (**b**) Excision defect and flap raised, (**c**) Flap transposed into defect, (**d**) Final closure with trimming of excess tissue, (**e**) Lesion upper side wall, (**f**) Excision defect and flap incisions, (**g**) Flap transposed into defect, (**h**) Final closure, (**i**) Markings for excision and flap, (**j**) Excision defect and flap raised, (**k**) Trial transfer into defect, (**l**) Closure of secondary defect, appropriate thinning of flap, (**m**) Final closure

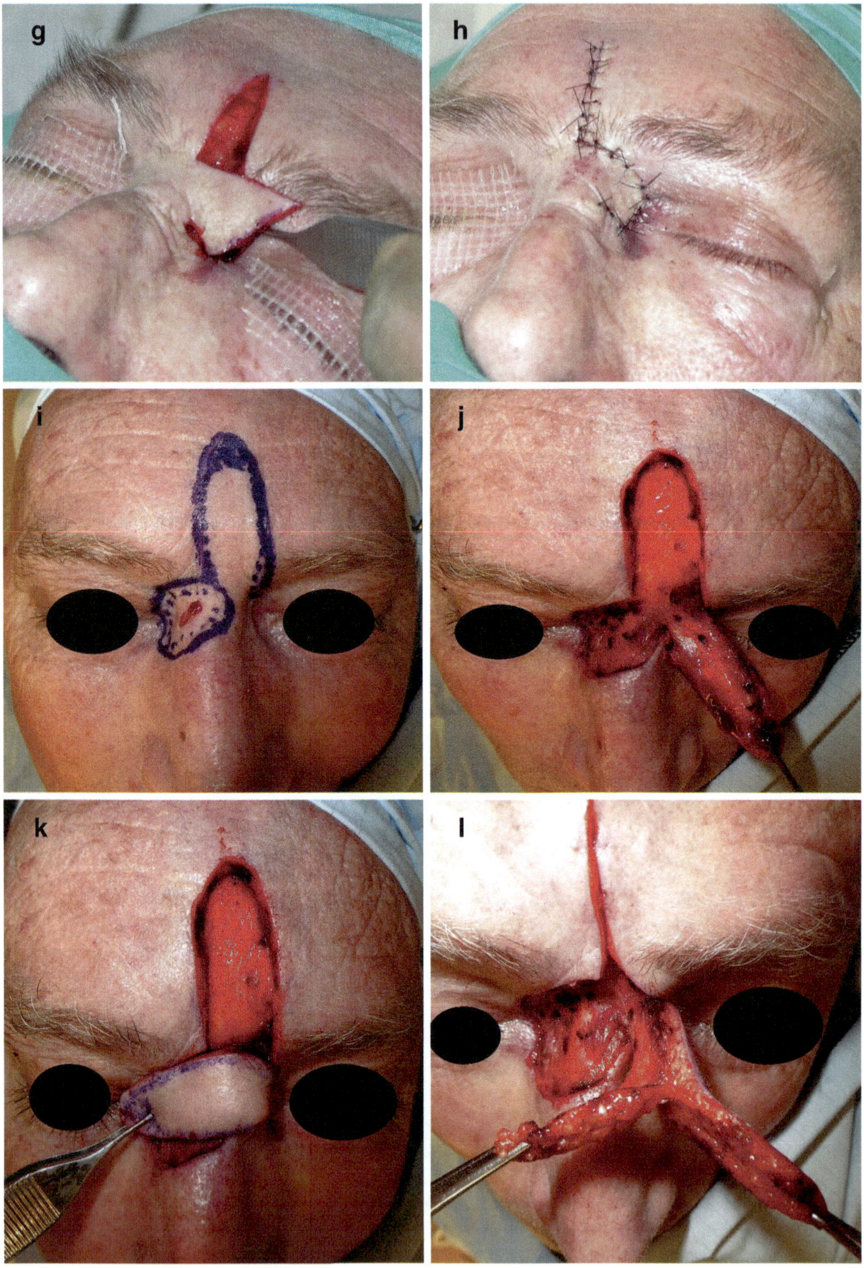

Fig. 7.9 (continued)

Fig. 7.9 (continued)

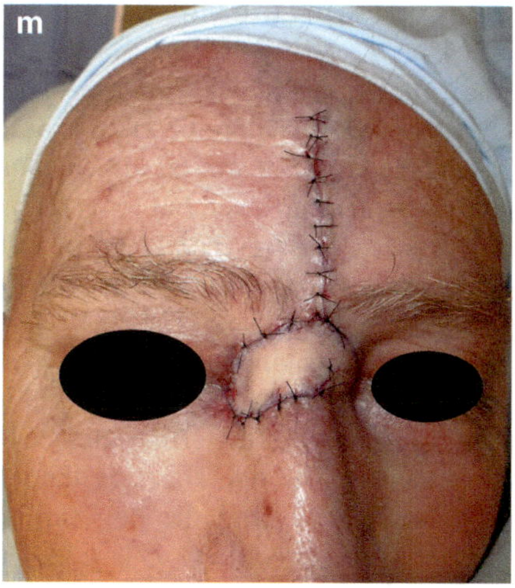

Bilobed Flap (Laterally Based)

Indications: Medium defect, lower/mid sidewall, nasal tip and alar.

Technique: The bilobed flap is best suited for circular defects. The first lobe is designed to be of similar dimensions to the defect, and the second lobe can be made slightly narrower, but longer to accommodate pointed ends on the summit, for primary closure. The angle of transfer between the defect and the second lobe is based on the site of tissue recruitment, which is often the remaining nasal sidewall/medial cheek. The flap is raised in the sub-muscular plane over the nose and subcutaneous plane in the cheek. The wound margins are widely undermined, and the defect is closed in layers. Closure is best carried out in an orderly sequence; the tertiary defect is closed first, followed closure of the primary defect. The flap covering the secondary defect is appropriately trimmed and closed next, and the dog ear is addressed last. (Fig. 7.10a–i, also see Fig. 3.5).

Tips: Wide undermining of the wound margins is necessary for tension free closure. There is a tendency for "pin cushioning" of the flap. This can be partly mitigated by modifying the defect and flap margin to include right-angled corners and parallel wound margins.

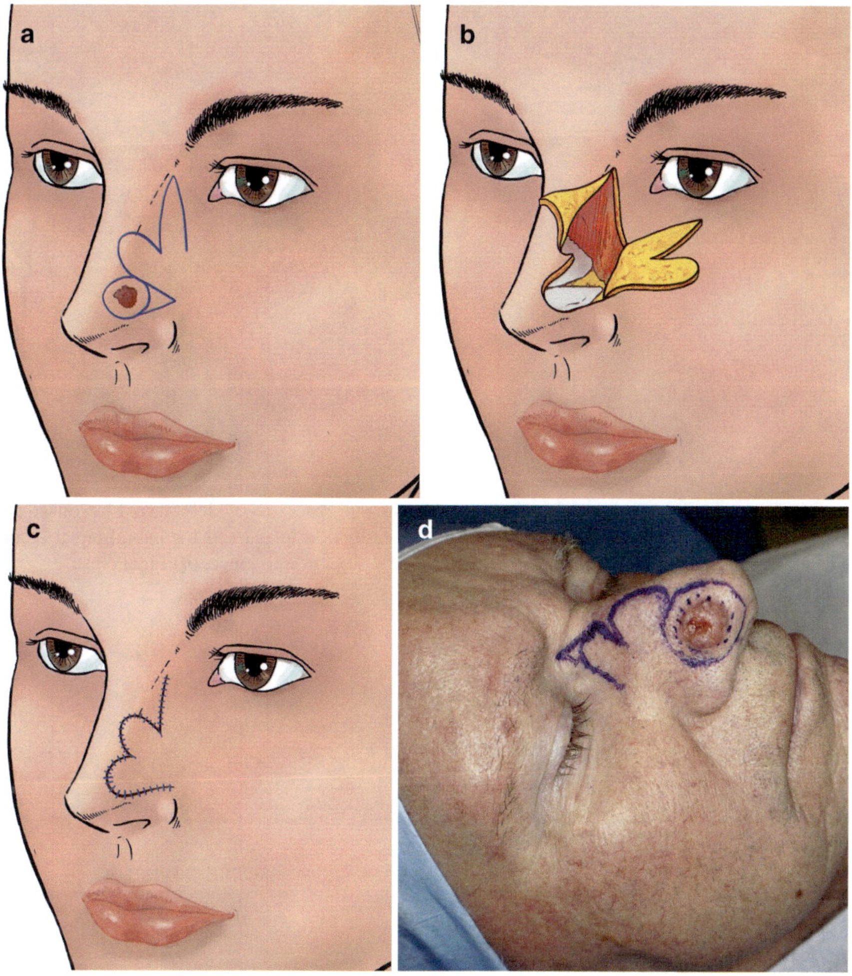

Fig. 7.10 Laterally based bilobed flap. (**a**) Markings for excision and flap, (**b**) Excision defect and flaps raised, (**c**) Final closure, (**d**) Markings for excision and flap, (**e**) Excision defect, (**f**) Flap raised, (**g**) Wide undermining, (**h**) Trial transposition, (**i**) Final closure

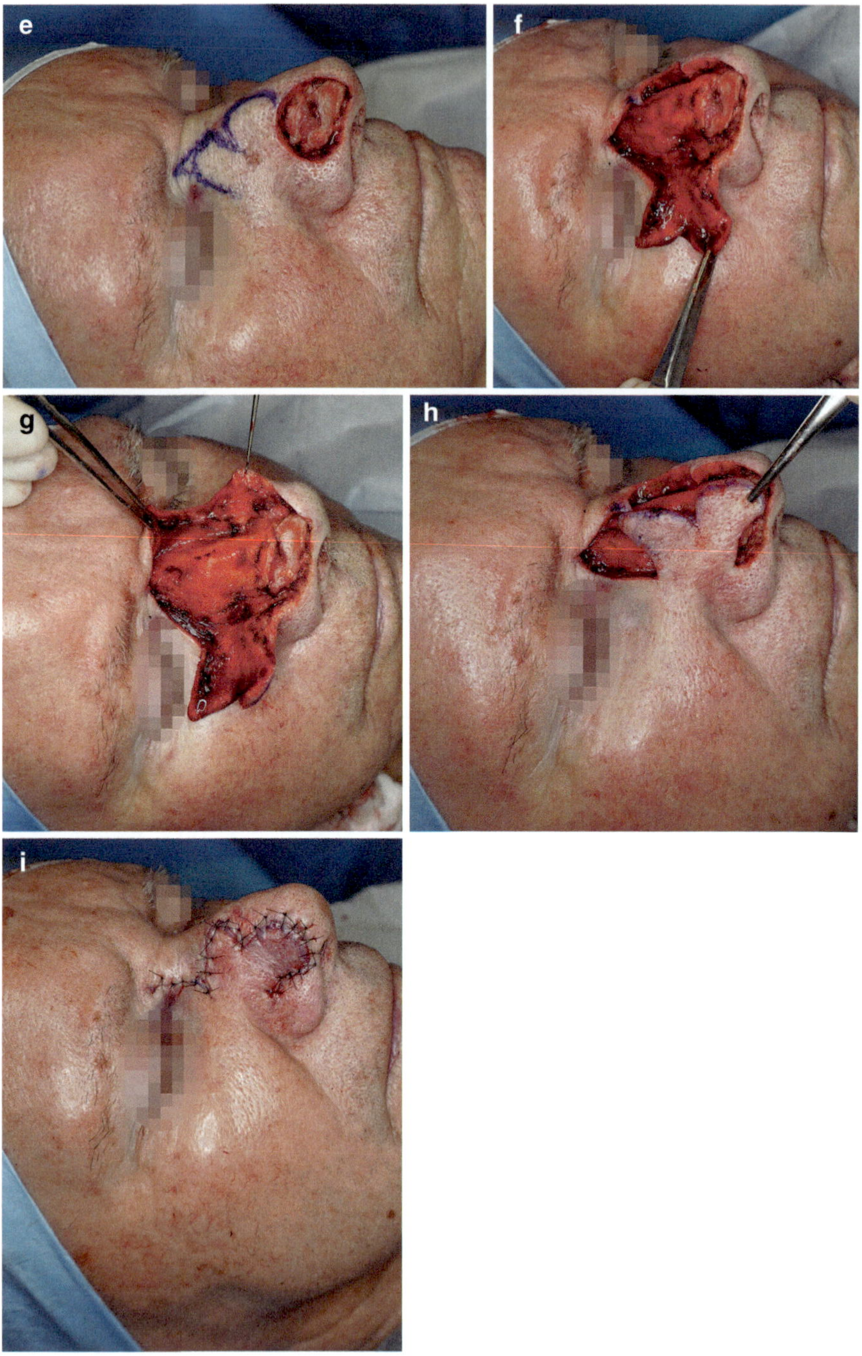

Fig. 7.10 (continued)

Bilobed Flap (Medially Based)

Indications: Small and medium defects, lateral inferior sidewall.

Technique: The bilobed flap is best suited for circular defects. The first lobe is designed to be of similar dimensions to the defect, and the second lobe can be made slightly narrower, but longer to accommodate pointed ends on the summit, for primary closure. The angle of transfer between the defect and the second lobe is based on the site of tissue recruitment, which is often the remaining nasal sidewall/glabella. The flap is raised in the sub-muscular plane. The wound margins are widely undermined, and the defect is closed in layers. Closure of the primary defect often results in a dog ear at the base, which is corrected across the nasal tip. The additional length of the second limb has to be excised, and the second lobe defect is closed primarily along the dorsum/sidewall junction (Fig. 7.11a–k).

Tips: Bilobed flaps work best when the defect is at least 5 mm away from the alar rim. Wide undermining of the wound margins is necessary for tension free closure. Any tension will result in distortion of the alar margin. Approximation of the second lobe defect to begin with makes subsequent wound closure easier. There is a tendency for "pin cushioning" of the flap. This can be partly mitigated by modifying the circular defect and flap margin to include right-angled corners and parallel wound margins.

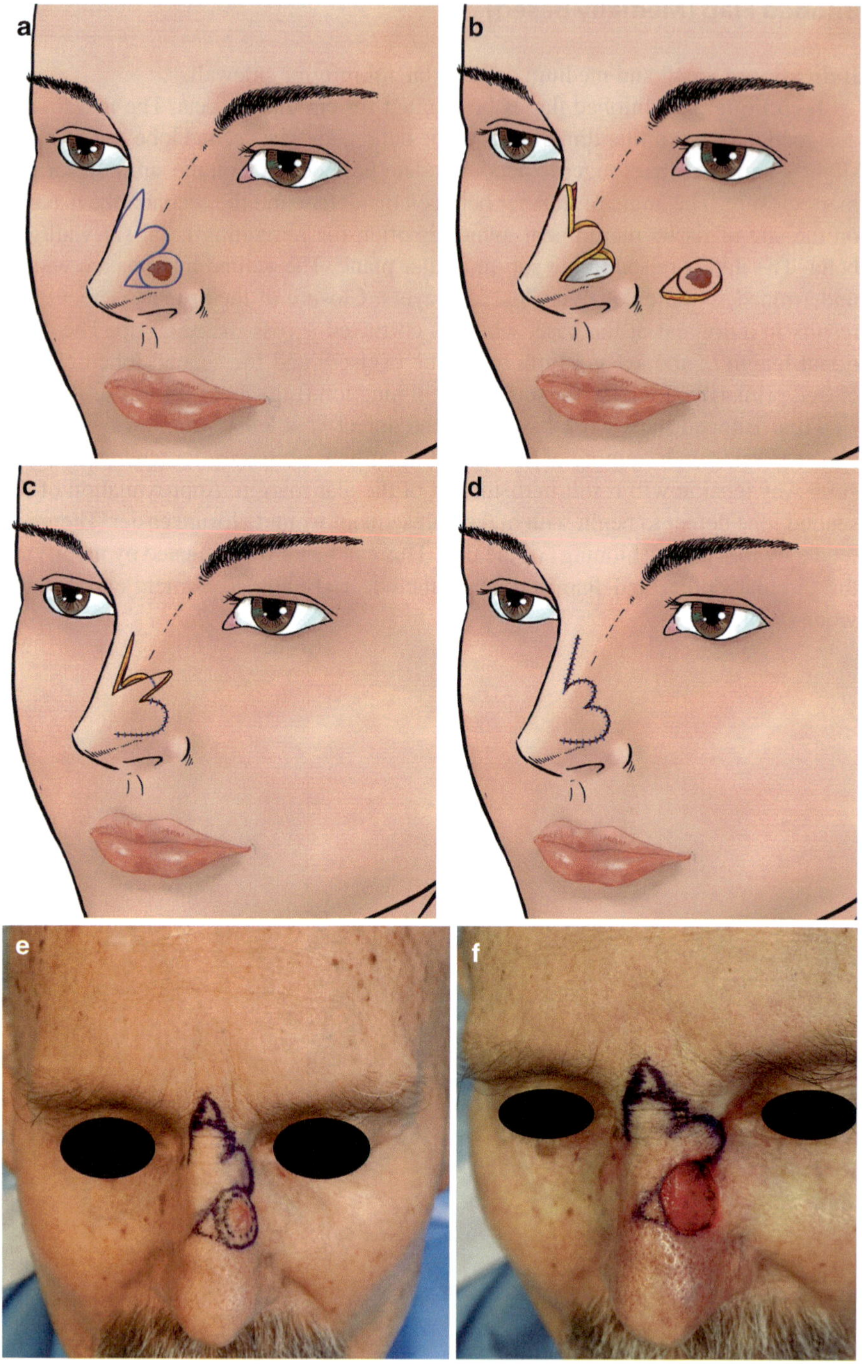

Fig. 7.11 Medially based bilobed flap. (**a**) Markings for excision and flap, (**b**) Excision defect and flaps raised, (**c**) Flaps transposed into defect, (**d**) Final closure, (**e**) Markings for excision and flap, (**f**) Excision defect, (**g**) Flap incisions, (**h**) Flaps raised with wide undermining, (**i**) Flap transposed into defect, (**j**) Final closure, (**k**) Late appearance with no revisions

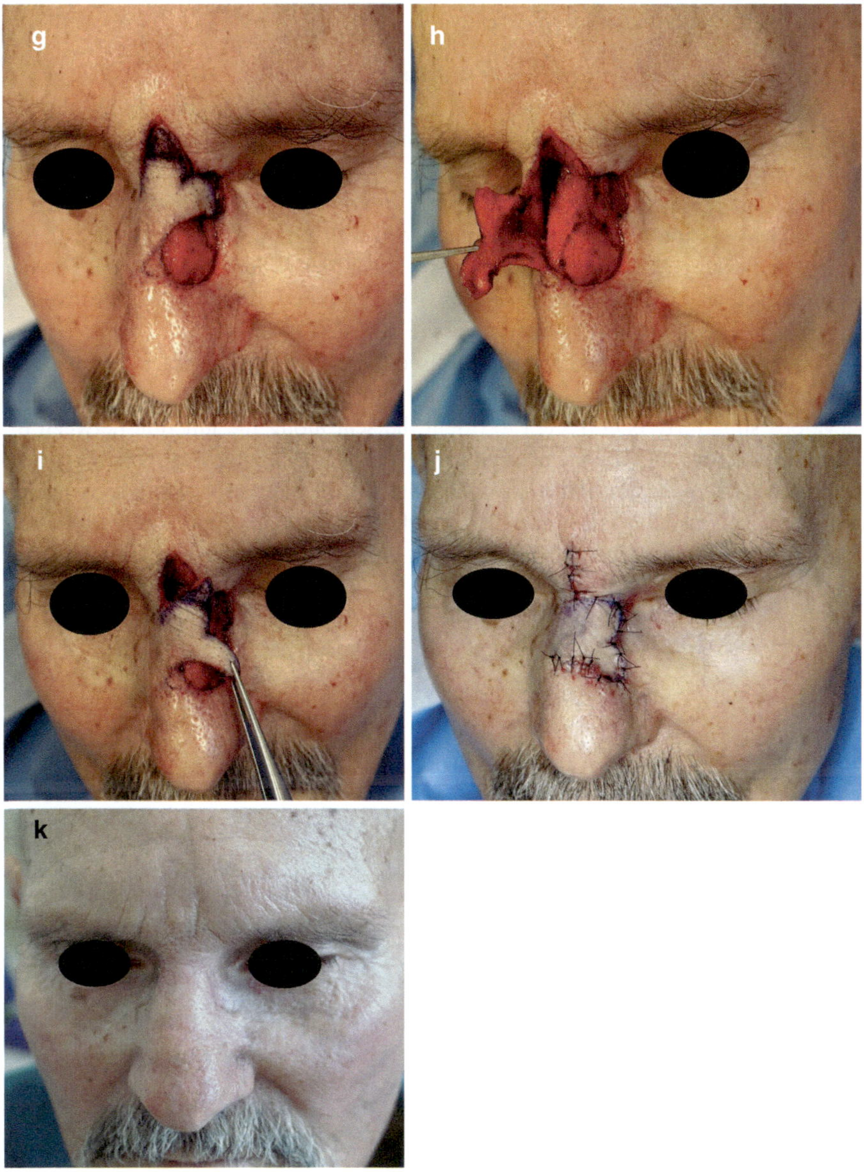

Fig. 7.11 (continued)

Apron Flap

Indications: Medium defects, lower sidewall, alar defects.

Technique: The defect is converted into a triangle with the base along the alar groove and the apex superiorly. An incision is made laterally from the base of the defect along the alar groove and extended inferiorly along the melolabial skin crease. A further incision is made superiorly from the apex, parallel to the nasofacial crease, taking care to maintain adequate width to retain vascularity. The flap is raised in the subcutaneous plane and the wound edges widely undermined. The flap is mobilised into the defect, and excess tissue trimmed along the alar groove and superiorly. The wound is closed in layers (Fig. 7.12a–m).

Tips: The cheek wound edge is mobilised to lie along the nasofacial skin crease, and additional deep sutures are placed to anchor it into place. The dog ear that develops superiorly is corrected to orient the scar along the junction between the dorsum and sidewall. The facial/angular vessels lie beneath the flap, and meticulous haemostasis is mandatory. The apron flap can be considered for alar defects when a staged interpolated flap is not suitable/considered. Cartilage support will be required, and smaller revision surgery might have to be undertaken at a later date (Fig. 7.12n–r).

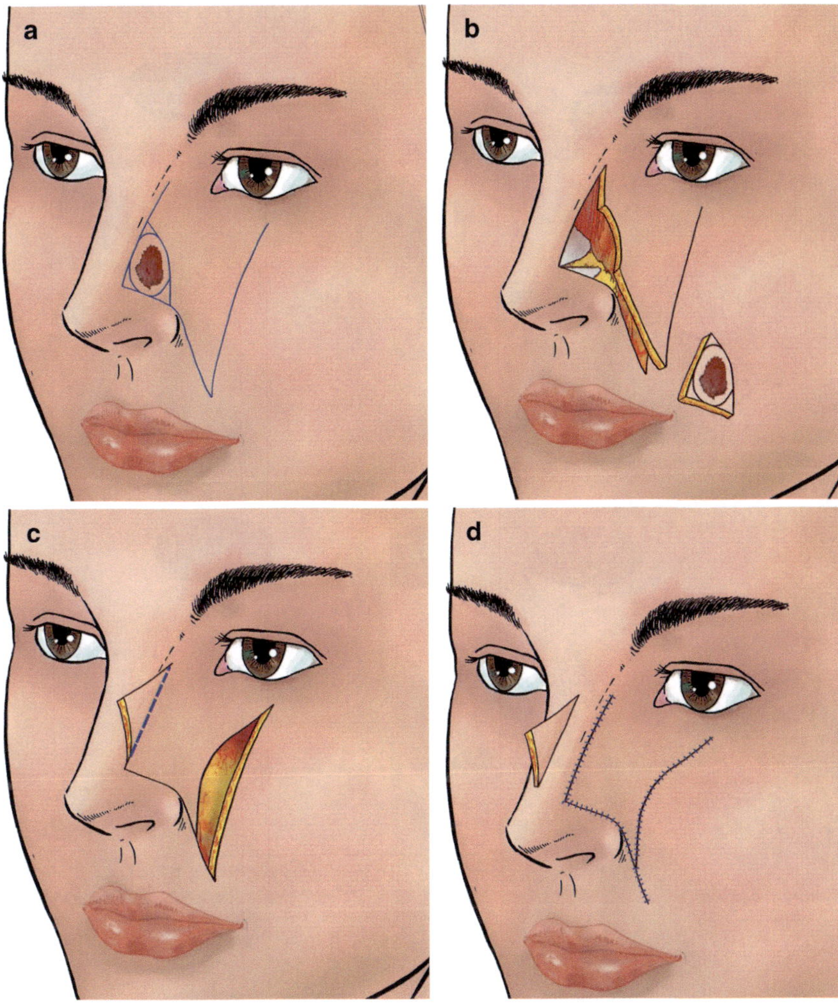

Fig. 7.12 Apron flap. (**a**) Markings for excision and flap, (**b**) Excision defect and flap raised, (**c**) Flap transposed into defect, (**d**) Final closure, (**e**) Markings for excision and flap, (**f**) Excision defect, (**g**) Flap incisions, (**h**) Flap transposed into defect, (**i**) Final closure, (**j**) Early post operative apperanace with no revisions, (**k**) Markings for excision and flap, (**l**) Excision defect and flap raised, (**m**) Final closure, (**n**) Markings for composite resection, (**o**) Excision defect and markings for flap, (**p**) Ear conchal cartilage harvest, (**q**) Final closure nose/ear, (**r**) Final closure nose

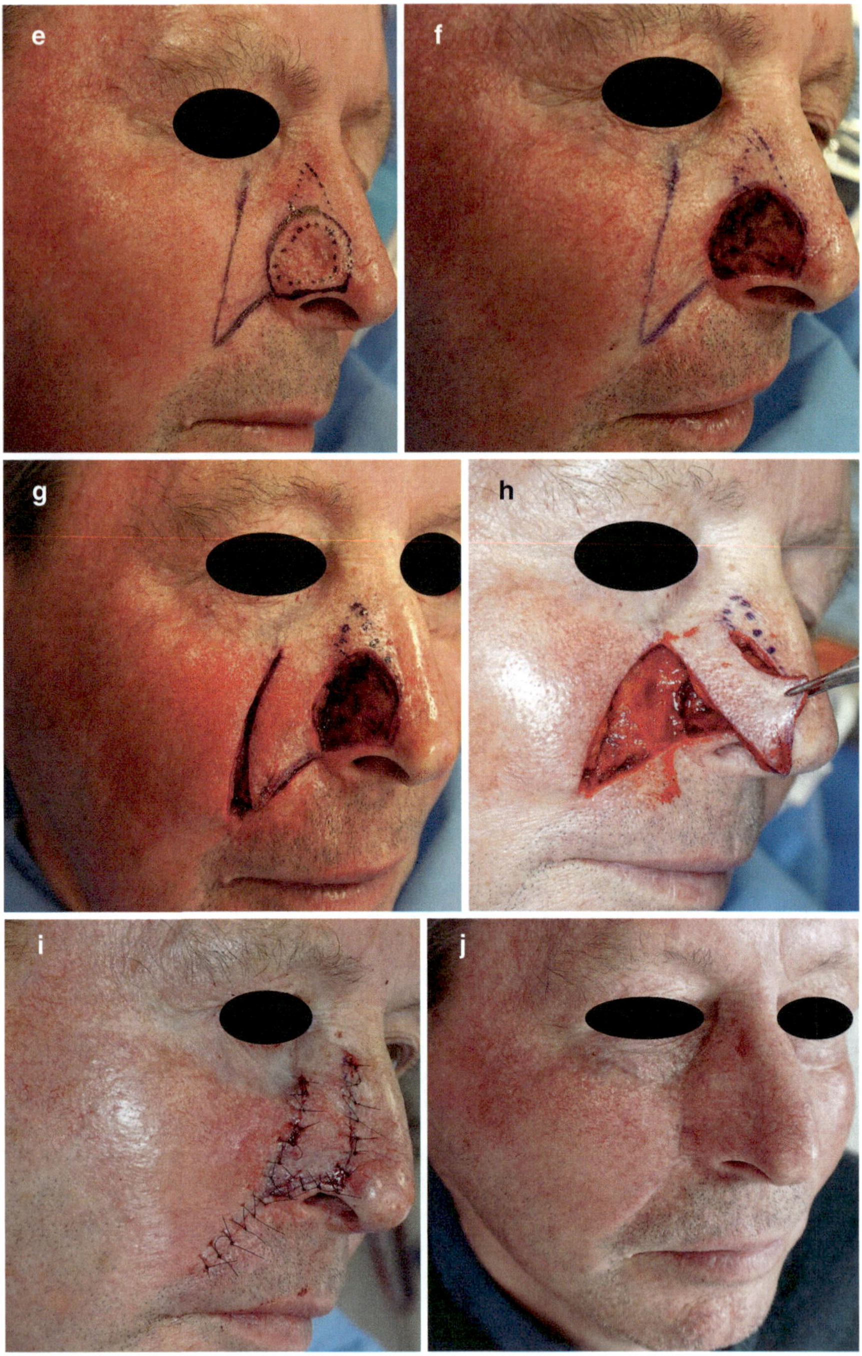

Fig. 7.12 (continued)

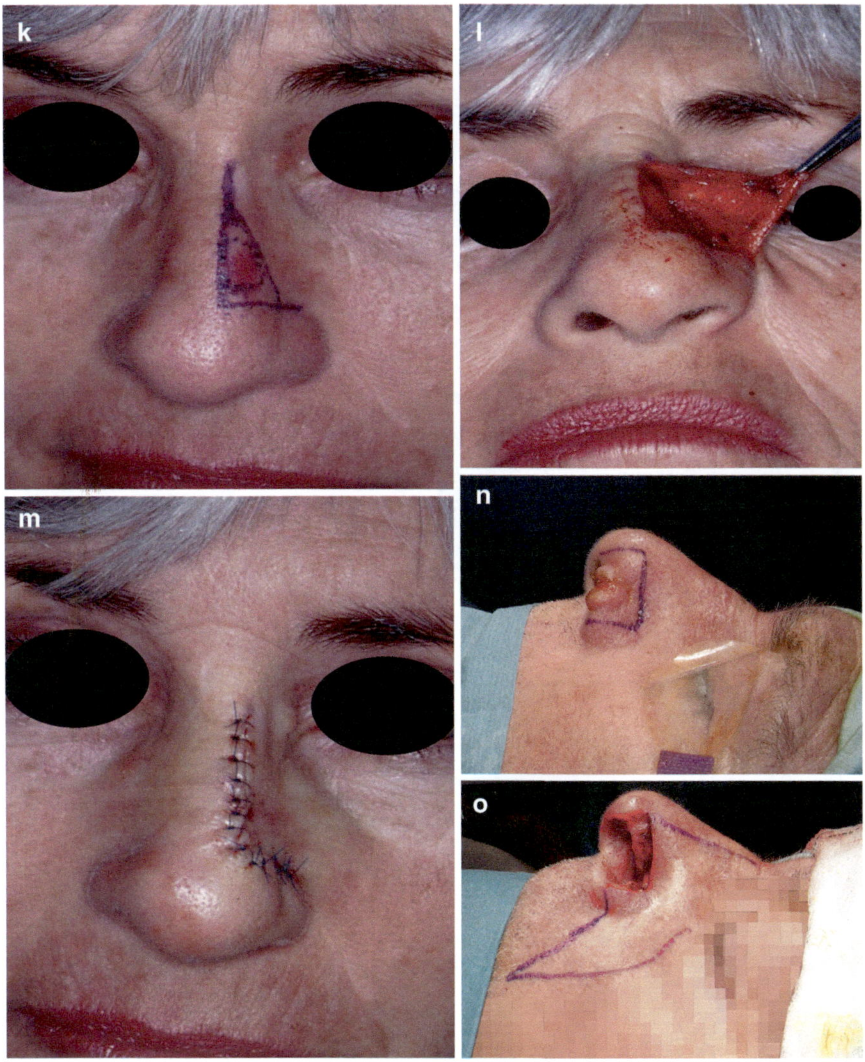

Fig. 7.12 (continued)

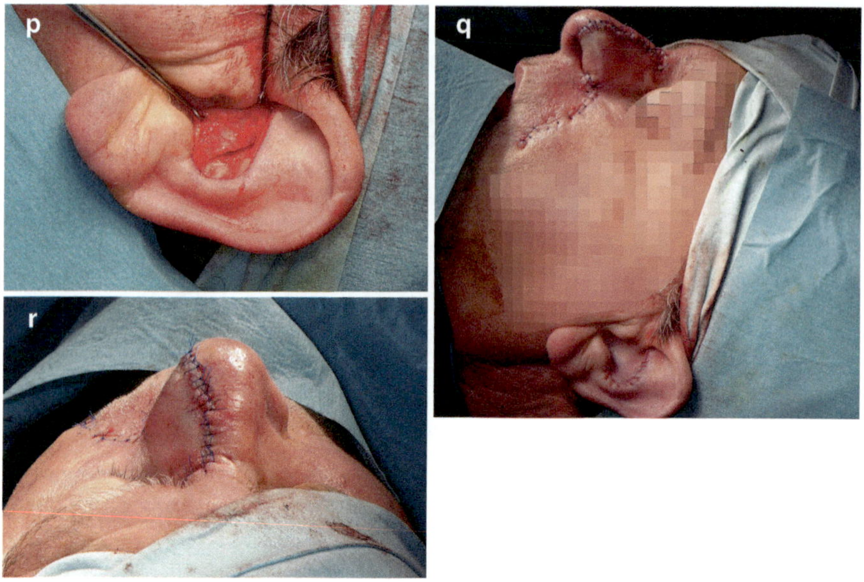

Fig. 7.12 (continued)

Ala Defects

Island Advancement Flap

Indications: Small medial alar, small/medium sidewall defects.

Technique: The defect is converted to obtain parallel wound edges. Curvilinear incisions are made from the cephalic and caudal margins of the defect, to delineate a triangular skin island, at least 2–3 times the length of the defect. The flap is oriented along the alar groove. The incision is deepened down to the perichondrium along the entire outline of the flap. The central deep tissue attachment, including the nasalis muscle, beneath the flap is preserved to provide the vascularity. The surrounding deep tissue closest and furthest from the defect is released incrementally to obtain the necessary mobility. The adjacent wound margins are widely undermined, and the flap is mobilised into the defect and closed in layers (Fig. 7.13a–g).

Tips: Judicious use of diathermy for haemostasis and avoidance of tension is necessary to prevent damage to the pedicle.

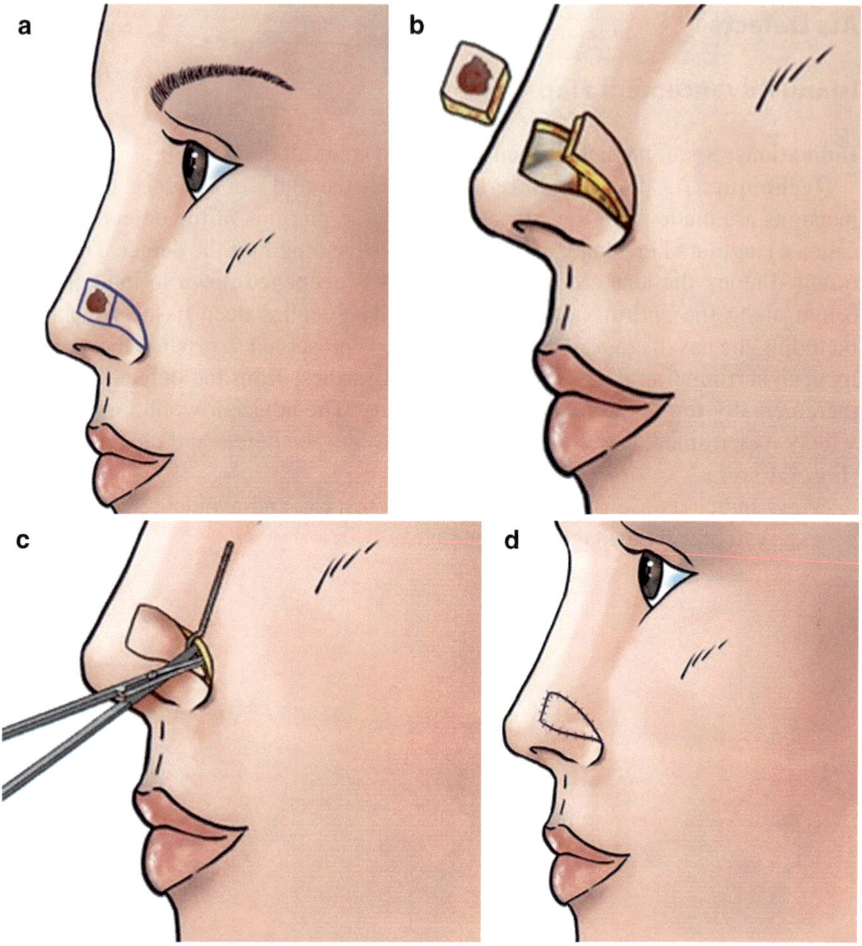

Fig. 7.13 Island advancement flap. (**a**) Markings for excision and flap, (**b**) Excision defect and flap raised, (**c**) Undermining around pedicle, (**d**) Final closure, (**e**) Markings for excision and flap, (**f**) Excision defect and flap raised, (**g**) Final closure

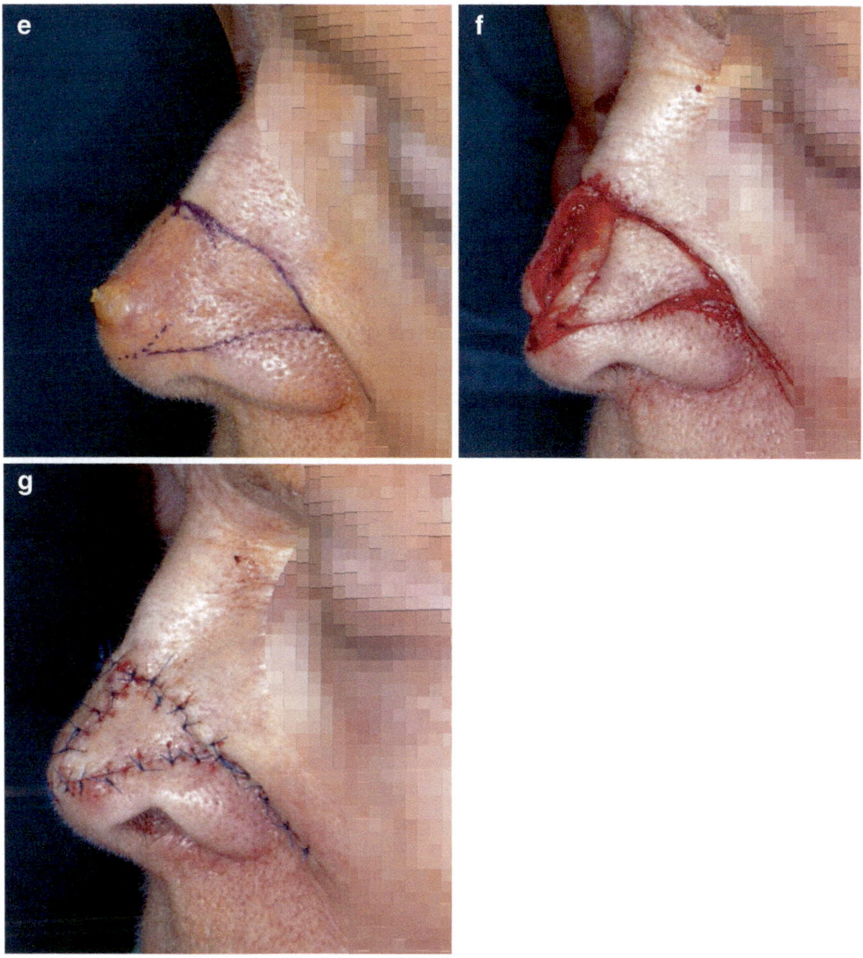

Fig. 7.13 (continued)

Bilobed Flap (Laterally Based)

Indications: Small, medium defect.

Technique: The bilobed flap is best suited for circular defects. The first lobe is designed to be of similar dimensions to the defect, and the second lobe can be made slightly narrower, but longer to accommodate pointed ends on the summit, for primary closure. The angle of transfer between the defect and the second lobe is based on the site of tissue recruitment, which is often the remaining nasal sidewall/medial cheek. The flap is raised in the sub-muscular plane over the nose and subcutaneous plane in the cheek. The wound margins are widely undermined, and the defect is closed in layers. Closure of the primary defect often results in a dog-ear at the base, which is corrected along the alar groove. The additional length of the second limb has to be excised, and the tertiary defect is closed primarily along the nasofacial crease (Fig. 7.14a–c, also see Fig. 7.10).

Tips: Bilobed flaps work best when the defect is at least 5 mm away from the alar rim. Wide undermining of the wound margins is necessary for tension free closure. Any tension will result in distortion of the alar margin. Approximation of the second lobe defect to begin with makes subsequent wound closure easier. There is a tendency for "pin cushioning" of the flap. This can be partly mitigated by modifying the circular defect and flap margin to include right-angled corners and parallel wound margins.

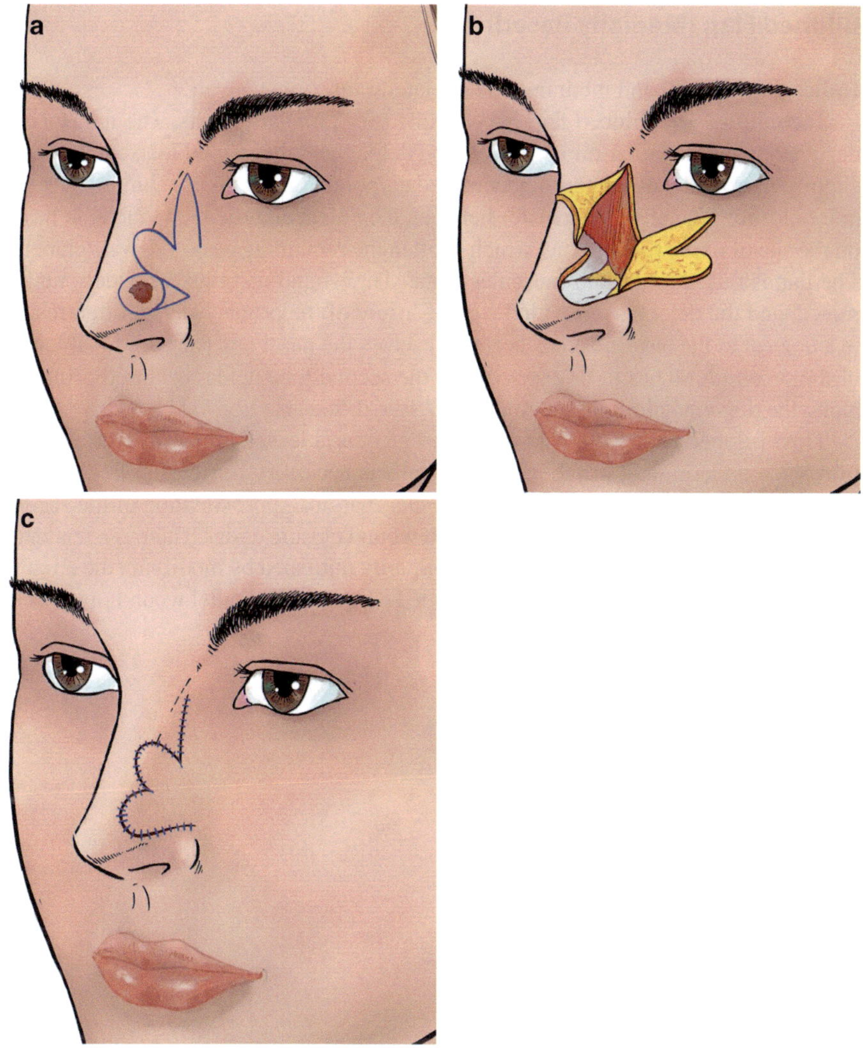

Fig. 7.14 Laterally based bilobed flap. (**a**) Markings for excision and flap, (**b**) Excision defect and flaps raised, (**c**) Final closure

Bilobed Flap (Medially Based)

Indications: Small and medium defects, lateral inferior sidewall.

Technique: The bilobed flap is best suited for circular defects. The first lobe is designed to be of similar dimensions to the defect, and the second lobe can be made slightly narrower, but longer to accommodate pointed ends on the summit, for primary closure. The angle of transfer between the defect and the second lobe is based on the site of tissue recruitment, which is often the remaining nasal sidewall/glabella. The flap is raised in the sub-muscular plane. The wound margins are widely undermined, and the defect is closed in layers. Closure of the primary defect often results in a dog ear at the base, which is corrected across the nasal tip. The additional length of the second limb has to be excised, and the second lobe defect is closed primarily along the dorsum/sidewall junction (Fig. 7.15a–d, see also Fig. 7.11).

Tips: Bilobed flaps work best when the defect is at least 5 mm away from the alar rim. Wide undermining of the wound margins is necessary for tension free closure. Any tension will result in distortion of the alar margin. Approximation of the second lobe defect to begin with makes subsequent wound closure easier. There is a tendency for "pin cushioning" of the flap. This can be partly mitigated by modifying the circular defect and flap margin to include right-angled corners and parallel wound margins.

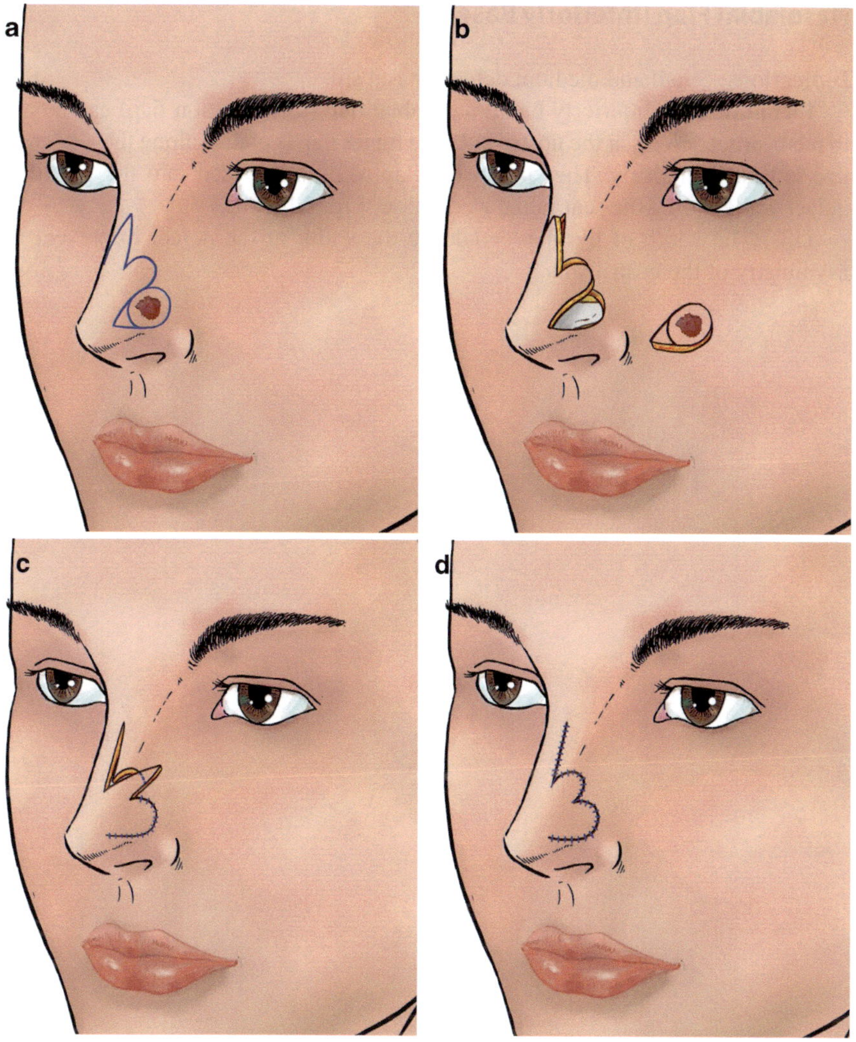

Fig. 7.15 Medially based bilobed flap. (**a**) Markings for excision and flap, (**b**) Excison defect and flap raised, (**c**) Flap transposed into defect, (**d**) Final result

Nasolabial Flap (Inferiorly Based)

Indications: Small and medium defects, nasal sill.

Technique: An inferiorly based nasolabial flap (transposition flap) can be used to reconstruct defects at the nostril sill. The finger flap is placed along the alar crease and is based inferiorly. This allows the flap to be transposed into the nostril sill defect while hiding the scar in the alar crease (Fig. 7.16a–d).

Tips: The width of the flap should be the width of the defect to prevent any asymmetry of the nostril sills.

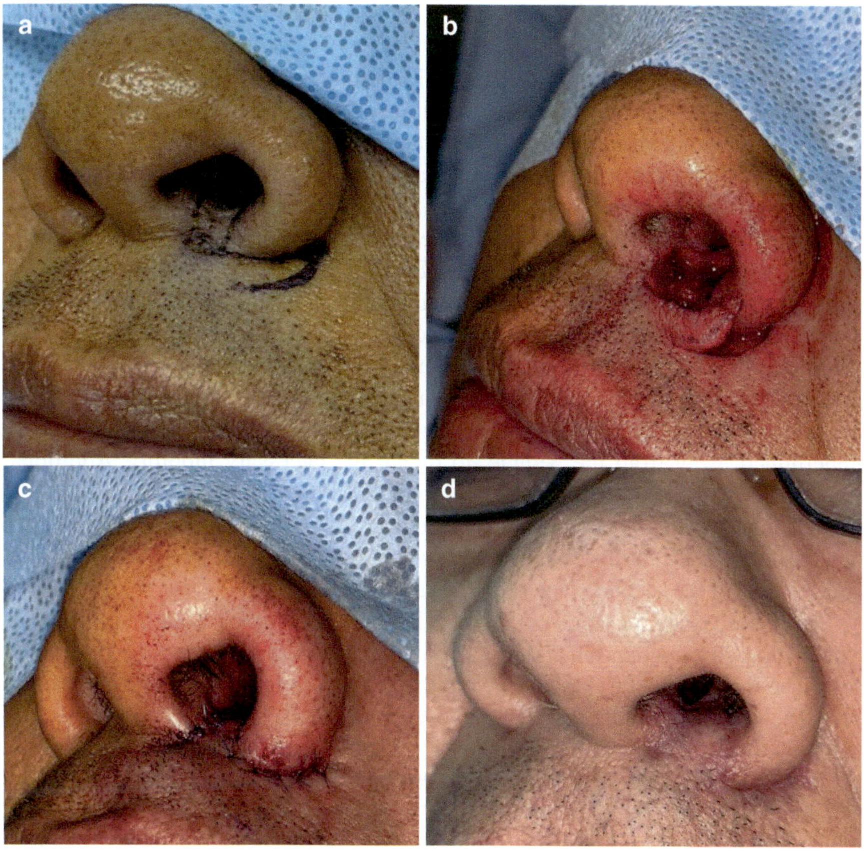

Fig. 7.16 Inferiorly based nasolabial flap. (**a**) Markings for excision and flap, (**b**) Excision defect and flap raised, (**c**) Final closure, (**d**) Early post operative appearance

Two-Stage Melolabial Flap

Indications: Medium ala defects, Columella defects.

Technique: The ala defect is enlarged, if involving more than half of the subunit, to occupy the whole ala subunit. An accurate template is made of the ala defect, if necessary from the contralateral ala. A suitably contoured auricular cartilage graft is sutured into the defect to provide support. The donor site is marked accurately with the template to mostly lie lateral and superior to the commissure, with the medial border to lie along the melolabial fold. Two triangles are marked inferiorly and superiorly from the donor site to facilitate primary closure. The superior ellipse should stop about 1 cm short of the alar facial sulcus to preserve this landmark.

An incision is made all along the skin marking and the distal portion of the flap elevated first in the subcutaneous plane. The plane of dissection is deepened, as one progress medially, down to the underlying muscle. The wound margins are widely undermined away from the pedicle, to obtain the necessary mobility. Additional deep tissue is released incrementally, till the flap is transferred into the defect without tension. The flap is sutured into the defect. The distal skin triangle is excised, and the donor defect is closed primarily. The proximal triangle can be left in situ and excised during the second stage (Fig. 7.17a–d).

The second stage is carried out 4 weeks later, and the pedicle detached at its base. The medial cheek wound is undermined and closed in layers along the melolabial fold. The margins of the flap attached to the nose are released laterally and superiorly. The excess subcutaneous fat is removed, and the flap contoured accurately and sutured into place (Fig. 7.17e, f).

Tips: The direction of transfer is clockwise for left and counter clockwise for right-sided defects. This will have to be taken into account when orienting the template and designing the flap. The medial skin triangle can often be left in situ during the initial flap transfer and removed during the second stage. Any lateral alar skin present following the initial excision can be retained and removed during the second stage (the template and flap are however designed from the beginning to replace the whole ala subunit). It is often advantageous to retain a rim of ala laterally, close to the alar facial sulcus, for ease of suturing.

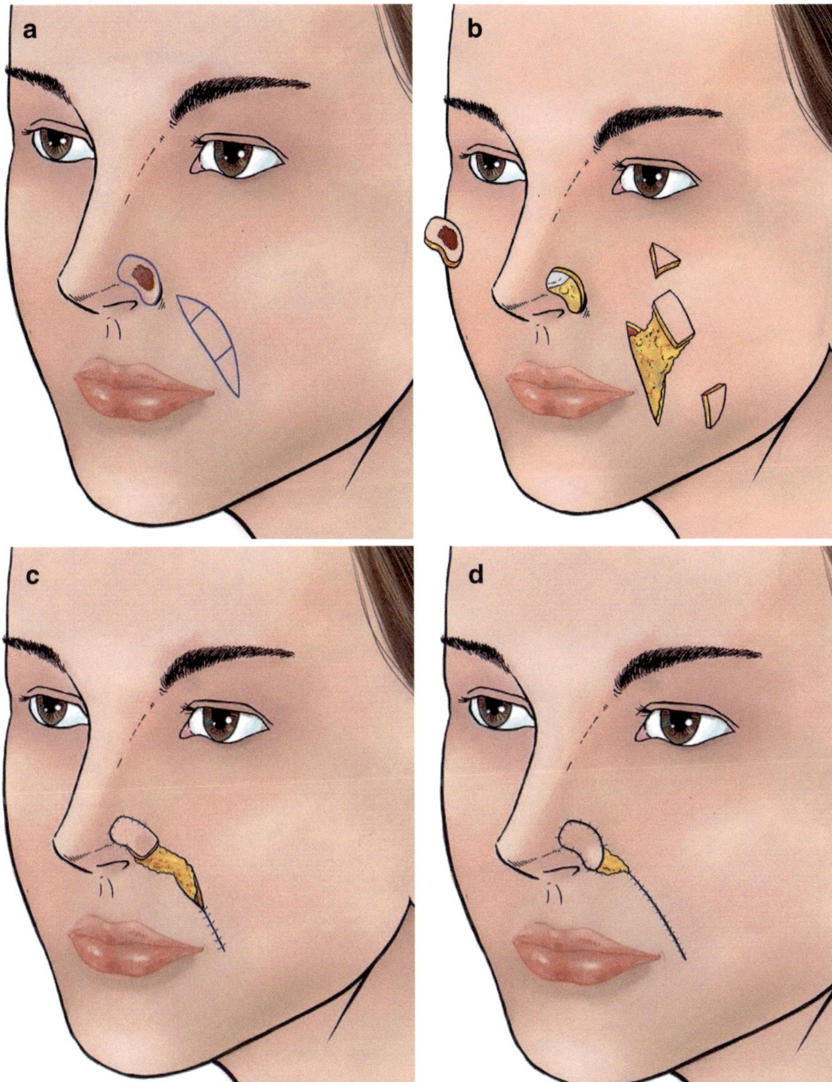

Fig. 7.17 Two stage melolabial flap. (**a**) Markings for excision and flap, (**b**) Excision defect and flap raised, (**c**) Flap sutured into defect with intact subcutaneous pedicle, (**d**) First stage closure with intervening pedicle bridge, (**e**) Second stage division of pedicle bridge, (**f**) Final flap inset

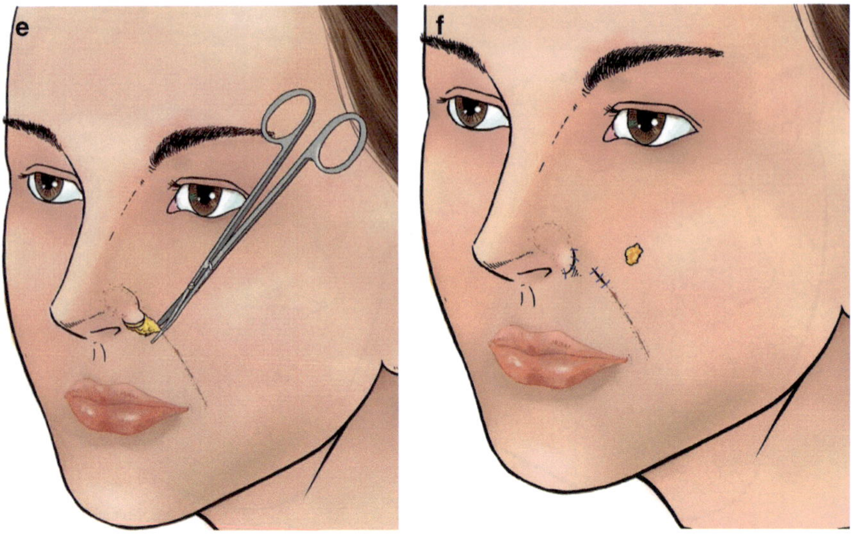

Fig. 7.17 (continued)

Paramedian Forehead Flap

Indications: Medium/large defects—tip, ala, side wall, dorsum, multiple subunits.

Technique: The defect is modified to encompass the whole subunit, if it occupies more than half the subunit. An accurate template is made from the marking, prior to modification of the defect if necessary from the contralateral side. A trial transfer is carried out to determine the location of the donor site and reach the flap. Additional factors that have to be taken into account include the hair line and size of the defect. The course of the supra-orbital artery is marked out with a Doppler, if available. The supra-orbital vessels run vertically towards the vertex, 2 cm from the midline, emerging from the orbit at the medial end of the eyebrow. The flap is marked out using the template in the upper forehead along the course of the supra-orbital vessels. The width of the proximal pedicle can be restricted to about 2 cm, to facilitate ease of closure and pivoting. The flap is raised in the supra-periosteal plane, taking care not to damage the vessels in the deep aspect. Inferiorly, the supra-orbital vessels course through the orbicularis oculi and corrugator supercilii, after emerging from the orbit, before entering the flap pedicle. The incision inferiorly is therefore restricted to skin initially, and blunt dissection is undertaken in the supra-periosteal plane and the required mobility continuously assessed. Addition sectioning of the corrugator might be necessary to obtain mobility.

The donor site is closed in layers after wide undermining, if necessary up to the lateral orbital margins. Larger defects in the upper forehead are left to heal by secondary intention, rather than using additional flaps.

The mobilised flap consists of skin, subcutaneous tissue and frontalis muscle. The distal muscle and the subcutaneous tissue are trimmed carefully, to obtain the necessary thickness for inset, taking care to preserve the sub-dermal vascular plexus. The flap is sutured into the defect without tension. The exposed deep surface of the pedicle is covered with a skin graft for ease of care. The sutures are removed in 1 week.

The second stage repair is carried out 3–4 weeks later. The pedicle is divided midway between the defect and base, taking care to maintain the requisite length proximally to reconstruct any additional tissue that might be excised in the cephalic nose. The tubed pedicle is opened to reconstitute a "flat" flap. Any additional skin in the superior nose is excised, and the superior wound margins of the inset flap undermined widely. Additional trimming of the flap is carried out at this stage. We prefer to insert the cartilage support during the second/third stage of the procedure.

The base of the flap is excised as a "V", and the adjacent wound margins are widely undermined. The wound is closed in layers taking care to accurately orient the position of the eyebrows.

Tips: Time taken to create an accurate template of the proposed defect is well spent. Care is taken to avoid damage to the pedicle, especially near the orbit margins. Thinning of the flap can be done in the second stage, and an additional stage used for division and inset, if there are any concerns regarding the vascularity especially in heavy smokers. Tracing the pedicle down to the orbital margins and extending the skin incision through the eyebrow can gain additional length. In smaller defects, the pedicle can be based on the dorsal nasal vessels, which enable harvesting a flap with longer reach. Aggressive thinning of the flap in the second/third stage, and insertion of the supporting cartilage can help recreate the contours of the nose (Fig. 7.18a–n).

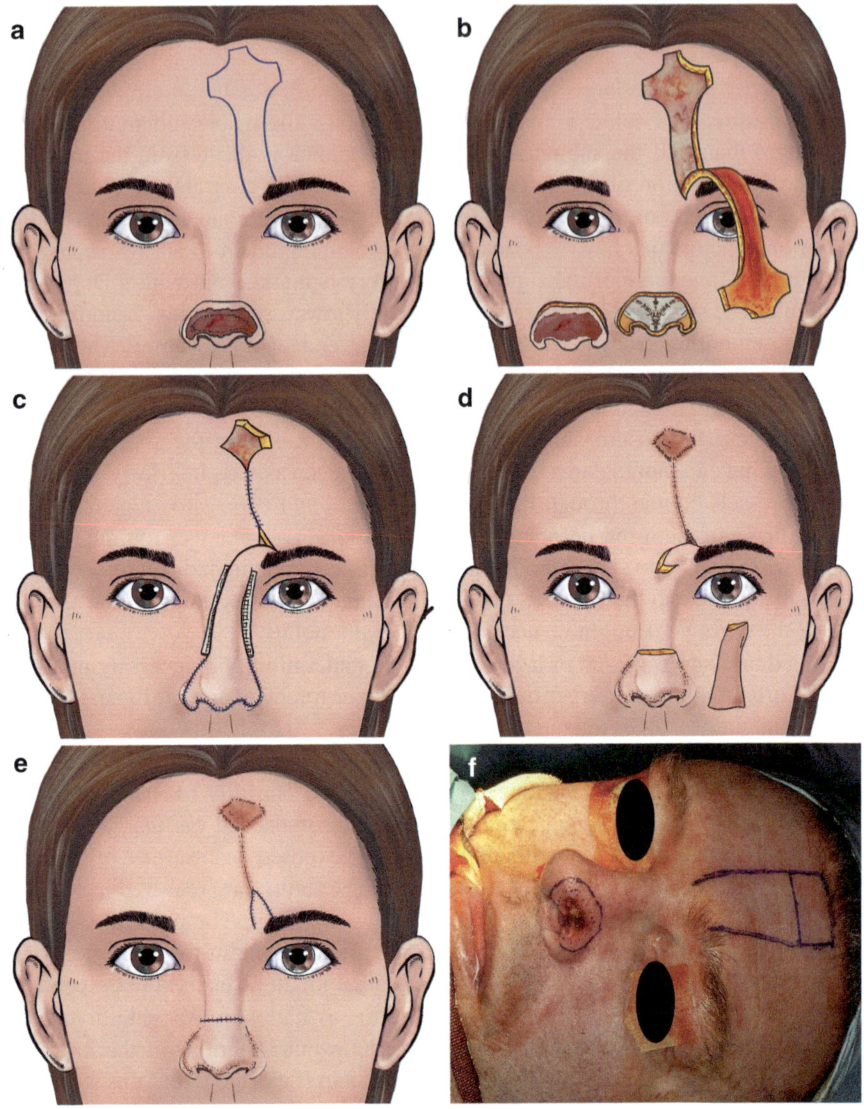

Fig. 7.18 Paramedian forehead flap. (**a**) Markings for excision and flap, (**b**) Excision defect and flap raised, (**c**) Flap inset and closure of forehead defect, (**d**) Second stage flap division, (**e**) Inset of flap and pedicle base, (**f**) Markings for excision and flap, (**g**) Excision defect, (**h**) Pedicle delineated, (**i**) Falp raised, (**j**) First stage flap inset and closure of forehead defect - lateral view, (**k**) First stage flap inset and closure of forehead - superior view, (**l**) Early post operative appearance - first stage, (**m**) Second stage divsion of flap and inset of pedicle base, (**n**) Early post operative appearance after second stage with no revisions (Composite images)

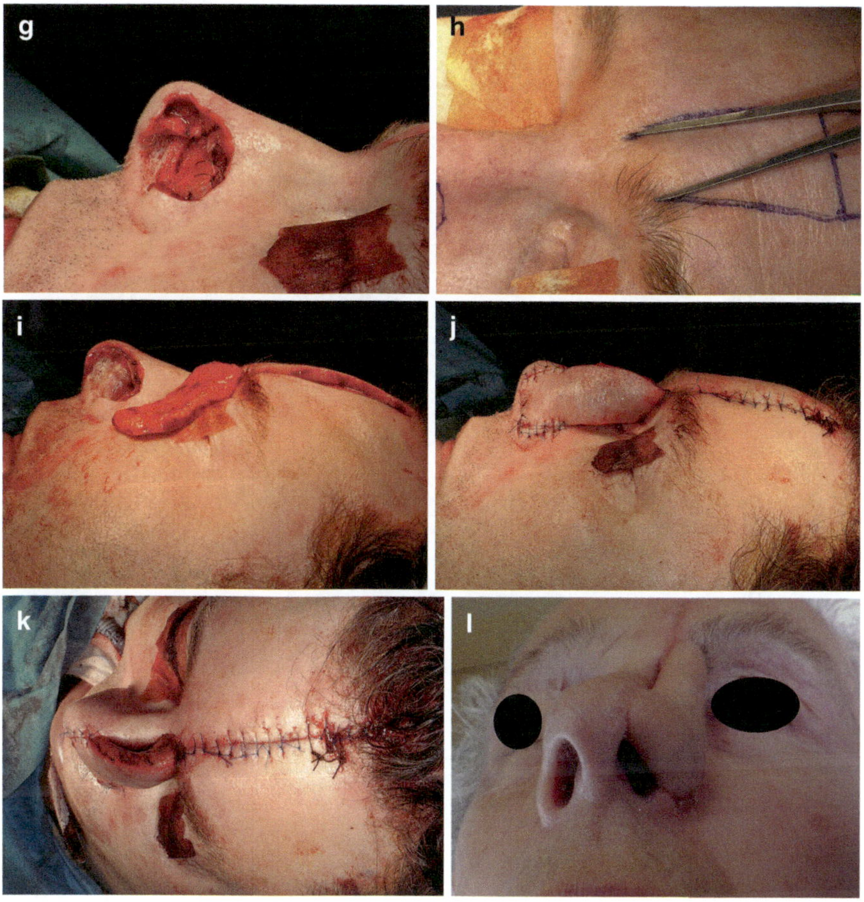

Fig. 7.18 (continued)

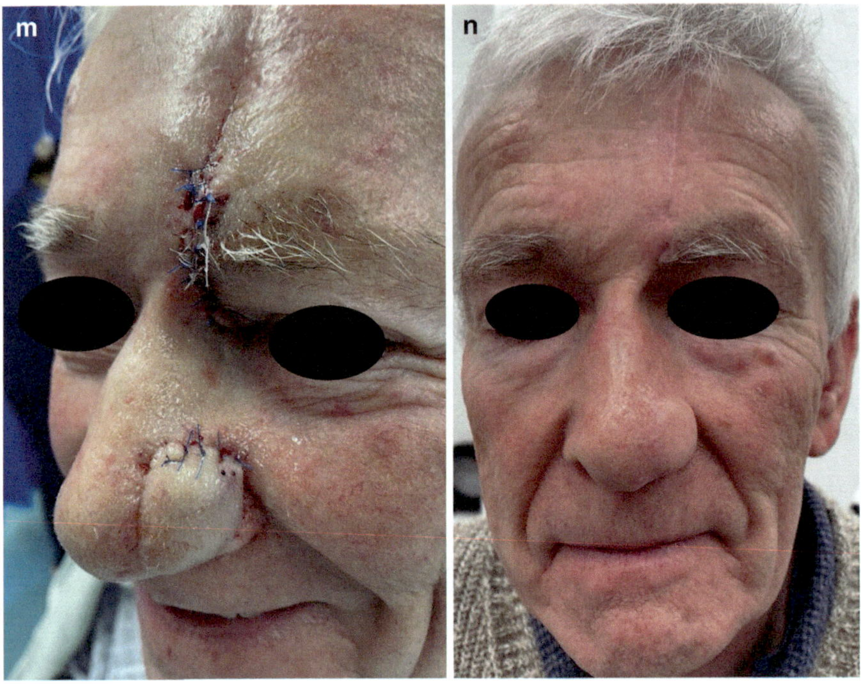

Fig. 7.18 (continued)

Apron Flap

(See Fig. 7.12).

Columella

Primary Closure (Vertical/Horizontal)

Indications: Small defects.

Technique: Depending on the orientation of the defect, availability of tissue for closure and the likely distortion of the nasal tip, the wound is closed with a horizontal or vertical orientation.

Skin Graft

Indications: Medium defects.

Technique: An accurate template is made of the defect, which is transferred to the donar site to harvest a full-thickness skin graft. The "defatted" graft is sutured to the defect, with additional "long" sutures that can be used for "tying" over the bolus. The graft can be "quilted" to the base, to decrease the risk of haematoma and dead space. A non-adherent dressing is laid over the sutured graft, over which a cotton wool ball/sponge soaked in proflavin or a suitable antibiotic ointment is placed. The tie-over bolus sutures are now used to hold the dressing in place. The sutures and pack are removed in 7–10 days time (see Fig. 7.19a–e).

Tips: A more acceptable result is obtained in individuals with thin skin and superficial defects. A forehead donar site can be considered, as the tissue match is closer than that of the neck.

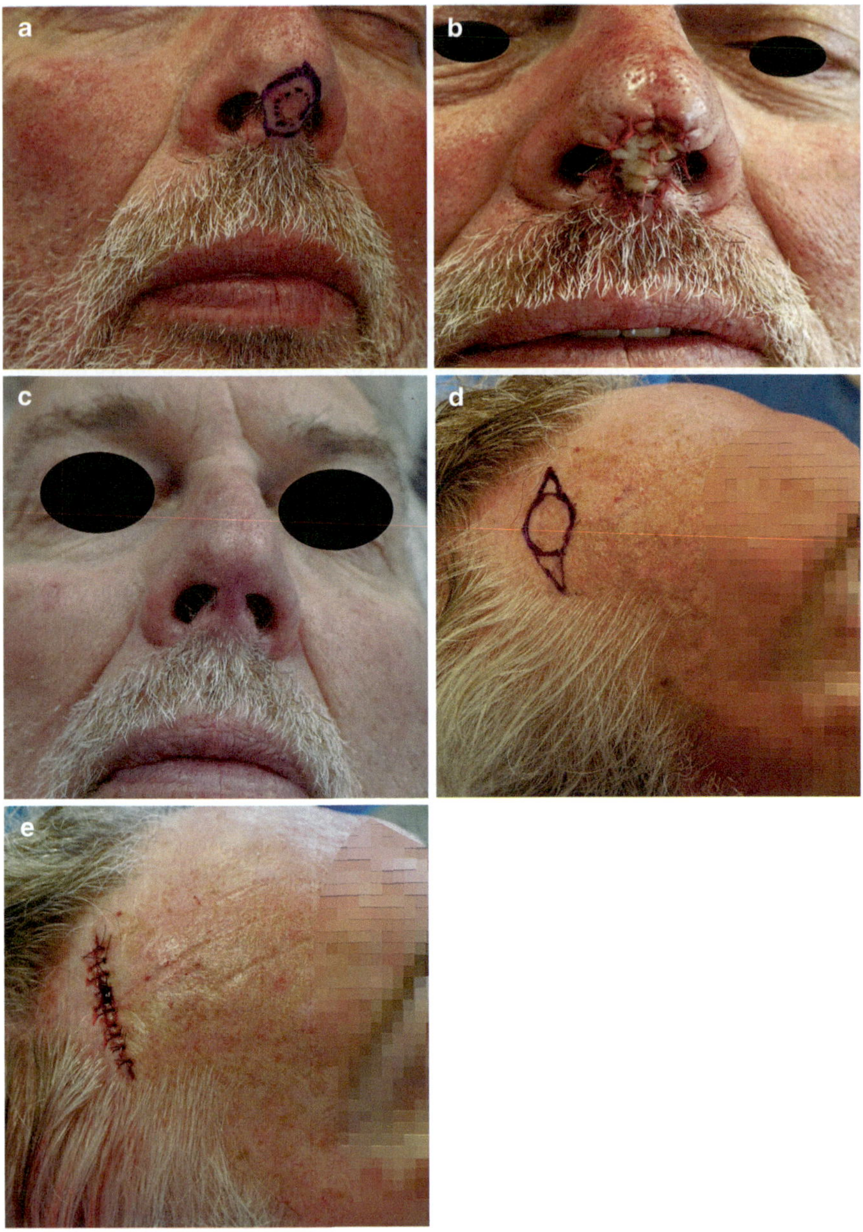

Fig. 7.19 Skin graft. (**a**) Markings for excision, (**b**) Skin graft sutured in place, (**c**) Post operative appearance, (**d**) Template skin graft harvest forehead, (**e**) Closure of donar site

Two-Stage Melolabial Flap

(See Fig. 7.17).

Suggested Algorithm

Dorsum

Small

1. Primary closure (vertical/horizontal).

Medium

1. Glabella advancement flap.
2. Glabella transposition flap.
3. Skin graft.

Nasal Tip

Small

1. Primary closure (Vertical/horizontal).

Medium

1. Glabella advancement flap.
2. Bilobed flap.
3. Skin graft.

Columella

1. Primary closure.
2. Skin graft.
3. Two-stage melolabial flap.

Side Wall

Small

1. Primary closure (vertical).
2. Healing by secondary intention (upper).

Medium

1. Skin graft.

Upper side wall

1. Glabella transposition flap.

Lower side wall

1. Bilobed flap.
2. Apron flap.

Ala

Small

1. Island advancement flap.

Medium

1. Bilobed flap (laterally based).
2. Bilobed flap (medially based).
3. Two-stage melolabial flap.
4. Apron flap.

Paramedian Forehead Flap

1. Large nasal defects involving multiple nasal subunits.
2. Large nasal tip defects.
3. Large ala defects.
4. Large dorsal defects.
5. Large side wall defects.

8 Eyelids

Subunits and Anatomical Considerations

Eyelids perform many important functions, which include protection of the eye and maintaining an adequate tear film. The aesthetic eyelid unit is defined by the lower margin of the eyebrow, lateral and inferior orbital rims and the nasojugal fold. A sound understanding of anatomy and function is essential for eyelid reconstruction and should only be attempted by an appropriately trained clinician.

The eyelids are complex multilayered structures supported by cartilaginous tarsal plates. The free lid margin contains eyelashes and secretory glands, and the extension of the tarsal plates forms the medial and lateral canthal tendons.

Reconstruction could be more easily understood if the eyelids were considered to consist of an **anterior lamella** composed of skin and orbicularis oculi and a **posterior lamella** composed of conjunctiva, tarsal plate, orbital septum and the lid retractors. The orbital septum is occasionally considered the middle lamella, and the "grey line" along the lid margin represents the junction between the anterior and posterior lamellae.

The eyelid aesthetic unit can be further subdivided from a reconstructive point of view into upper lid, lower lid, medial canthus and lateral canthus subunits (Fig. 8.1).

The skin of the eyelid is the thinnest in the body, and the RSTLs around the eyelids are horizontally oriented (Fig. 8.2). However, excision parallel to the RSTLs, especially in the lower eyelid, runs the risk of eyelid retraction and ectropion. It is therefore preferable to orient excisions to be perpendicular to the lid margins, unless there is significant skin redundancy. Excisions along the RSTL in the adjacent lateral and medial canthus, eyebrow and glabella regions can be performed and will provide relatively unobtrusive scars.

V. Ilankovan et al., *Local Flaps in Facial Reconstruction*,
https://doi.org/10.1007/978-3-031-49464-2_8

Full-thickness defects require reconstruction of both the anterior and posterior lamella, in which case it is mandatory that at least one of the reconstructed lamella should contain its own blood supply. Involvement of the lid margins is another important determinant of reconstruction.

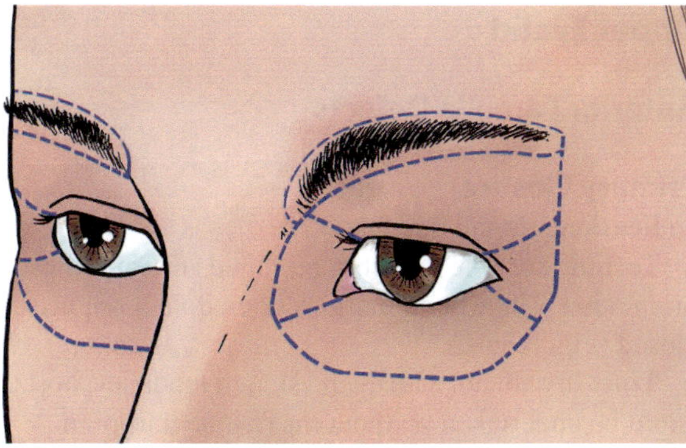

Fig. 8.1 Eyelid subunits

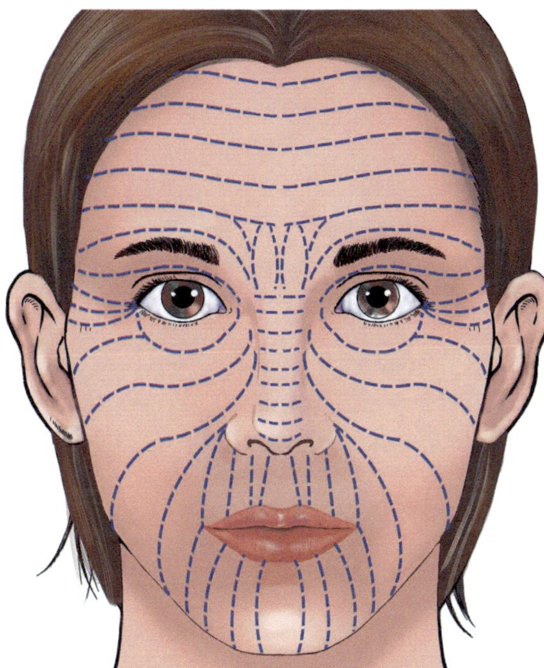

Fig. 8.2 Eyelid and surrounding RSTL's

Upper Eyelid

Anterior Lamella Defects

Primary Closure

Indications: Small defects.

Technique: The defect is modified into an ellipse with a vertical or horizontal orientation. The wound margins often do not require undermining, and the defect is closed (Fig. 8.3a–c).

Tips: In patients with eyelid skin redundancy, horizontal ellipse along the RSTLs could be undertaken, without the risk of ectropion.

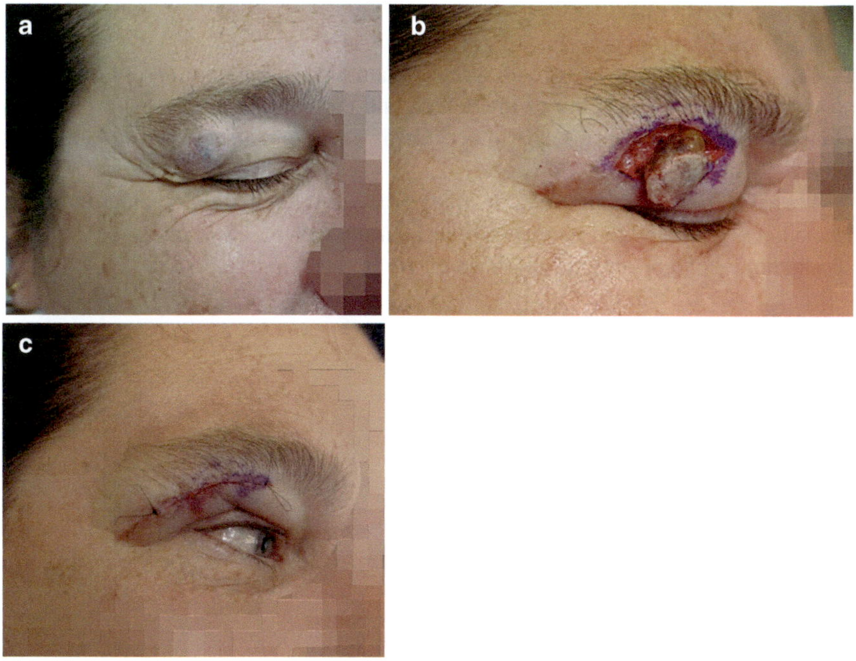

Fig. 8.3 Horizontal excision and primary closure. (**a**) Lesion upper eyelid, (**b**) Excision defect, (**c**) Final closure

Advancement Flap

Indications: Medium defects.

Technique: The defect is modified to obtain parallel wound margins. Incisions are made from the extremity of the defect, and the flap raised in the sub-muscular plane. The wound margins are undermined, and the defect is closed in layers (Fig. 8.4a–c).

Tips: The base of the flap can be made broader to maintain a satisfactory vascular pedicle. The flaps can be medially or laterally based and when based medially, should not extend beyond the confines of the eyelid skin.

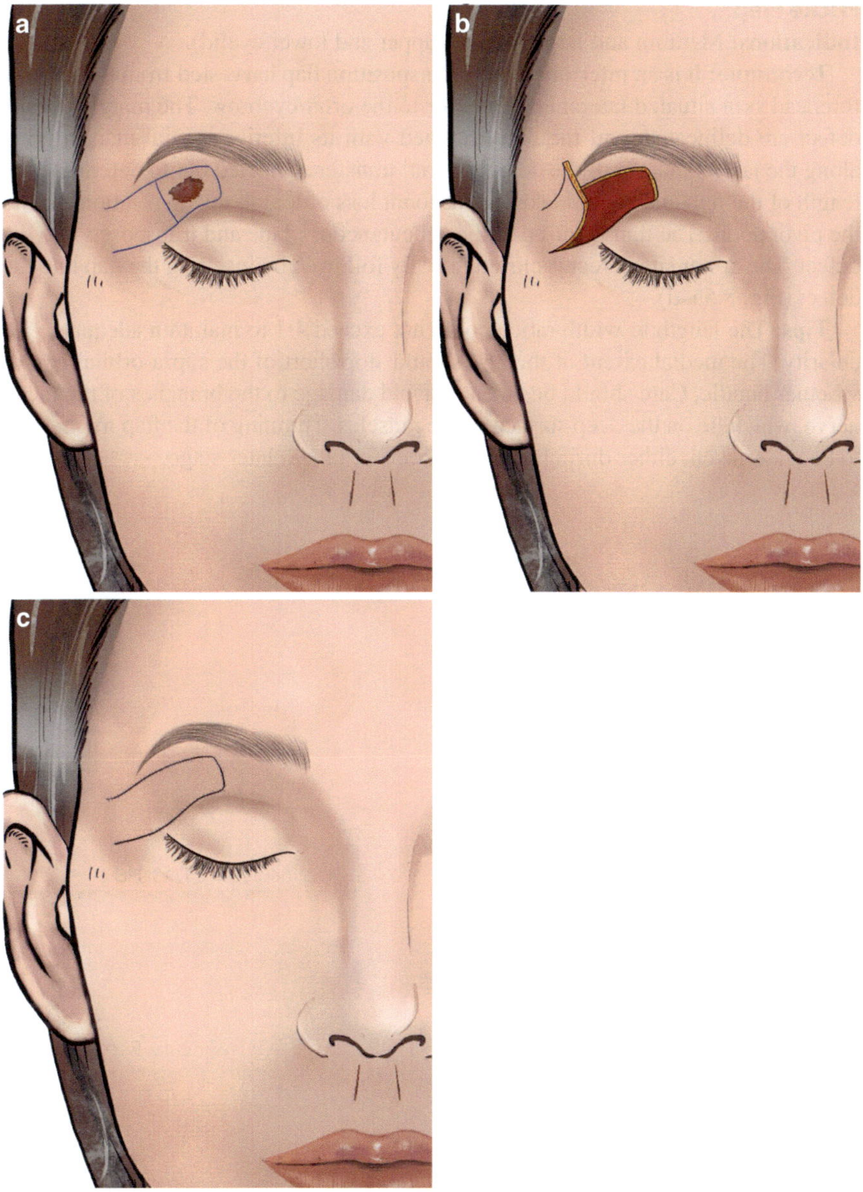

Fig. 8.4 Advancement flap. (**a**) Markings for excision and flap, (**b**) Excision defect and flap raised, (**c**) Final closure

Fricke Flap

Indications: Medium and large defects (upper and lower eyelid).

Technique: It is an inferiorly based transposition flap harvested from the temple/forehead skin situated lateral and superior to the orbit/eyebrow. The margins of the defect are delineated, and the flap designed with its inferior medial margin lying along the lateral margin of the defect. A trial transfer is carried out to determine the length of the flap and should take into account loss of length due to rotation around the pivot point. The flap is raised in the subcutaneous plane and transposed into the defect. The donor site defect is closed initially followed by insetting the flap into the defect (Fig. 8.5a–d).

Tips: The length to width ratio should not exceed 4:1 to maintain adequate vascularity. The medial extent of the flap should stop short of the supra-orbital neurovascular bundle. Care should be taken to avoid damage to the branches of the facial nerve, which lie on the deep surface of the muscles. Thinning of the flap might have to be undertaken, either during the initial transfer or at a later stage.

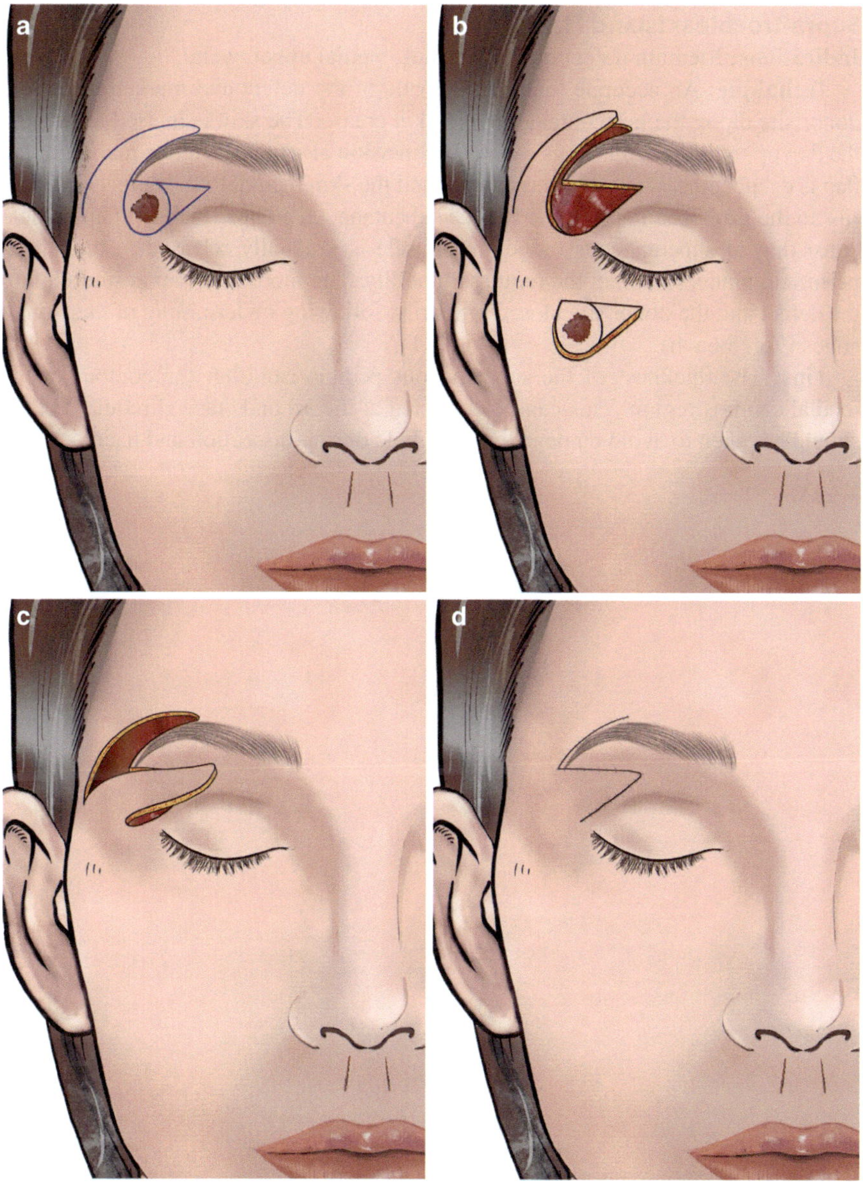

Fig. 8.5 Fricke flap. (**a**) Markings for excision and flap, (**b**) Excision defect and flap raised, (**c**) Flap transposed into defect, (**d**) Final closure

Supra-trochlear Island Flap

Indications: Medium defect medial canthus, medial upper eyelid.

Technique: An accurate template is made of the defect and marked out at the donor site along the horizontal glabellar skin crease. The skin is incised all around the flap up to the subcutaneous tissue. The incision along the superior margin of the flap is deepened down to the periosteum, and the skin medial to the defect and inferior to the proposed flap is raised in the subcutaneous plane. The deep flap pedicle consisting of subcutaneous tissue and muscle is gradually released in the supra-periosteal plane, to obtain the required mobility. The mobilised flap is sutured into the defect and the donor site closed primarily, following undermining of the wound edges (Fig. 8.6a–h).

Tips: The thickness of the subcutaneous pedicle can alter the contour of the medial canthus region. This can be corrected at the second stage if required. Care should be taken to avoid damage to the pedicle during dissection and haemostasis.

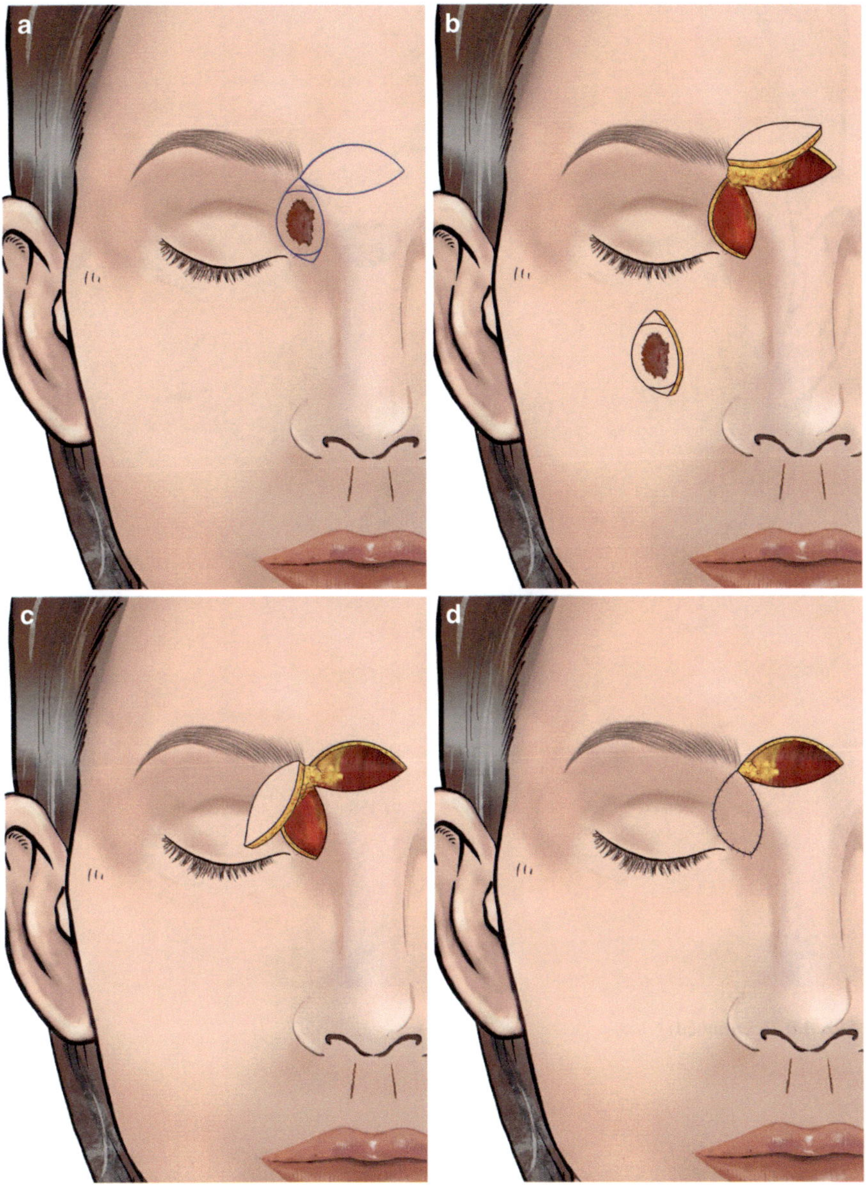

Fig. 8.6 Supra-troclear island flap. (**a**) Markings for excision and flap, (**b**) Excision defect and flap raised, (**c**) Flap transposed into defect, (**d**) Flap sutured into defect, (**e**) Final closure, (**f**) Markings for excision and flap, (**g**) Excision defect, (**h**) Final closure

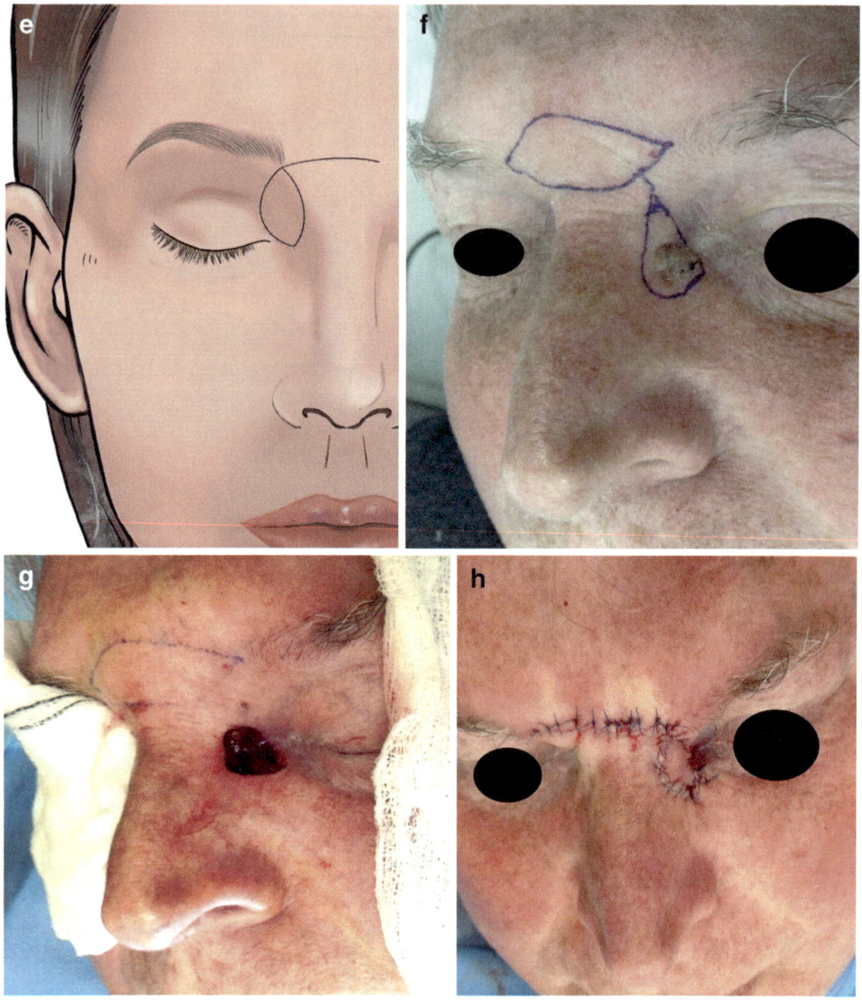

Fig. 8.6 (continued)

Glabella Transposition Flap

Indications: Medium defects medial canthus/jugum nasi.

Technique: The defect is modified into a triangle with the base placed laterally. A curvilinear incision is made from the superior edge of the defect and extended superiorly into the glabella skin crease. A back cut is made from the summit, across to the contralateral medial canthus. The nasal component of the flap is raised in the sub-muscular plane and the glabellar component in the subcutaneous plane. The wound margins are widely undermined and closed in layers. The secondary glabellar/nasal root defect is closed primarily and any excess skin in the superior aspect of the flap discarded. Dog ear at the primary defect is corrected as required (Fig. 8.7a–d, e–h, i–m).

Tips: The flap often has to be thinned, to match the defect margins. Primary closure of the glabella defect medialises the eyebrows and would have to be taken into account, when considering this flap. Variations to the design of the flap can be utilised to best accommodate the defect and the eventual scar (Fig. 8.7e–h, i–m).

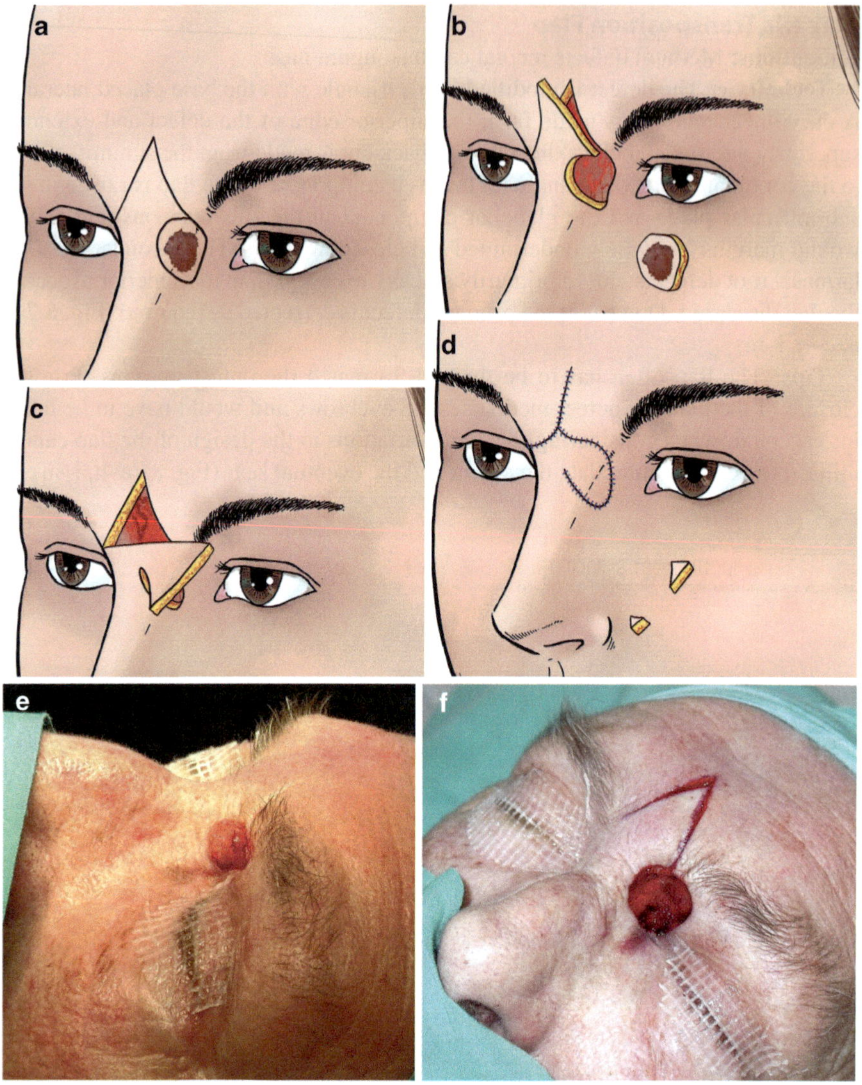

Fig. 8.7 Glabella transposition flap. (**a**) Markings for excision and flap, (**b**) Excision defect and flap raised, (**c**) Flap transposed into defect, (**d**) Final closure (**e**) Lesion medial canthus area, (**f**) Excision defect and flap incision, (**g**) Flap transposed into defect, (**h**) Final closure, (**i**) Markings for excision and flap, (**j**) Excision defect and flap raised, (**k**) Trial transfer of flap, (**l**) Appropriate thining of flap, (**m**) Final closure

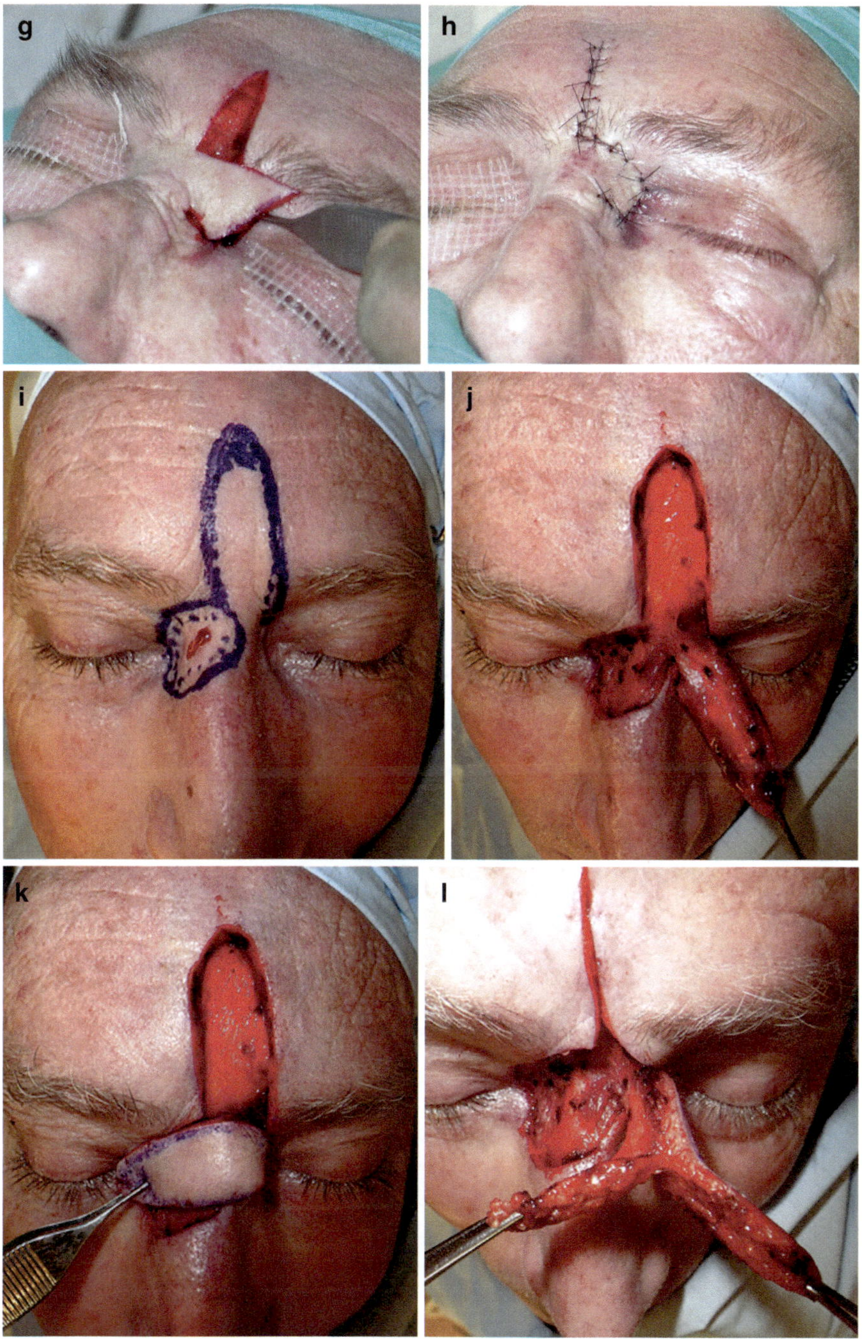

Fig. 8.7 (continued)

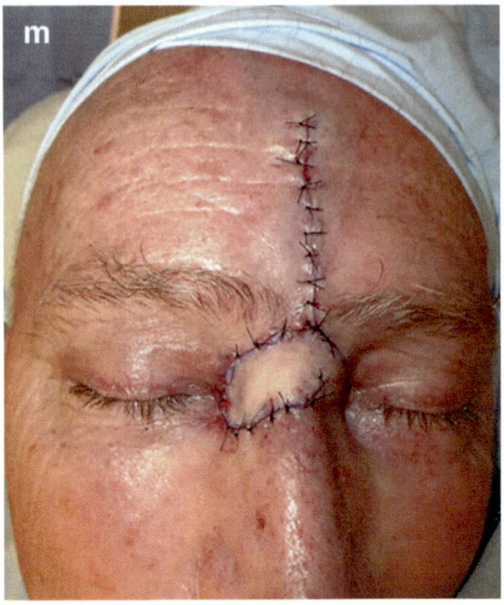

Fig. 8.7 (continued)

Full-Thickness Defects

Primary Closure (See Lower Eyelid)

Indications: Small defects.

Technique: The lesion is excised to leave a shield-shaped defect, with parallel sides towards the lid margin. The wound is closed in layers with sutures placed in the tarsal plate, avoiding going through the palpebral conjunctiva. The orbicularis oculi and skin layers are then closed.

Tips: Accurate approximation of the lid margin is essential to prevent notching and can be helped with vertical mattress sutures along the grey line. It is often helpful to place all the sutures in the tarsal plate, prior to tightening.

Primary Closure with Lateral Canthotomy and Cantholysis (See Lower Eyelid)

Indications: Medium defect.

Technique: The lesion is excised to leave a shield-shaped defect. A 1-cm incision is made through the skin and orbicularis muscle overlying the lateral canthus. The lateral canthus is next divided (Canthotomy) horizontally between the upper and lower limbs, up to the bony orbital rim. The upper lid is put under tension and the superior limb of the lateral canthus transected (cantholysis) vertically, till it is completely released from its lateral attachments. The primary defect is closed in layers as is the skin incision overlying the lateral canthus.

Tips: The position of the lateral canthus can be easily identified / felt by putting the lid margins under stretch. Completion of the cantholysis can be confirmed by medial displacement of the lid margins with forceps, while vertically transecting the canthal limb. Free movement of the lid margin is obtained, once the cantholysis is complete. There is often webbing in the lateral extremity of the lid margin at the site of cantholysis.

Cutler-Beard Flap

Indications: Large defects.

Technique: The upper lid defect is modified to obtain wound margins that are perpendicular to the lid margin. The upper eyelid wound defect is measured, following medial displacement of the wound edges with forceps. A horizontal incision, about 2 mm longer than the defect is made on the lower eyelid, 5 mm away from the lid margin. Two parallel vertical incisions are then made inferiorly from the extremities of the horizontal incision, up to the conjunctival fornix. These incisions are through the full thickness of the lower eyelid and care should be taken to avoid injury to the globe.

The flap is advanced beneath the lower eyelid bridge and suture into the upper eyelid defect in layers.

The second-stage release is carried out 6–8 weeks later. The flap is divided 2 mm below the anticipated upper lid margin. The conjunctiva along the cut margin is sutured to the skin margin. The remaining flap is returned to the lower eyelid and the wound margins freshened and sutured in layers (Fig. 8.8a–f, g–n).

Tips: The patient should be counselled appropriately about the two-stage procedure and "closure" of the eye during this period of time. A wider flap is designed to avoid tension during closure. In the second stage, a strip of orbicularis oculi muscle often has to be excised to permit conjunctival/skin approximation. Support for the upper eyelid can be provided in the form of a cartilage graft, as a third-stage procedure.

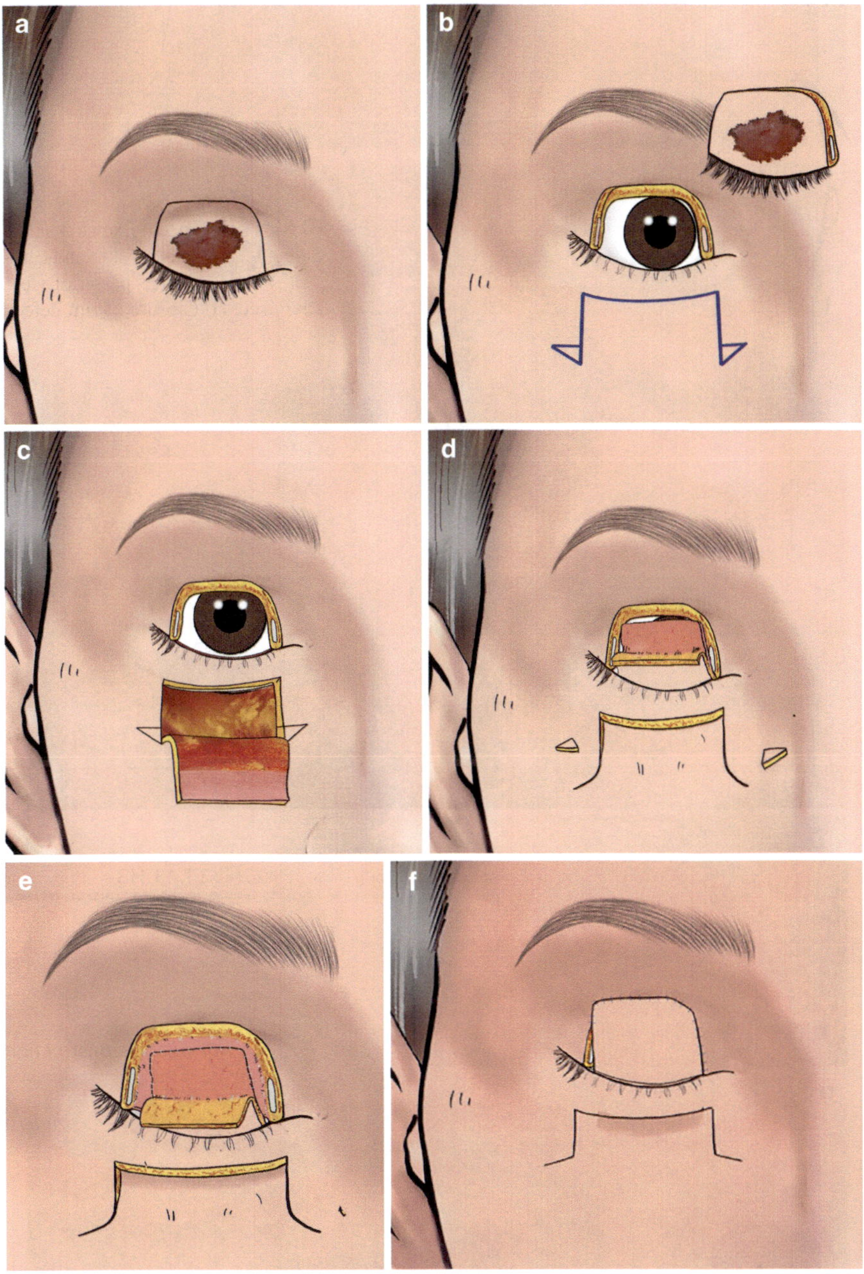

Fig. 8.8 Cutler beard flap. (**a**) Markings for excision, (**b**) Upper eyelid excision defect and markings for flap in lower eyelid, (**c**) Full thickness flap raised preserving lower lid margin, (**d**) Flap mobilised into defect, (**e**) Suturing of conjunctiva, (**f**) Suturing of skin margins, (**g**) Second stage division of lower eyelid pedicle, (**h**) Markings for excision and flap, (**i**) Excision defect and flap raised, (**j**) Flap advanced into upper eyelid defect, (**k**) Flap sutured into place, (**l**) External appearance prior to second stage division, (**m**) Internal appearance prior to second stage division, (**n**) Late apperance - eyes open, (**o**) Late appearance - eyes closed

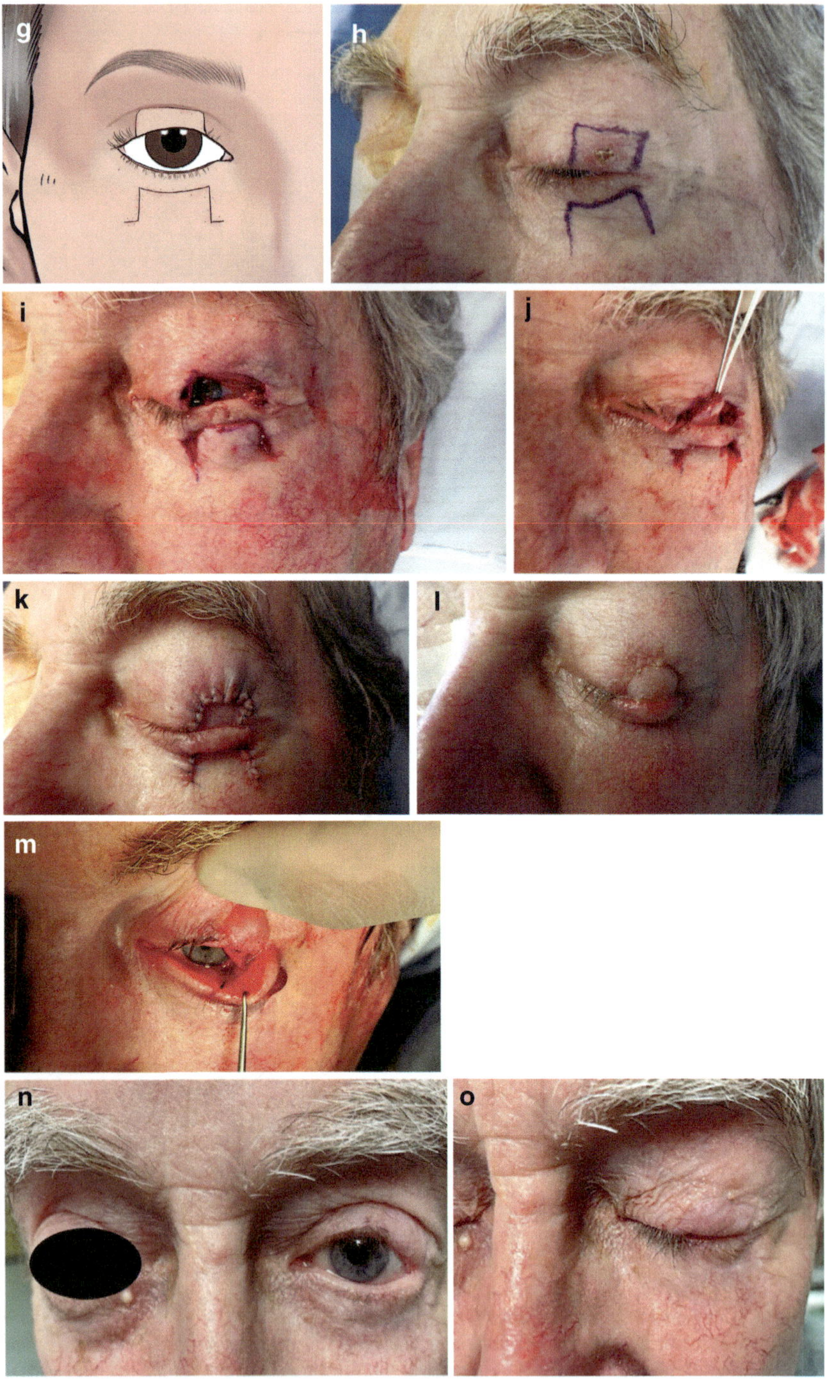

Fig. 8.8 (continued)

Lower Eyelid

Anterior Lamella Defects

Primary Closure

Indications: Small defects.

Technique: The defect is modified into an ellipse with a vertical orientation. The wound margins are undermined, and the defect is closed.

Tips: Tear-shaped excision with a broader superior margin can be undertaken. The inferior aspect is closed vertically and the superior margin horizontally to obtain a "T" shaped scar.

Tripier Flap

Indications: Medium/large defects.

Technique: It is an inferolaterally based transposition flap harvested from the upper eyelid. The margins of the defect are delineated, and the flap designed with its inferior medial margin lying along the lateral margin of the defect. A trial transfer is carried out to determine the length of the flap and should take into account loss of length due to rotation around the pivot point. The flap is raised as a skin only or musculocutaneous flap. The donor site defect is closed initially followed by insetting the flap into the defect (Fig. 8.9a–d, e–h, i–m).

Tips: The length to width ratio should not exceed 4:1 to maintain adequate vascularity. Adequate width should be incorporated in the flap to avoid the risk of ectropion. The amount of skin that can be safely harvested from the upper lid should be estimated by the "pinch" test. It can be designed as a bipedicle flap, with medial and lateral attachments.

Advancement Flap

Indications: Medium defects.

Technique: The defect is modified to obtain parallel wound margins. Incisions are made from the extremity of the defect, and the flap raised in the sub-muscular plane. The wound margins are undermined, and the defect is closed in layers (see Fig. 8.4).

Tips: The base of the flap can be made broader to maintain a satisfactory vascular pedicle. The flaps can be medially or laterally based and when based medially, should not extend beyond the confines of the eyelid skin.

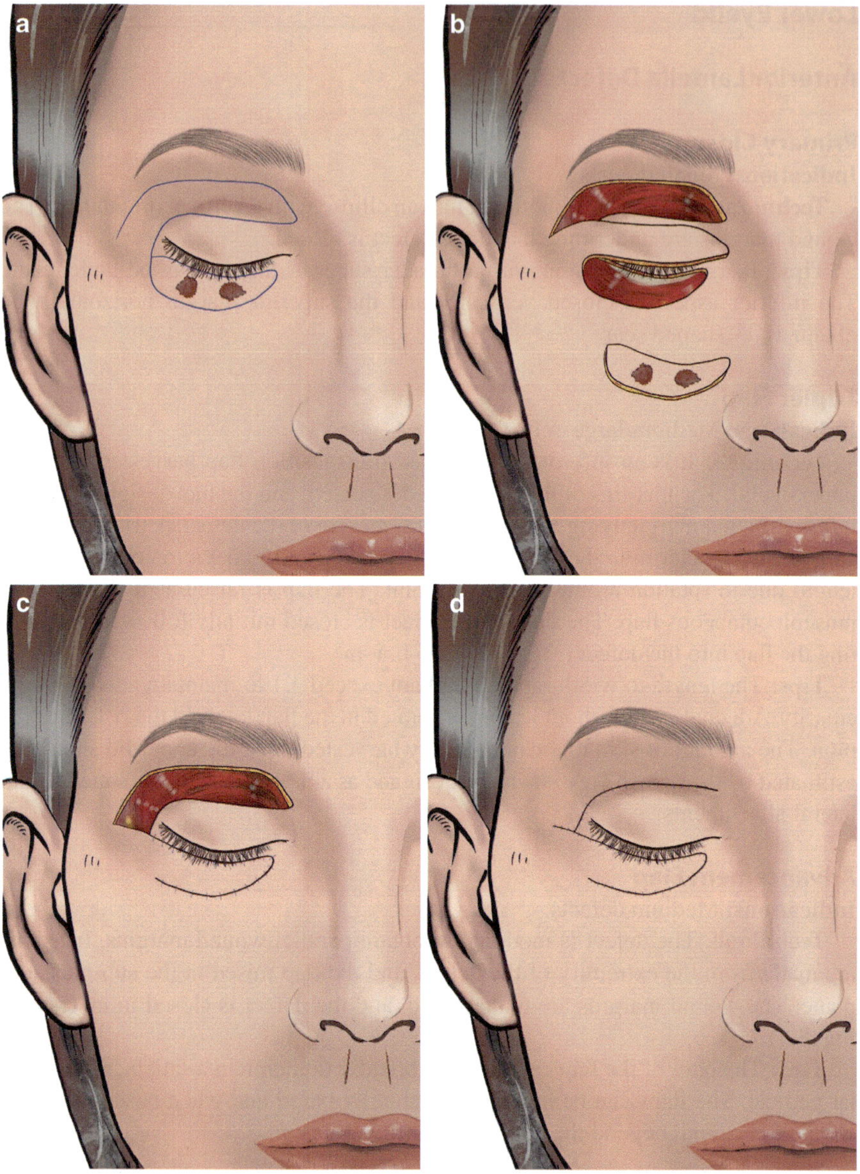

Fig. 8.9 Tripier flap. (**a**) Markings for excision and flap, (**b**) Excision defect and flap raised, (**c**) Flap transposed into defect, (**d**) Final closure, (**e**) Markings for excision and flap, (**f**) Excision defect, (**g**) Flap transposed into defect, (**h**) Final closure, (**i**) Markings for flap and lower eyelid release, (**j**) Lower eyelid defect, (**k**) Flap raised and transposed into defect, (**l**) Lateral canthopexy, (**m**) Final closure

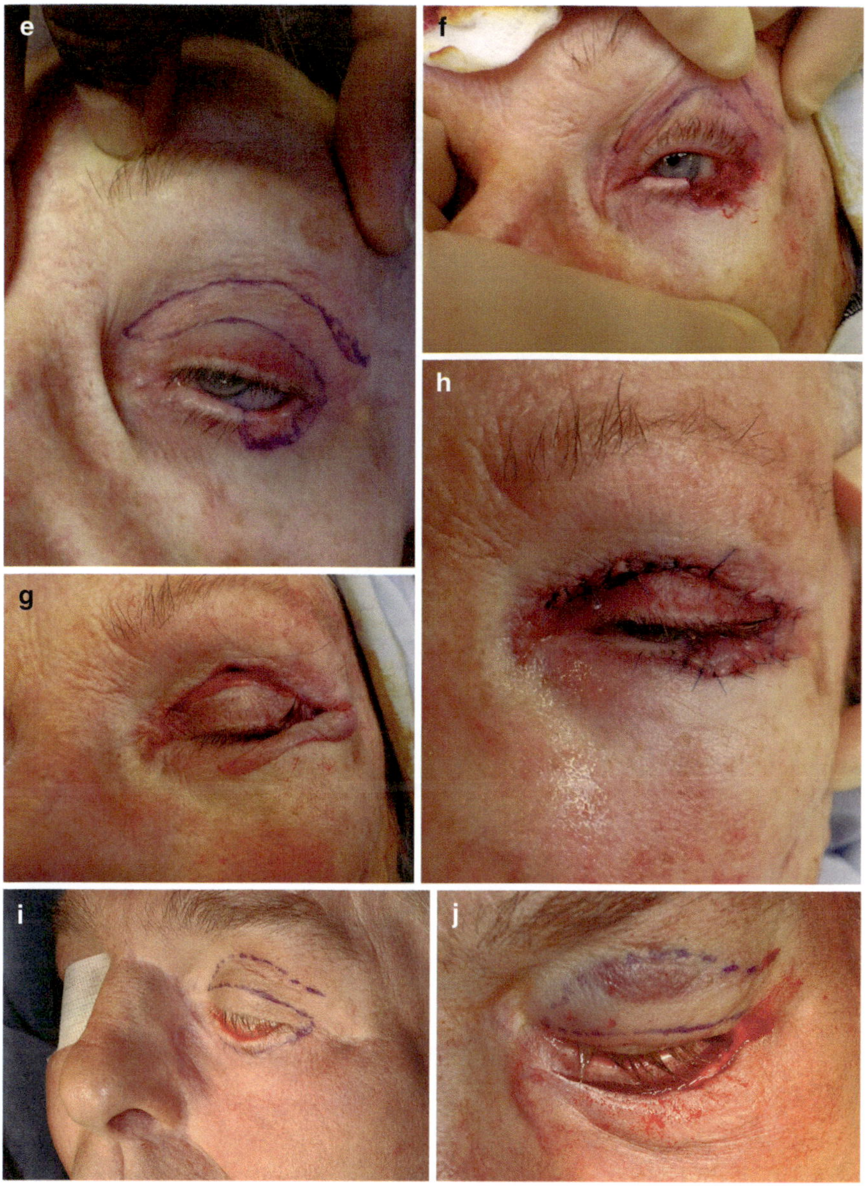

Fig. 8.9 (continued)

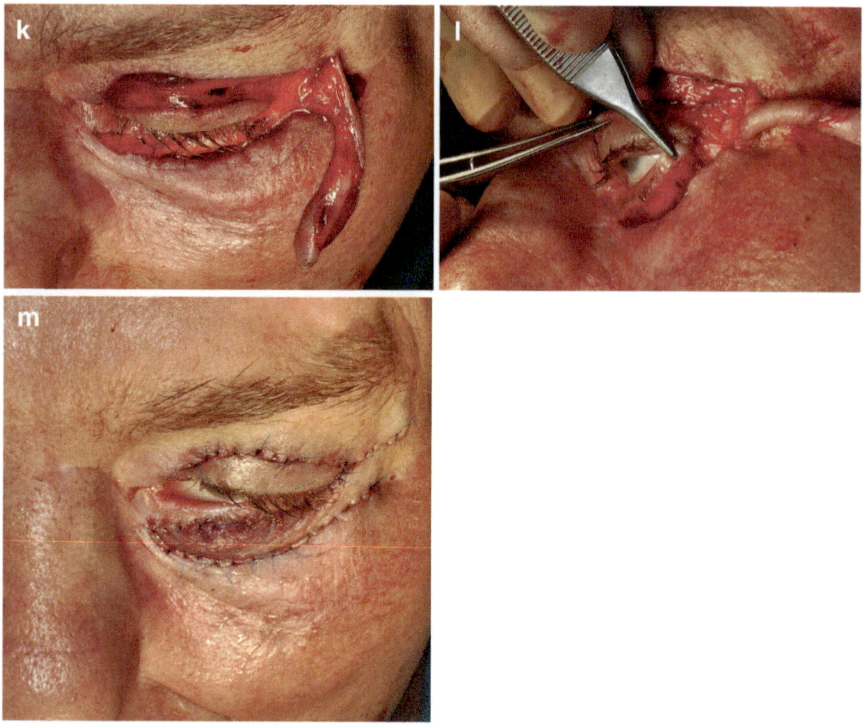

Fig. 8.9 (continued)

Rhombic Flap (Limberg Flap)

Indications: Medium defects. For defects that are rhomboid or can be converted into a rhombus. It offers the advantage of utilising the skin laxity adjacent to the lateral canthus.

Technique: Technically four flaps can be raised for any given defect, and the final decision is based on tissue laxity and orientation of the eventual scars. An incision is made by extending the short diagonal by a length equal to one side of the defect, and a further incision is made from its extremity parallel to the adjacent side of the defect, again of equal length. The incision and any undermining are best carried out in the subcutaneous plane in an attempt to avoid damage to branch of the facial nerve. The wound is closed in layers (Fig. 8.10a, b).

Tips: The amount of skin available in the adjacent area can be assessed using the "pinch test". With a rhomboid flap, some but not all the scars can be placed along the skin creases. It is often easier to close the secondary defect first followed by the primary defect. In the case of circular defects, it is not always necessary to remove additional tissue to convert the defect into a rhomboid.

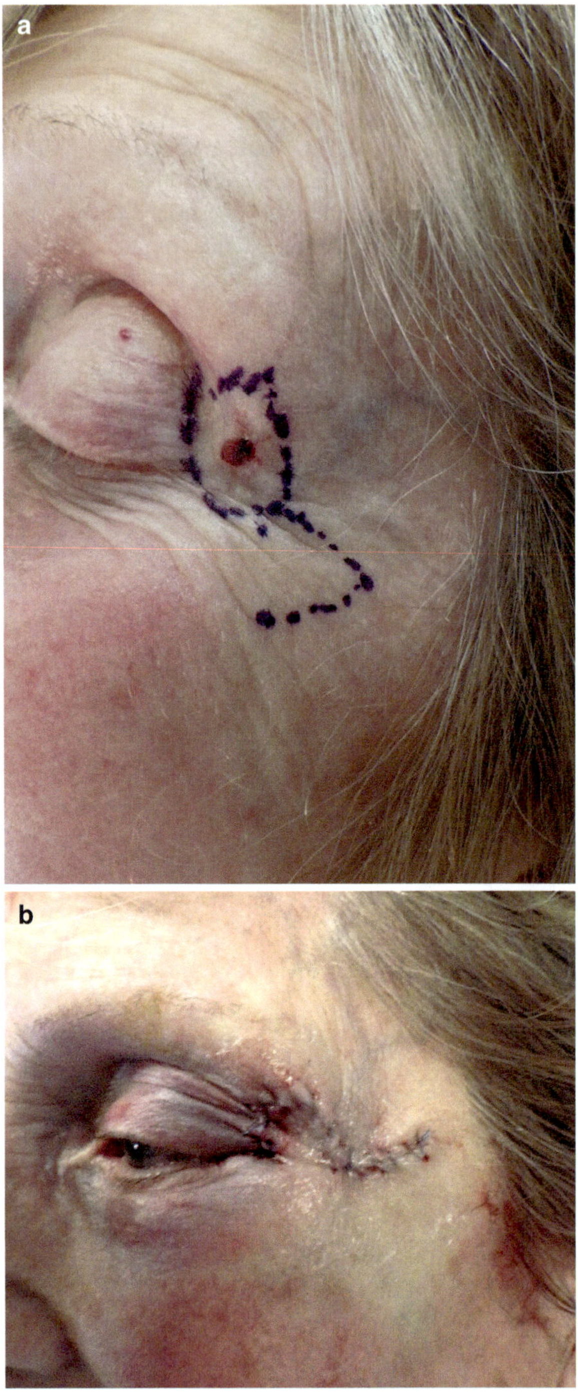

Fig. 8.10 Rhombic flap. (**a**) Markings for excision and flap (**b**) Final closure

Full-Thickness Defects

Primary Closure

Indications: Small defects.

Technique: The lesion is excised to leave a shield-shaped defect, with parallel sides towards the lid margin. The wound is closed in layers with sutures placed in the tarsal plate avoiding going through the palpebral conjunctiva. The orbicularis oculi and skin layers are then closed (Fig. 8.11a–c).

Tips: Accurate approximation of the lid margin is essential to prevent notching and can be helped with vertical mattress sutures along the grey line. It is often helpful to place all the sutures in the tarsal plate, prior to tightening.

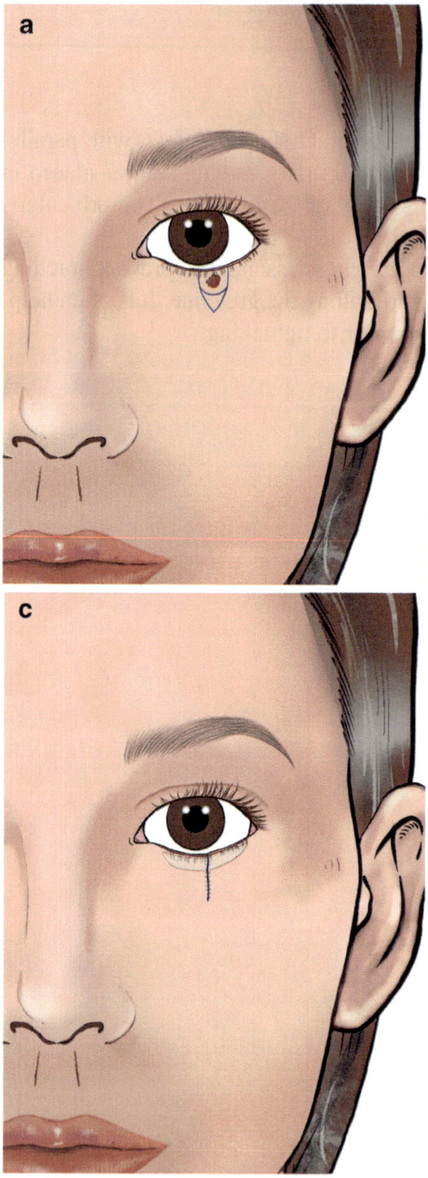

Fig. 8.11 Shield excision and primary closure. (**a**) Markings for excision, (**b**) Excision defect, (**c**) Final closure

Primary Closure with Lateral Canthotomy and Inferior Cantholysis

Indications: Medium defect.

Technique: The lesion is excised to leave a shield-shaped defect. A 1-cm incision is made through the skin and orbicularis muscle overlying the lateral canthus. The lateral canthus is next divided (Canthotomy) horizontally between the upper and lower limbs, up to the bony orbital rim. The lower lid is put under tension, and the inferior limb of the lateral canthus is transected (cantholysis) vertically, till it is completely released from its lateral attachments. The wound is closed in layers with sutures placed in the tarsal plate, avoiding going through the palpebral conjunctiva. The orbicularis oculi and skin layers are then closed, including the defect at the lateral canthus (Fig. 8.12a–e, f–m*). (*skin marking for a McGregor flap—not utilised).

Tips: An attempt made to approximate the wound edges after excision and if there is tension, one should proceed to a canthotomy/cantholysis. The position of the lateral canthus can be easily identified/felt by putting the lid margins under stretch. Completion of the cantholysis can be confirmed by medial displacement of the lid margins with forceps, while vertically transecting the canthal limb. Free movement of the lid margin is obtained, once the cantholysis is complete. There is often webbing in the lateral extremity of the lid margin at the site of cantholysis.

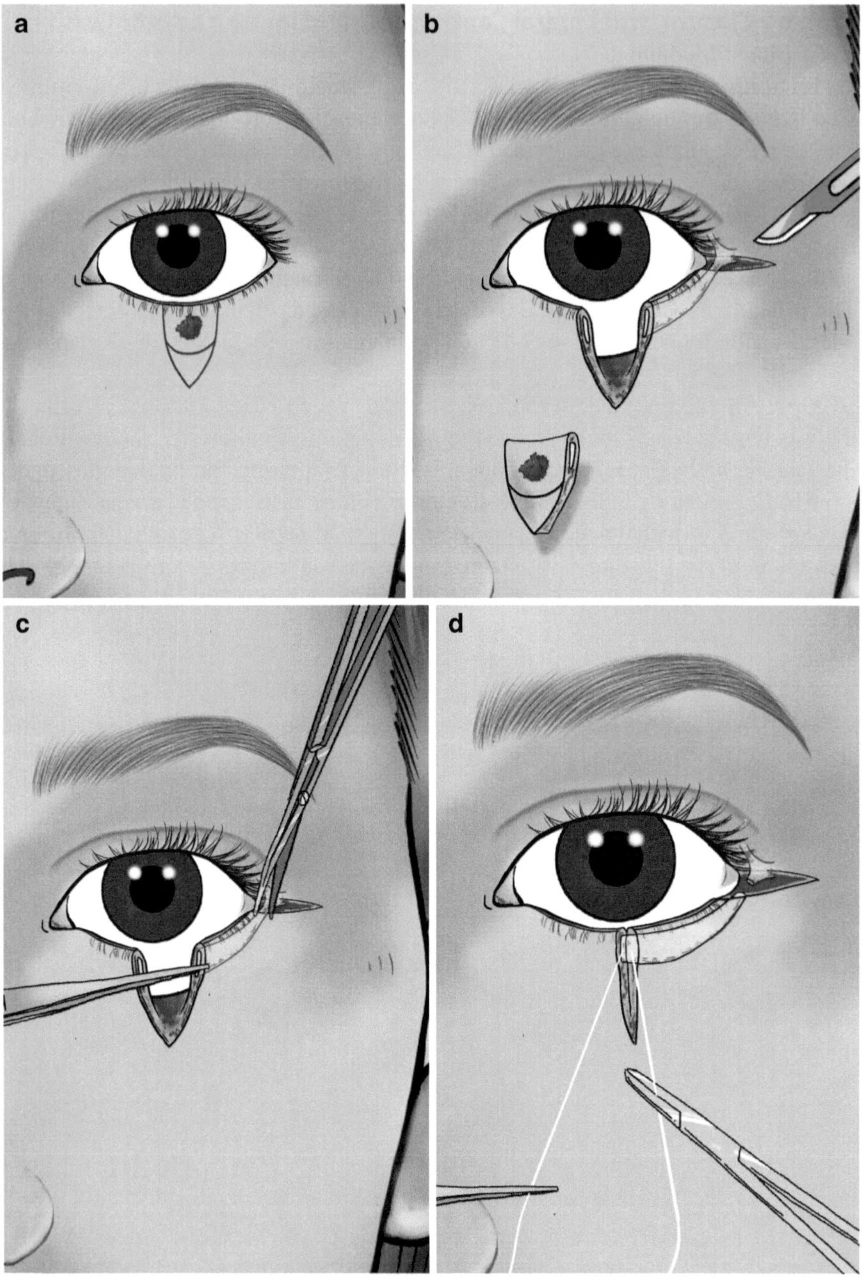

Fig. 8.12 Primary closure with lateral canthotomy and inferior cantholysis. (**a**) Markings for excision, (**b**) Excision defect and lateral canthotomy, (**c**) Inferior cantholysis, (**d**) Suturing of tarsal plate, (**e**) Final closure, (**f**) Lesion lower eyelid margin, (**g**) Markings for excision, (**h**) Markings for excision - eye open, (**i**) Excision defect, (**j**) Excision defect conjunctiva, (**k**) Lateral canthotomy and inferior cantholysis, (**l**) Additional mobility of eyelid following canthal release, (**m**) Final closure

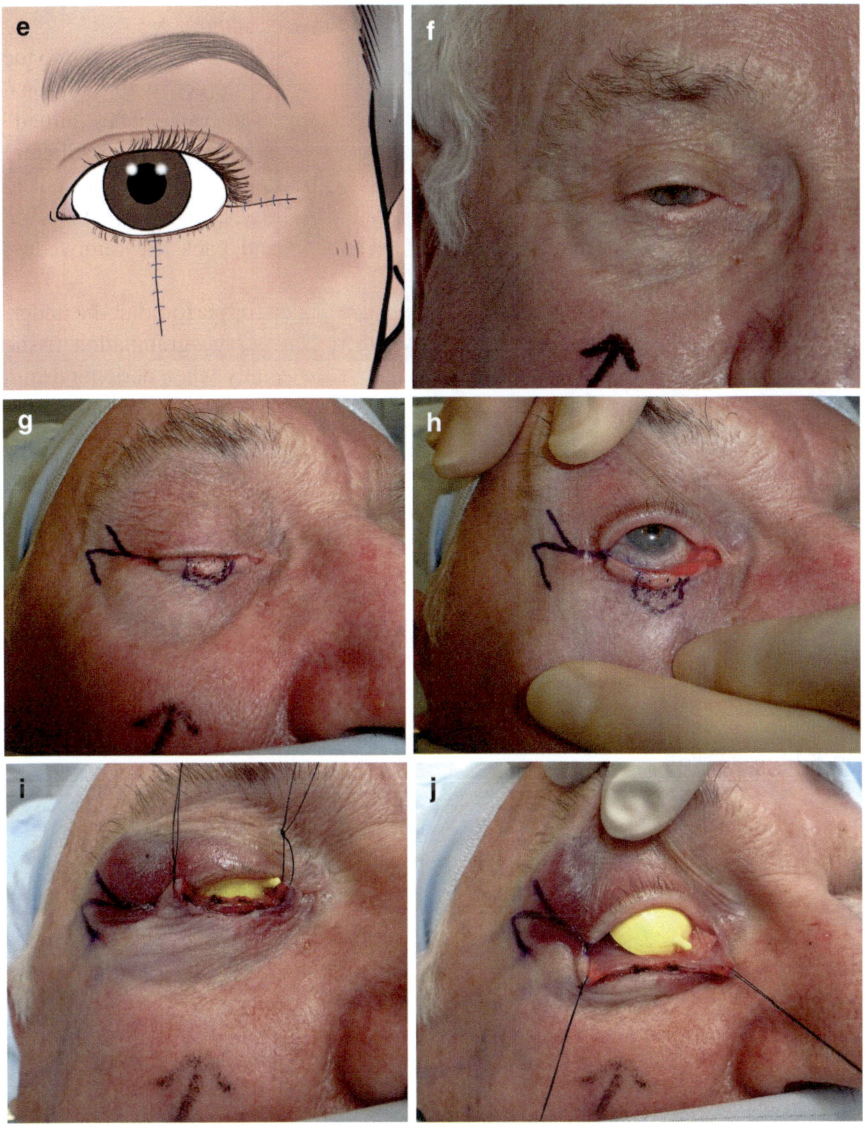

Fig. 8.12 (continued)

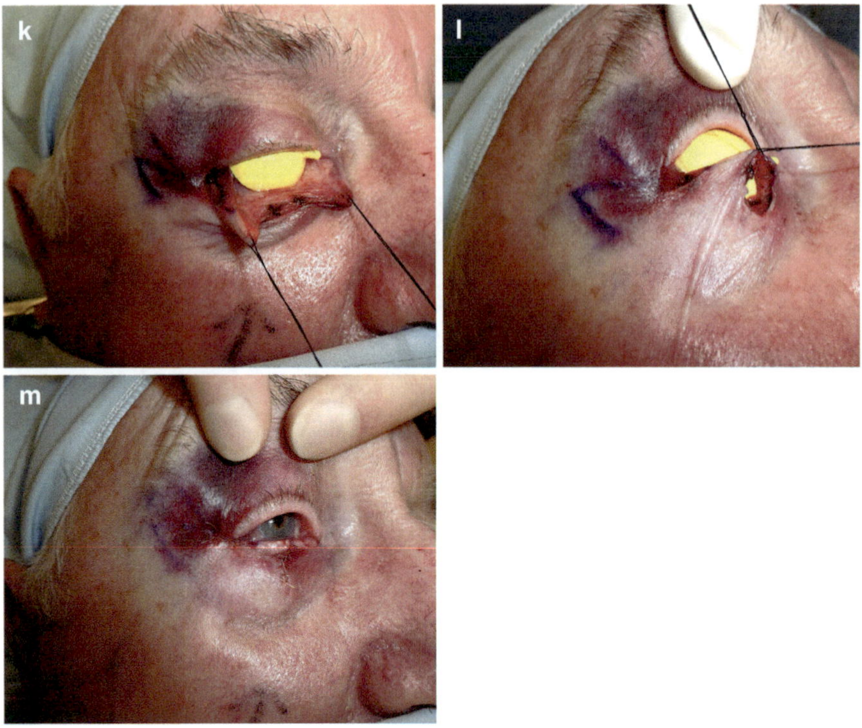

Fig. 8.12 (continued)

McGregor Flap

Indications: Medium/large defects.

Technique: The lesion is excised as a "V". An incision is made laterally from the lateral canthus into the pre-auricular region, following the upward curve of the lower eyelid margin. A further incision is made inferiorly from the lateral extremity of this incision, parallel to the lateral limb of the "V" shaped defect. A "Z" plasty is incorporated superiorly along the same lateral extension.

The lateral flap is raised in the subcutaneous plane and more medially, deep to the orbicularis oculi. A lateral canthotomy and inferior cantholysis are then performed to obtain the required mobilisation of the lower eyelid. The primary defect is closed in layers, and the skin/muscle layer approximated to the conjunctiva in the area of the lateral canthotomy. The secondary defect in the pre-auricular region is closed by a "Z" plasty (Fig. 8.13a–e, see also Fig. 10.7i–l).

Tips: The lateral extension along the curve of the lower eyelid margin and the additional "Z" plasty helps decrease the risk of ectropion, as the associated scar contracture is predominantly in a lateral and upward vector. For large flaps, anchoring sutures can be placed in the region of the zygomatic prominence for additional support. In the case of a full-thickness defect, the posterior lamella is reconstructed with a chondro-mucosal or palatal graft.

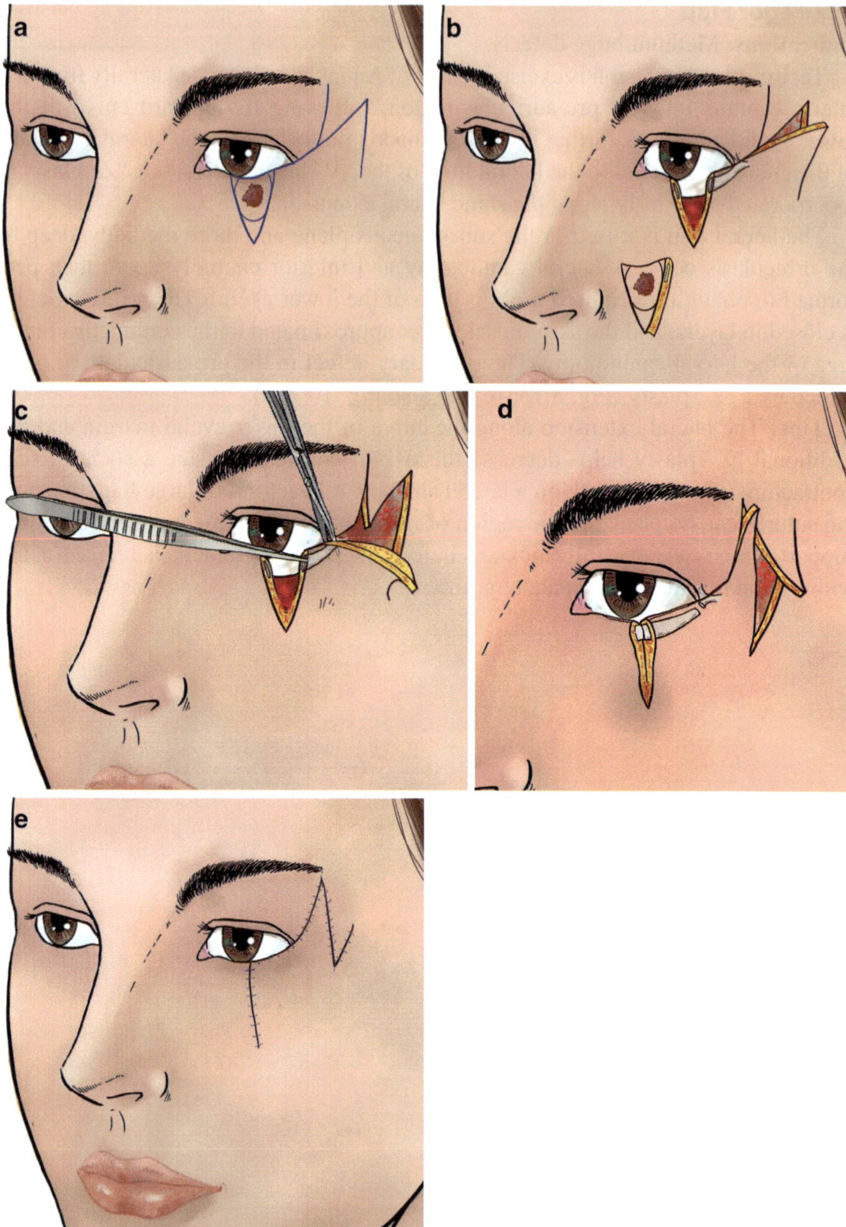

Fig. 8.13 Macgregor flap. (**a**) Markings for excision and flap, (**b**) Excision defect and flap raised, (**c**) Lateral canthotomy and inferior cantholysis, (**d**) Flap mobilsied into defect and "Z" plasty of lateral extension, (**e**) Final closure

Mustardé Flap

Indications: Large defects.

Technique: The defect is modified into a "V" with a vertical medial limb and a more oblique lateral limb. A curvilinear incision is made from the lateral canthus region, following the upward curve of the lower eyelid, up to the pinna and inferiorly along the pre-auricular skin crease. The flap is raised laterally in a subcutaneous plane and medially deep to the orbicularis oculi muscle. The flap is mobilised into the defect and sutured in layers (Fig. 8.14a–c, d–h, see also Fig. 10.7a–h).

Tips: The oblique lateral limb of the "V" along with the upward curve of the flap enables additional height to be created to the lower lid and decreases the risk of ectropion. Anchoring sutures should be placed in the region of the zygomatic prominence for additional support and prevent inferior decent of the flap. Drains are placed as necessary. Care should be taken to avoid damage to the branches of the facial nerve. Tension during wound closure and a thin flap can increase the risk of flap necrosis. In the case of a full-thickness defect, the posterior lamella is reconstructed with a chondro-mucosal or palatal graft.

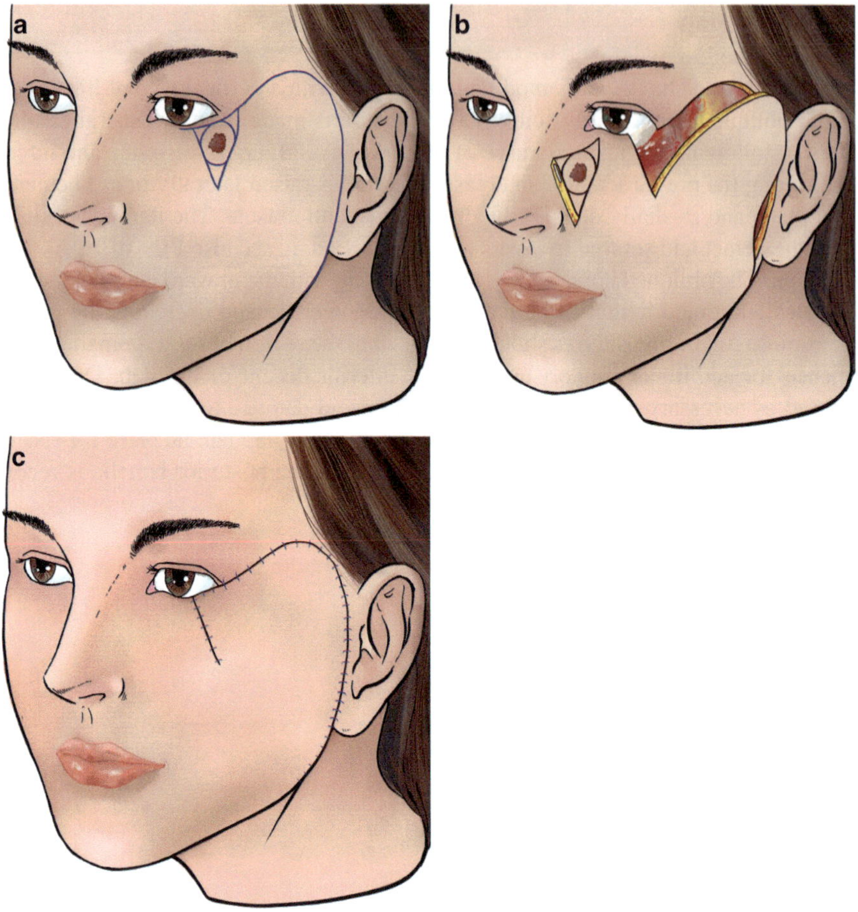

Fig. 8.14 Mustard'e flap. (**a**) Markings for excision and flap, (**b**) Excision defect and flap raised, (**c**) Final closure

Tenzel Flap

Indications: Medium defects (lower/upper eyelid).

Technique: The defect is modified to obtain perpendicular wound edges to the lid margin. A semi-circular incision is made from the lateral canthus, extending upwards to the eyebrow and terminating at the level of the lateral canthus. A musculo-cutaneous flap is raised on the deep surface of the orbicularis oculi. A lateral canthotomy and cantholysis carried out if there is any remaining eyelid, lateral to the defect. The wound is closed in layers with sutures placed in the tarsal plate, avoiding going through the palpebral conjunctiva. The orbicularis oculi and skin layers are then closed (Fig. 8.15a–g).

If there is no remaining eyelid lateral to the defect, a medially based periosteal flap is raised, from the lateral orbital rim to reconstruct the posterior lamella. The periosteal flap is sutured to the cut edge of the tarsal plate in the medial wound edge (Fig. 8.15d–f). The mobilised flap is sutured in layers.

Tips: An exaggerated upward extension of the Tenzel flap is preferable to avoid the risk of ectropion. The width of the flap is designed to be within the lateral orbital rim for best scars. The periosteal flap is designed to be at least 10 mm in width and raised with a superior inclination to follow the upper ward slant of the upper eyelid. This also helps decrease the risk of ectropion.

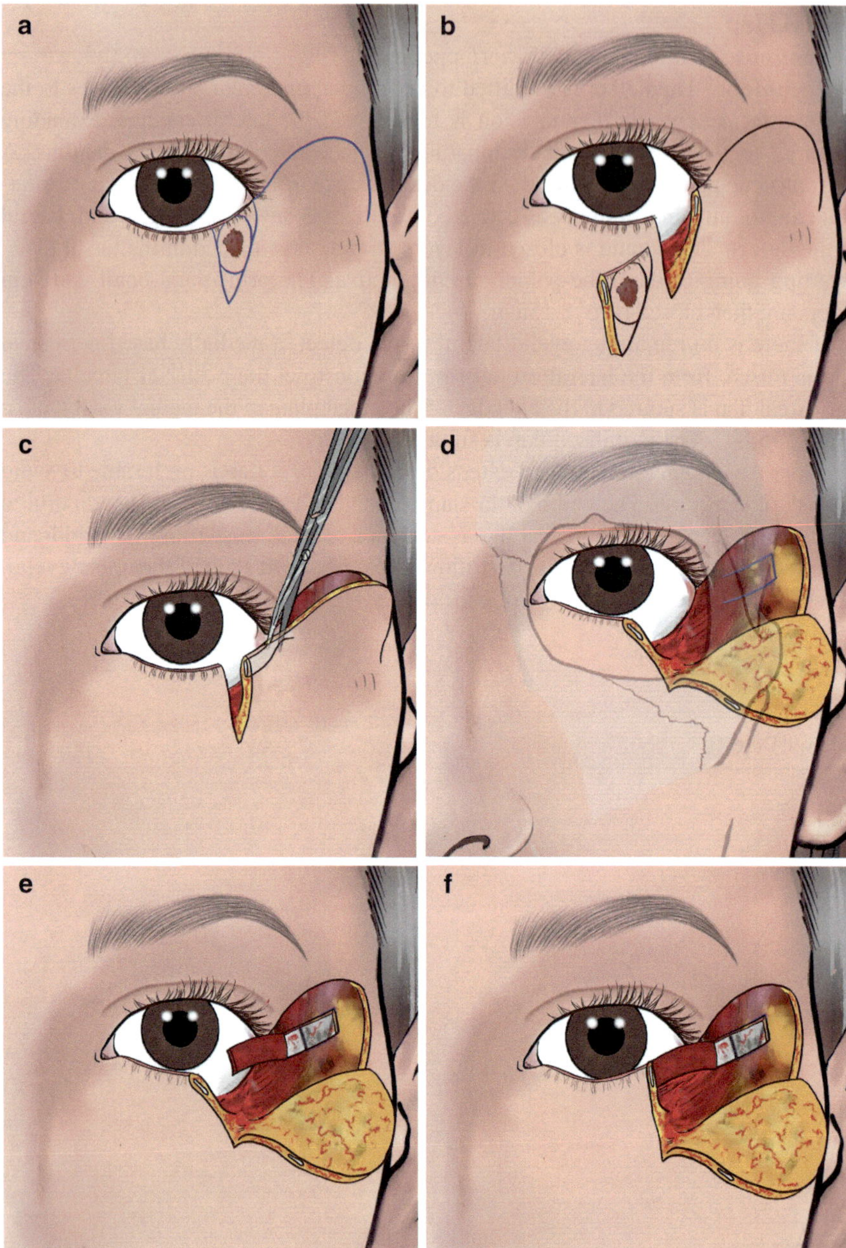

Fig. 8.15 Tenzel flap. (**a**) Markings for excision and flap, (**b**) Excision defect, (**c**) Flap raised and lateral canthotomy and inferior cantholysis, (**d**) Periosteal strip marked for lateral tarsal reconstruction, (**e**) Periosteal strip raised, (**f**) Periosteal strip sutured into place, (**g**) Final closure

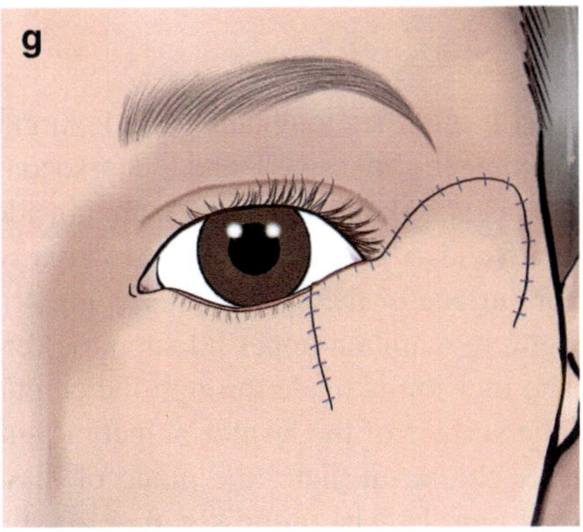

Fig. 8.15 (continued)

Hughes Flap

Indications: Large defects.

Technique: The defect is modified to obtain wound margins that are perpendicular to the lid margin. The defect is measured, and the tarsoconjunctival flap from the upper eyelid designed to be marginally shorter to maintain adequate tension following closure. The upper eyelid is everted with Desmarres retractors and the flap marked on the posterior surface of the eyelid, preserving 4 mm of the tarsal plate adjacent to the lid margin, to maintain upper lid support. Vertical marking is made from its extremities. The incision is made through the conjunctiva and tarsal plate and the flap raised on the surface of the levator palpebrae superioris, which is preserved. Superiorly, above the tarsal plate, the plane of dissection is between the conjunctiva and Muller's muscle. The mobilised flap is sutured into the lower lid defect in layers, with particular attention paid to approximation of the tarsal plates. The anterior lamella is reconstructed with a musculo-cutaneous advancement flap (Fig. 8.16a–g, i–o).

The second stage is performed about 4 weeks later. The flap is divided about 2 mm above the intended lower lid margin. The new lower lid margin is freshened, and the conjunctiva sutured to the skin margin (Fig. 8.16h). The remaining flap is sectioned at its attachment to the upper lid, and the defect left to continue to heal by secondary intention.

Tips: The patient should be counselled appropriately about the two-stage procedure and "closure" of the eye during this period of time. Periosteal flaps will have to be considered if there is no remaining lower lid at the extremities of the defect (See Fig. 8.15d–f). Skin graft can be used to reconstruct the anterior lamella.

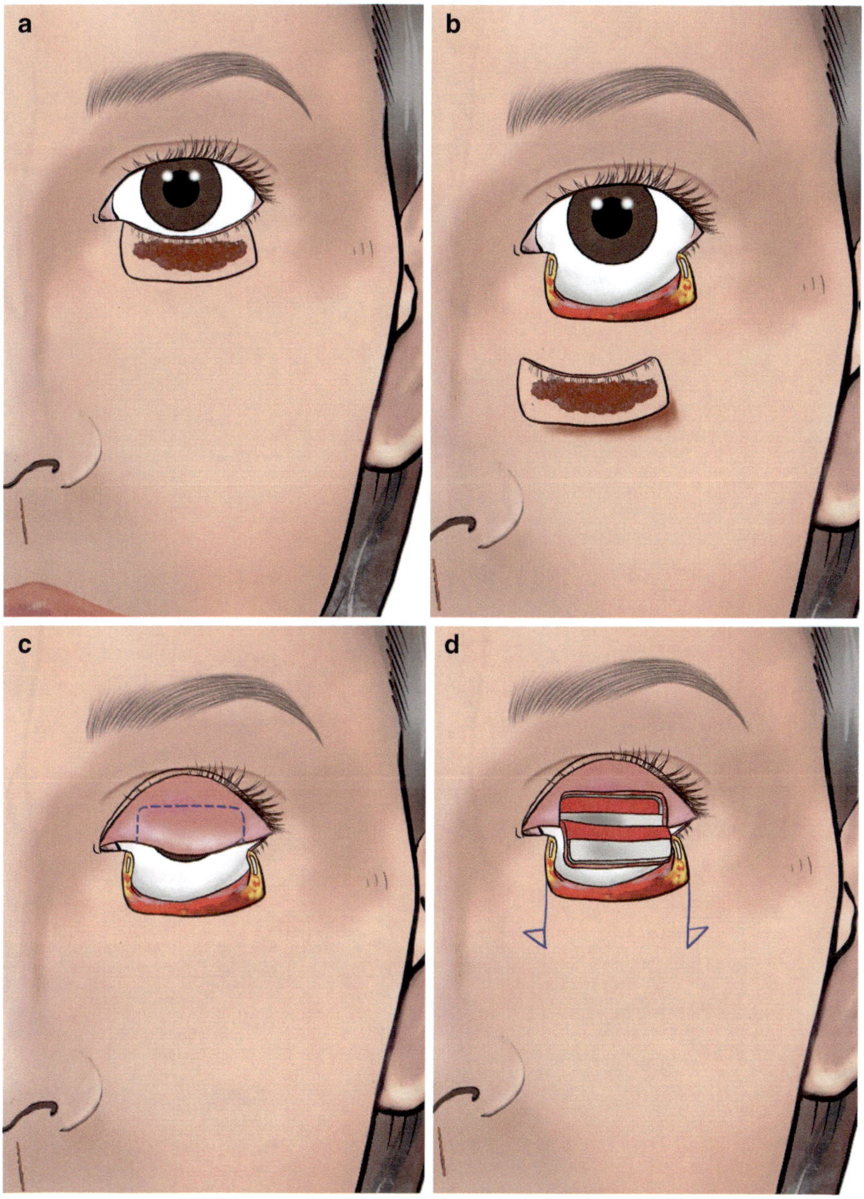

Fig. 8.16 Hughes flap. (**a**) Markings for excision, (**b**) Excision defect, (**c**) Markings for tarsoconjunctival flap in upper eyelid, (**d**) Flap transposed into lower eyelid defect to reconstruct posterior lamella defect, (**e**) Skin advancement flap to reconstruct anterior lamella defect, (**f**) Tarsoconjunctival flap sutured in situ, (**g**) Skin closure with intact upper eyelid pedicle, (**h**) Final result after second stage division of pedicle, (**i**) Markings for excison and lateral transposition flap, (**j**) Excision defect, (**k**) Upper eyelid tarsoconjunctival flap sutured insitu, (**l**) Lateral transposition flap sutured in situ, (**m**) Early post operative appearance of first stage procedure, (**n**) Appearance after second stage division - eyes open, (**o**) Appearance after second stage division- eyes closed

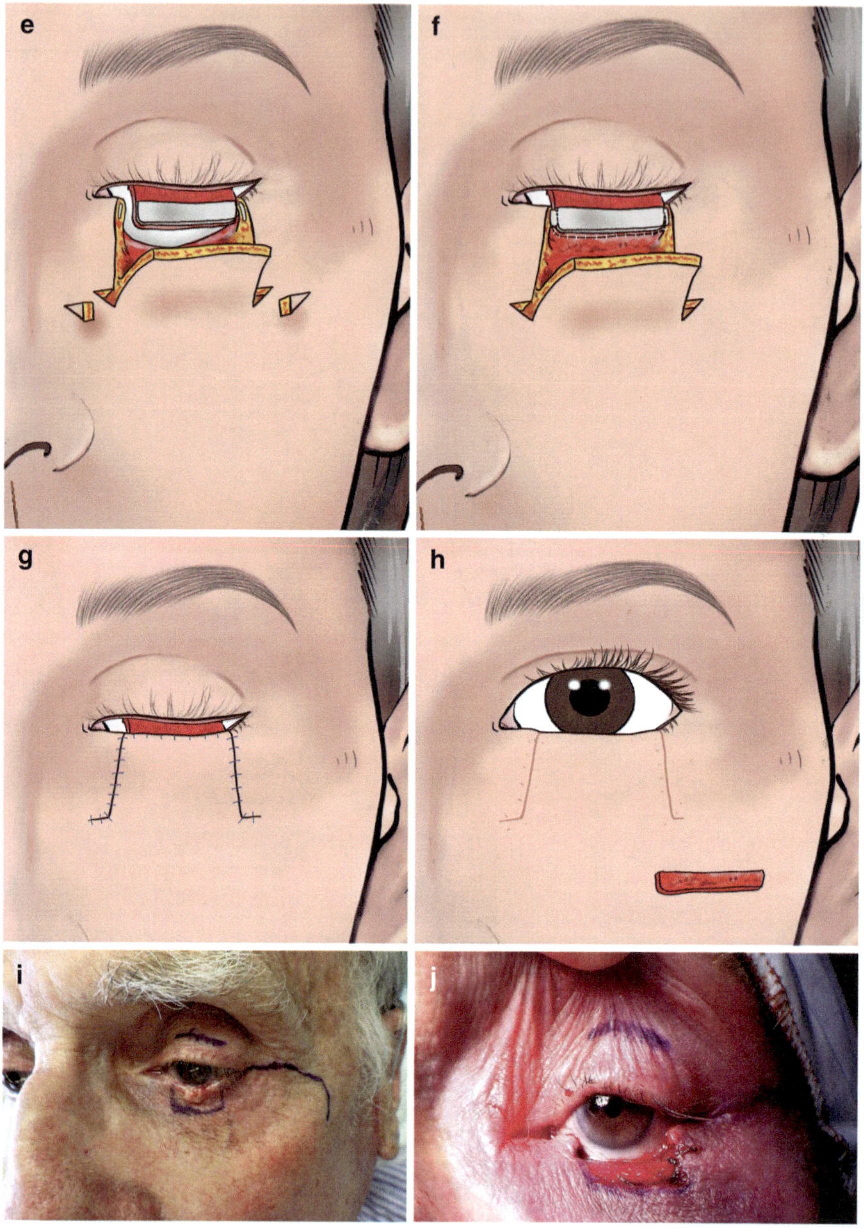

Fig. 8.16 (continued)

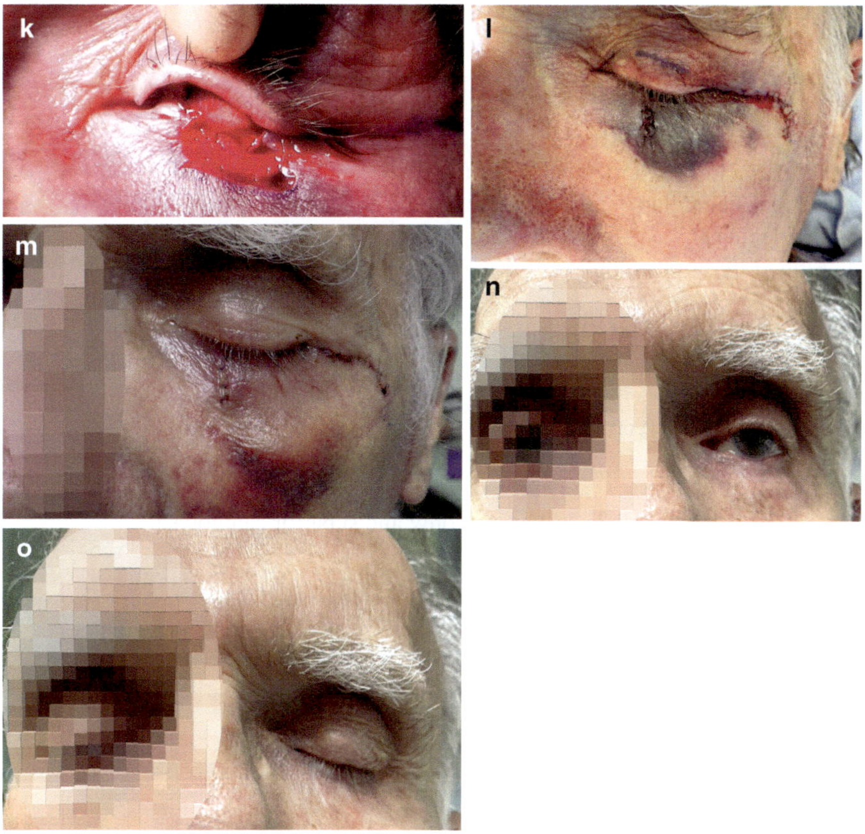

Fig. 8.16 (continued)

Suggested Algorithm

Upper Eyelid

Anterior Lamellar Defects

1. Primary closure (horizontal/vertical)
2. Advancement flap
3. Fricke flap
4. Skin graft

Full-thickness Defects

Small

1. Primary closure (vertical)

Medium

1. Primary closure with lateral canthotomy and superior cantholysis
2. Tenzel flap

Large

1. Cutler beard flap

Medial Canthus

1. Healing be secondary intention
2. Glabella transposition flap
3. Glabella island flap
4. Skin graft

Lower Eyelid

Anterior Lamella Defects

Small

1. Primary closure (vertical)
2. Tear drop

Medium

1. Advancement flap
2. Tripier flap
3. Rotation/transposition flap

Large

1. McGregor flap
2. Mustarde' flap

Full-Thickness Defects

Small

1. Primary closure

Medium

1. Primary closure with lateral canthotomy and inferior cantholysis
2. Tenzel flap

Large Defects

1. Hughes flap
2. McGregor flap
3. Mustarde' flap

Auricular Reconstruction

9

Subunits and Anatomical Considerations

The pinna is a structure made up of a complex three-dimensional cartilaginous framework and draped by skin on the lateral and medial aspects. The underlying elastic cartilage principally determines the shape of the ear. The skin on the *anterior* aspect is firmly adherent to the underlying cartilage and reveals the contours of the underlying cartilage, with minimal subcutaneous tissue. The skin of the *posterior* aspect is more loosely attached and contains more subcutaneous tissue.

The pinna lies between horizontal lines drawn from the superior orbital rim and the nasal spine. It protrudes from the scalp at an angle of 25°–35°.

The skin on the lateral surface is thin and densely adherent to the underlying cartilage, whereas the posterior skin in thick and more mobile. The auricular cartilage is supple and can be easily deformed by wound tension and scar contracture. Scars can be camouflaged in the many undulations of the pinna. Local flap reconstruction often results in a decreased height of the pinna, but when the shape is maintained, is surprisingly inconspicuous.

V. Ilankovan et al., *Local Flaps in Facial Reconstruction*,
https://doi.org/10.1007/978-3-031-49464-2_9

The goal of reconstruction is to try and preserve the shape, size and position of the pinna. Knowledge of the different parts of the pinna is essential for reconstruction (Fig. 9.1). When it comes to reconstructing auricular defects, it is more practical to analyse it in terms of (1) location, (2) extent and (3) composition of the defect.

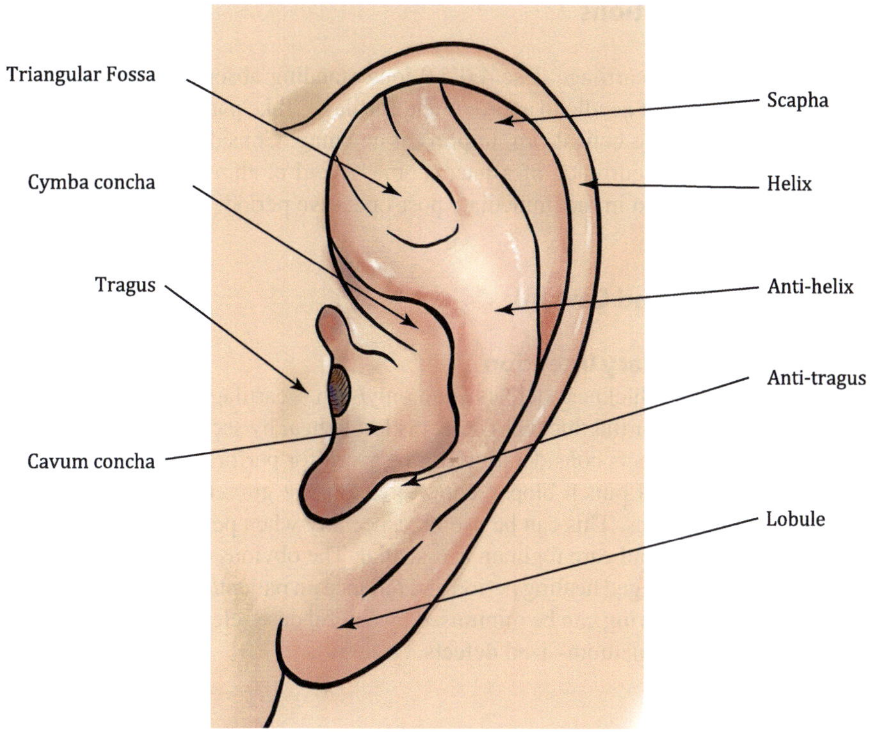

Fig. 9.1 Anatomical landmarks

Special Considerations

Care when handling cartilage. Use 4.0/5.0 long standing absorbable sutures, on a round bodied/tapercut needle to approximate cartilage. Take particular care to accurately approximate the helical rim, to prevent notching. Consider a pressure dressing to prevent the occurrence of a haematoma. Avoid clothing which need to be removed over the head in the immediate post-operative period.

Concha (Cymba and Cavum)

Healing by Secondary Intention

Indications: Partial thickness defects (skin only/skin + cartilage).

Technique: The partial thickness defect is left to heal by secondary intention. In case of skin only defects consideration can be given for perforating the underlying cartilage with a small punch biopsy core, to encourage granulation tissue ingress from the medial tissues. This can be useful, especially when perichondrium is lost.

Tips: A good wound care regimen is essential. The obvious disadvantage of this approach is the prolonged healing period and reliance on patient/career co-operation. Distortion due to scarring can be minimised by careful case selection and restricting its use to small- and medium-sized defects.

Skin Grafts

Indications: Partial thickness defects (skin only/skin + cartilage).

Technique: A suitable template is made of the defect, which is transferred to the donar site to harvest the graft. The graft is sutured to the defect, with additional "long" sutures that can be used for "tying" over the bolus. The graft can be "quilted" to the base, to decrease the risk of haematoma and dead space. A non-adherent dressing is laid over the sutured graft, over which a cotton wool ball/sponge soaked in proflavin or a suitable antibiotic ointment is paced. The tie-over bolus sutures are now used to hold the dressing in place. The sutures and pack are removed in 7–10 days time (Fig. 9.2a–d).

Tips: For skin only defects, consideration can be given for perforating the underlying cartilage with a small punch biopsy core, to encourage granulation tissue ingress from the medial tissues. This can be useful, especially when perichondrium is lost. Full-thickness grafts are preferred to split skin grafts.

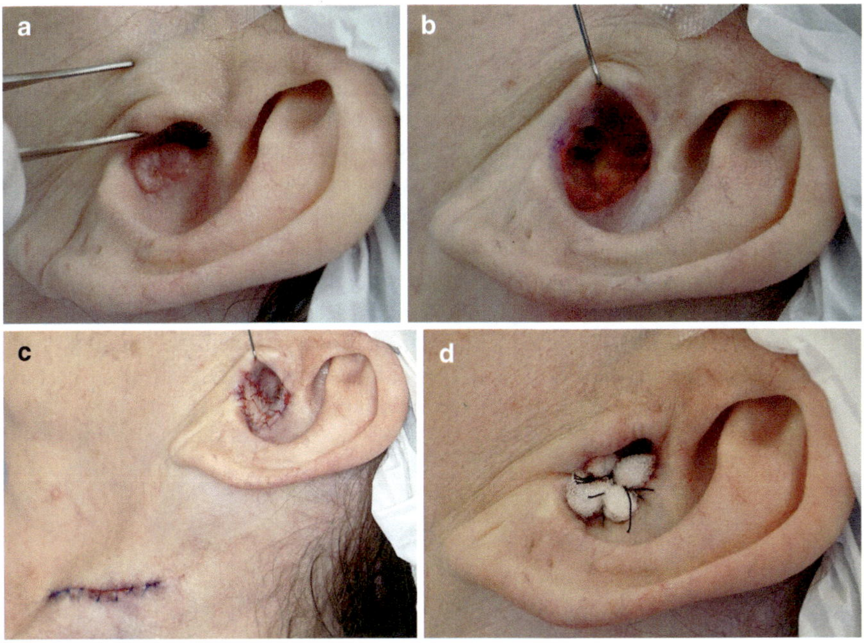

Fig. 9.2 Excision and skin graft. (**a**) Lesion concha, (**b**) Excision defect, (**c**) Skin graft and donar site sutured, (**d**) Tie over bolus dressing in situ

Revolving Door Flap

Indications: Medium and large skin + cartilage defects and posterior skin intact.

Technique: A template is made to accurately reflect the defect and the dimensions marked out in the posterior auricular surface/mastoid skin, with the base centred along the auriculocephalic sulcus. Skin is circumferentially incised and undermined anteriorly and posteriorly, taking meticulous care to maintain a central subcutaneous pedicle, along the auriculocephalic sulcus. The flap is pulled through the defect, like a revolving door and sutured into the defect. The secondary defect is closed primarily by undermining the surrounding tissues (Fig. 9.3a–j, k–s).

Tips: The anterior margin of the flap in the posterior auricular surface is marked out to overlap the underlying cartilage defect. The pinna will be "pinned" back when the secondary defect is closed. This can interfere with the fit of an existing hearing aid and would have to be discussed with the patient.

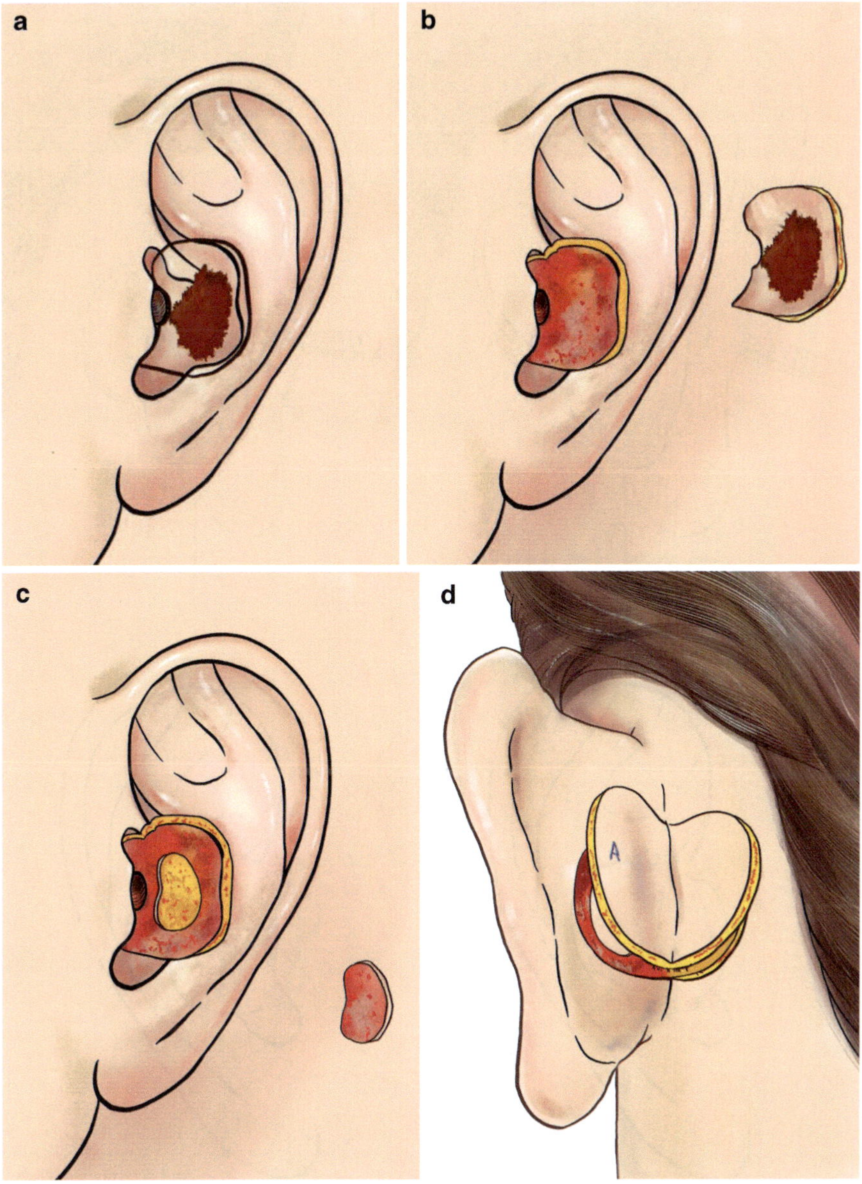

Fig. 9.3 Revolving door/flip-flop flap. (**a**) Markings for excision, (**b**) Excision defect, (cartilage intact), (**c**) Excision defect after removal of cartilage, (**d**) Flap incision with intact pedicle along auriculocephalic sulcus, (**e**) Anterior edge pulled through into defect, (**f**) Posterior edge pulled through into defect, (**g**) flap transferred into conchal defect, (**h**) Flap sutured into place, (**i**) Closure of posterior donar site, (**j**) Final closure, (**k**) Markings of excision, (**l**) Excision defect, (skin/cartilage), (**m**) Flap markings, (**n**) Anterior margin of flap raised, (**o**) Posterior margin raised maintaining pedicle along auriculocephalic sulcus, (**p**) Flap transfered into conchal defect, (**q**) Flap sutured in place, (**r**) Donar defect and auriculocephalic pedicle, (**s**) Final closure

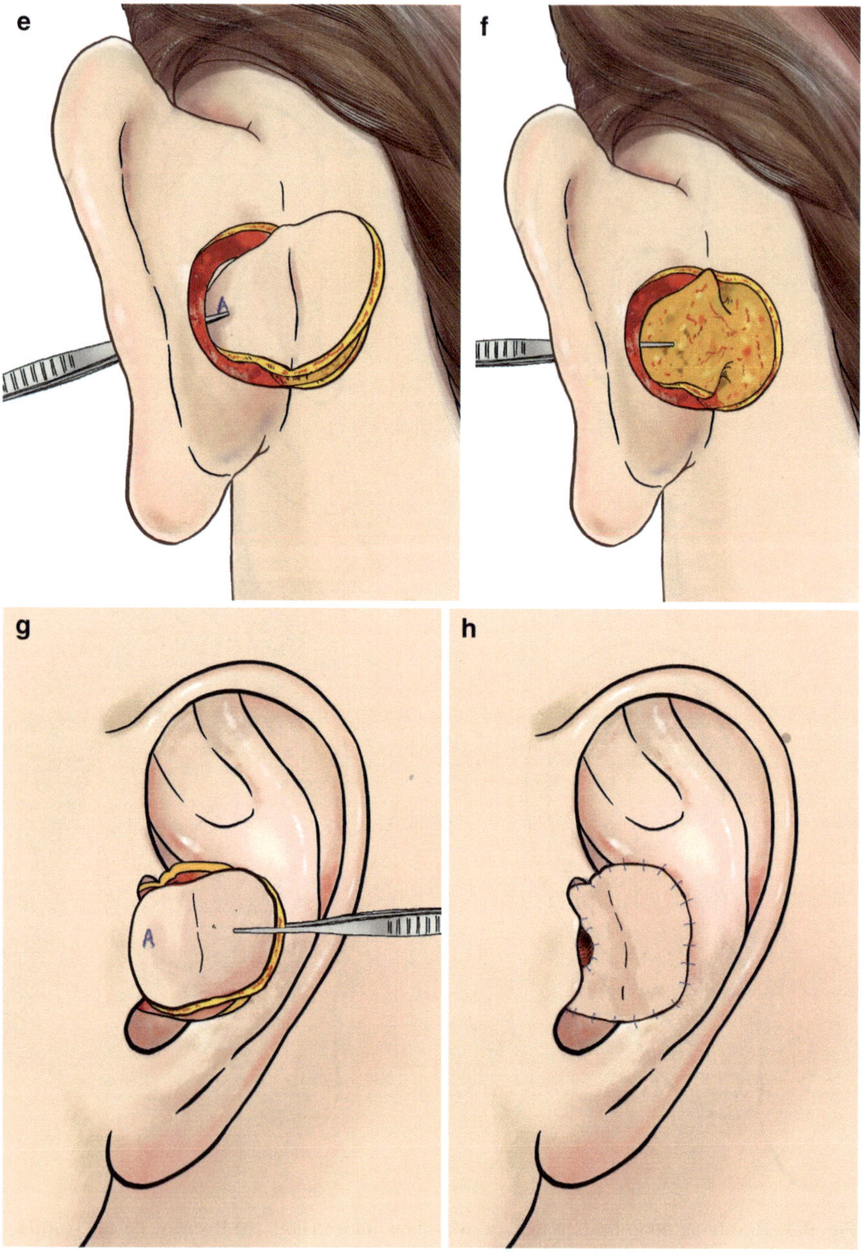

Fig. 9.3 (continued)

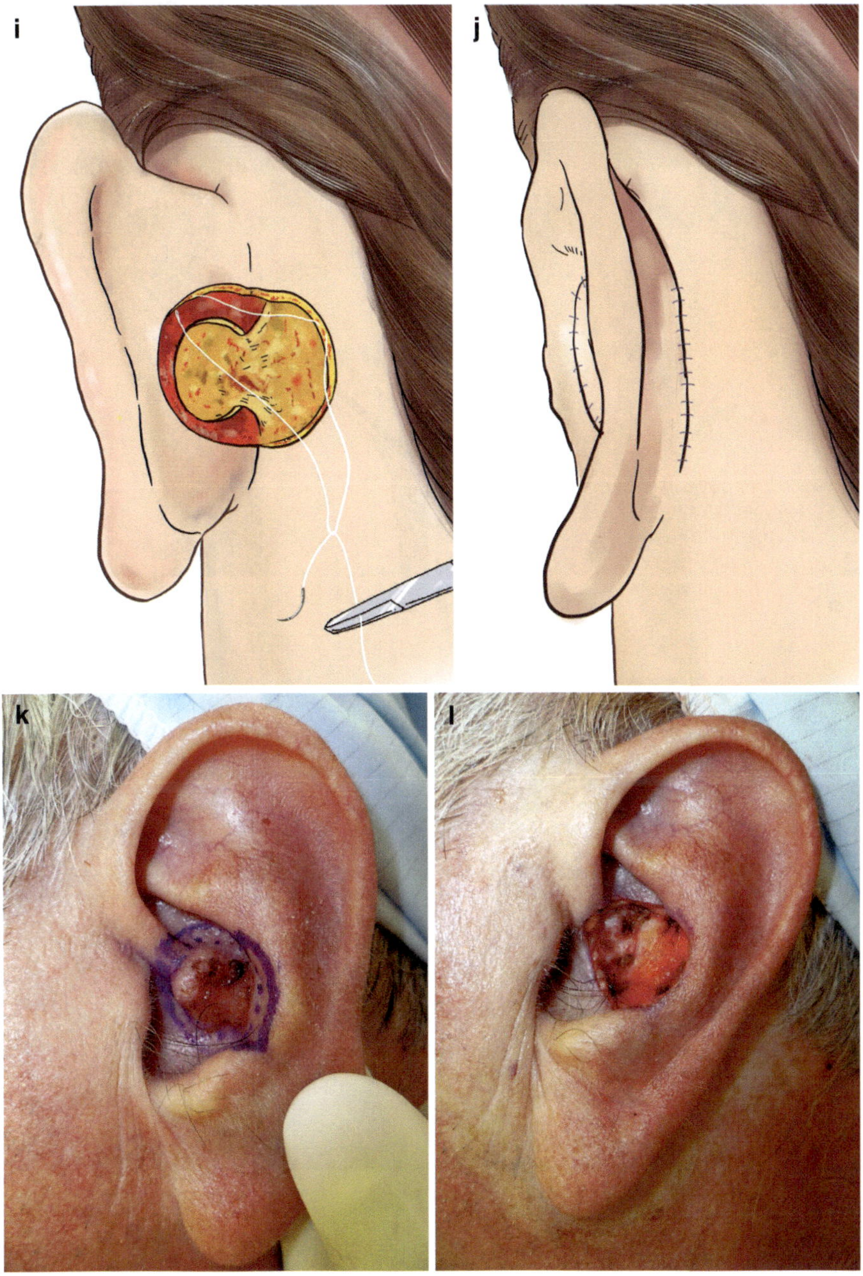

Fig. 9.3 (continued)

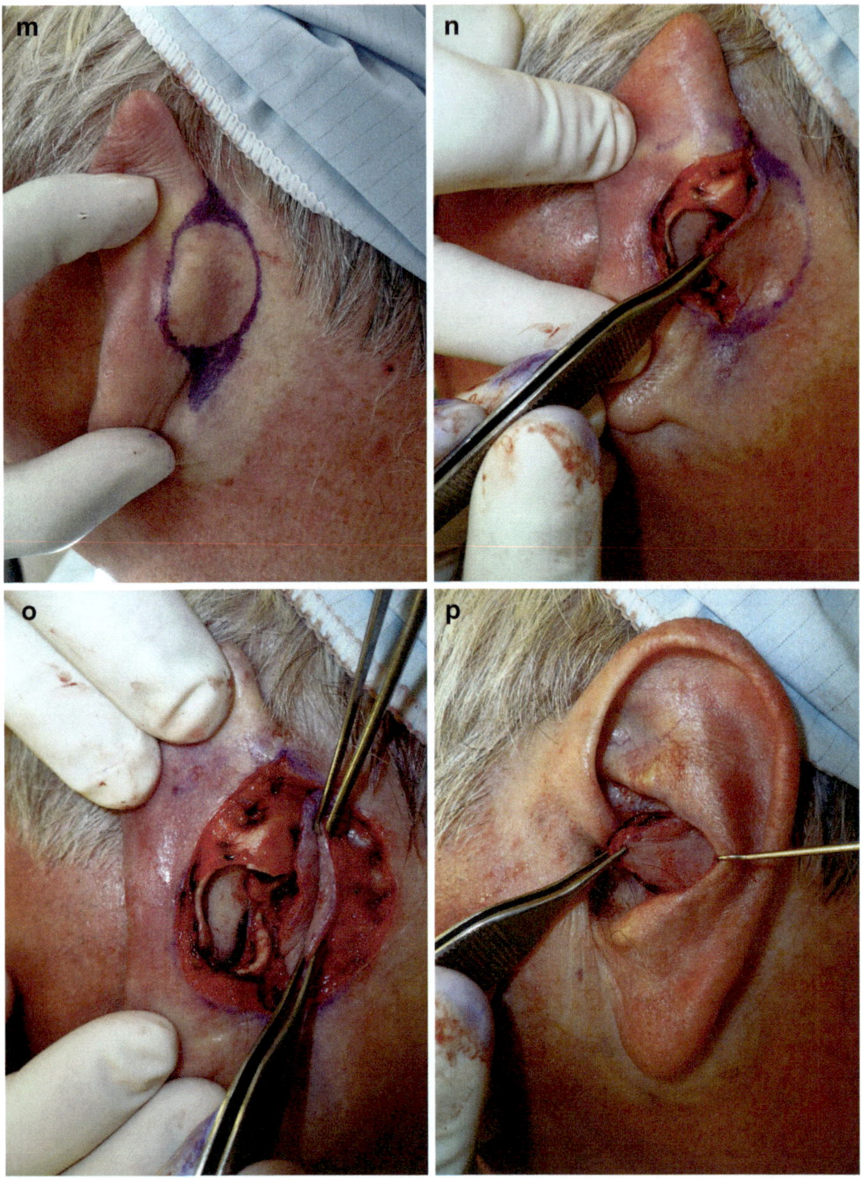

Fig. 9.3 (continued)

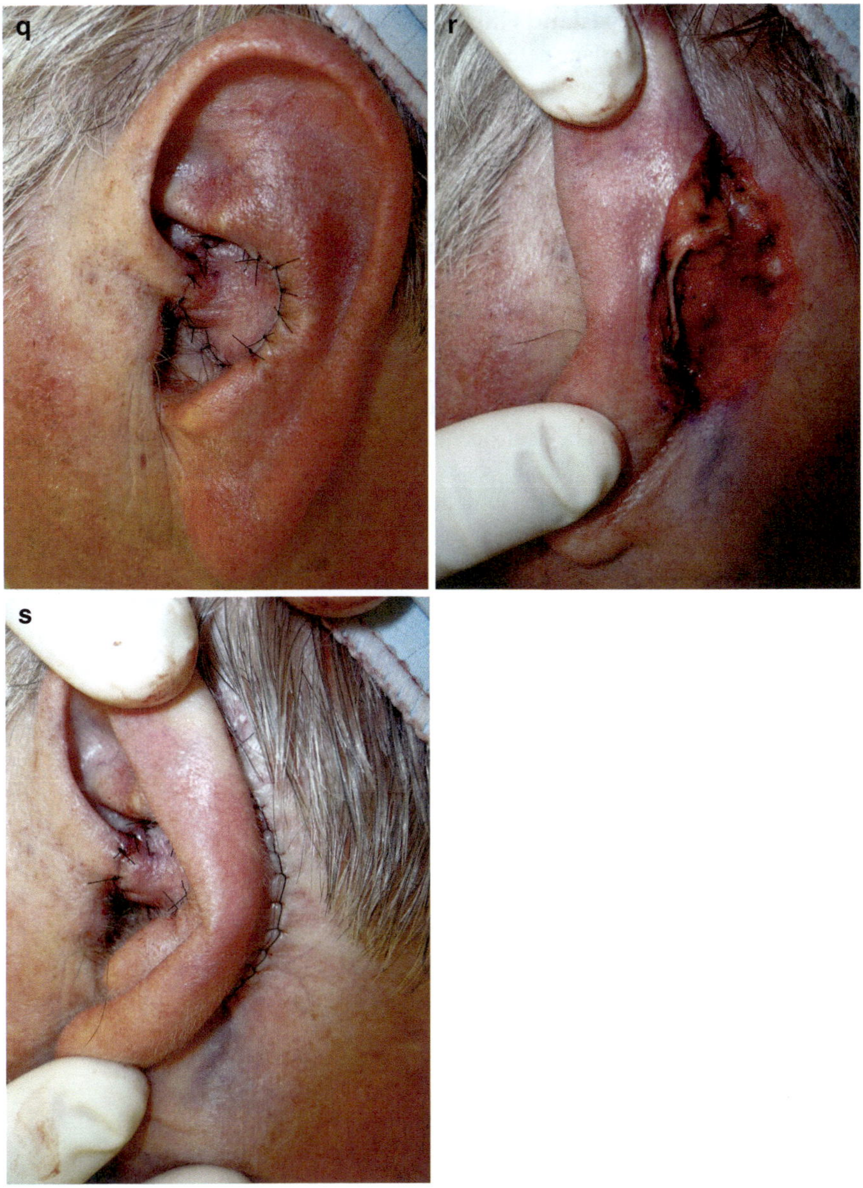

Fig. 9.3 (continued)

Post-Auricular Artery Island Flap

Indications: Skin + cartilage defects and posterior skin intact.

Technique: An accurate template is made of the defect and the dimensions marked on the posterior auricular surface/mastoid skin. The flap is incised laterally, superiorly and medially down to the periosteum, but only through the skin inferiorly, to maintain the vascular pedicle. Inferiorly the skin is raised in the subcutaneous plane and the island flap elevated deep to the vascular pedicle (post-auricular artery/post-auricular muscle), on the surface of the periosteum. The required mobility is obtained by undermining the flap inferiorly around the pedicle. A tunnel is created from the anterior margin of the flap into the defect. The flap is mobilised into the defect and sutured into place. The secondary defect is closed primarily by undermining the surrounding tissues (Fig. 9.4a–f).

Tips: Care should be taken to avoid damage to the pedicle during dissection and transfer. The tunnel should be of an adequate dimension to avoid compression of the pedicle. The pinna will be "pinned" back when the secondary defect is closed. This can interfere with the fit of an existing hearing aid and would have to be discussed with the patient.

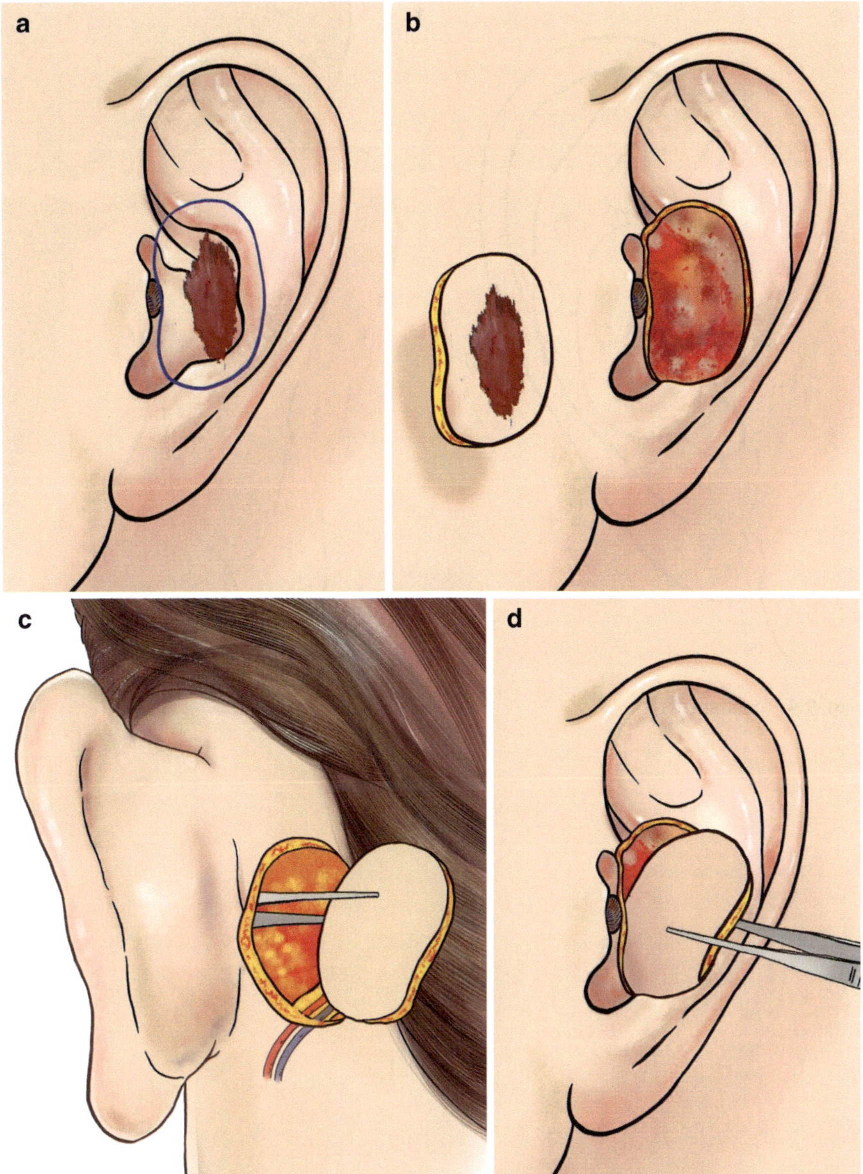

Fig. 9.4 Post auricular artery island flap. (**a**) Markings for excision, (**b**) Excision defect, (**c**) Falp raised on subcutaneous post auricular artery pedicle, (**d**) Flap transposed into defect, (**e**) Flap sutured into defect, (**f**) Closure of donar site

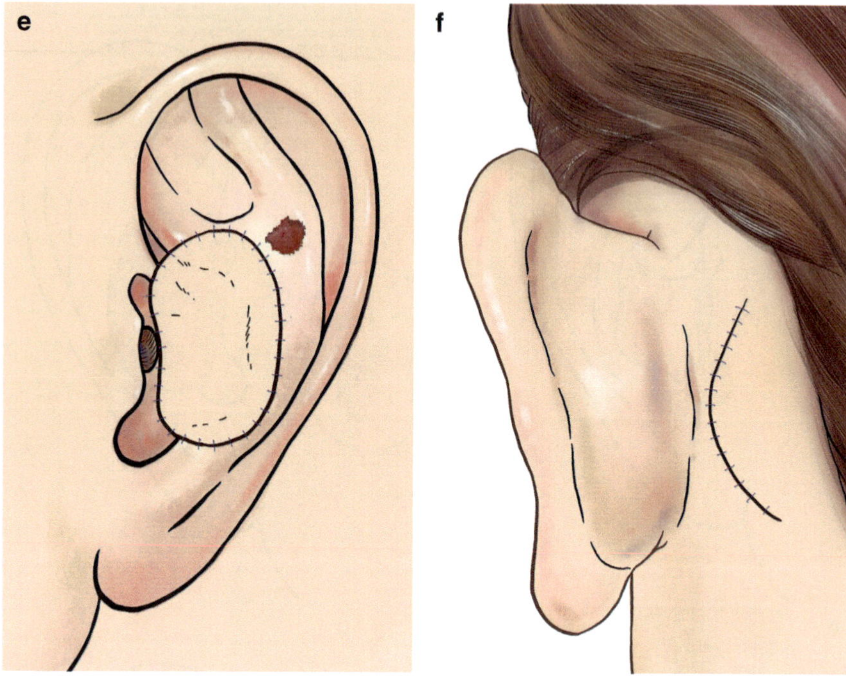

Fig. 9.4 (continued)

Post-Auricular Transposition Flap

Indications: Skin + cartilage defect and posterior skin intact.

Technique: A template is made to accurately reflect the defect, and the dimensions marked out in the posterior auricular/mastoid skin. The flap can be raised on a superior or inferiorly based pedicle, consisting of skin, subcutaneous tissue and post-auricular muscle (demonstration superiorly based flap). The margins of the flap are incised down to periosteum and the flap raised in the supra-periosteal plane. The flap is tunnelled anteriorly through to the conchal defect and sutured into place. The section of the flap passing through the tunnel can be de-epithelialised, in case of a one-stage reconstruction. Alternatively, the flap pedicle is left intact can be divided after 3 weeks as a two-stage procedure and inset into the defect. The secondary defect can be closed primarily by undermining the surrounding tissues (Fig. 9.5a–h, i–p).

Tips: The tunnel should be of an adequate dimension to avoid compression of the pedicle. The pinna will be "pinned" back when the secondary defect is closed. This can interfere with the fit of an existing hearing aid and would have to be discussed with the patient.

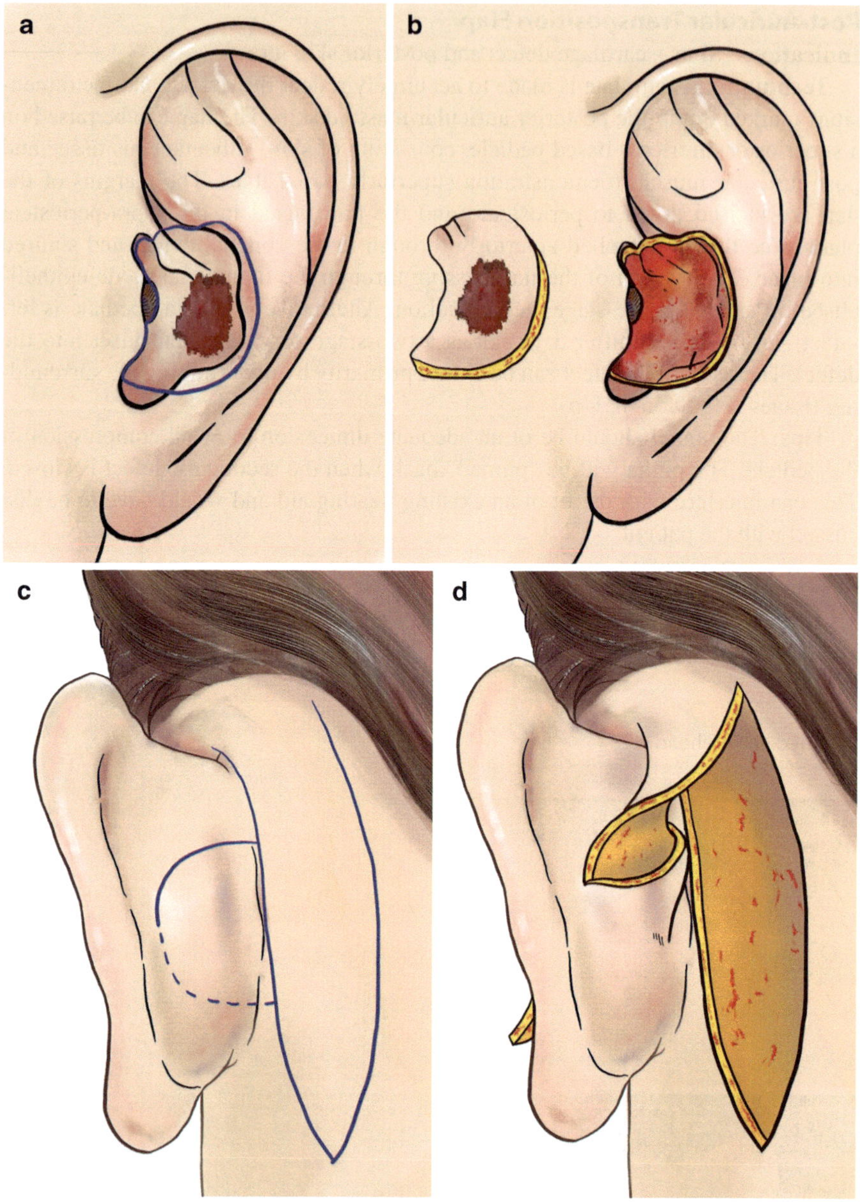

Fig. 9.5 Post auricular artery transposition flap. (**a**) Markings for excision, (**b**) Excision defect, (**c**) Superiorly based flap markings with incision for tunnel, (**d**) Flap raised and tunneled into defect, (**e**) Smal area of bridge de-epithelialised, (**f**) Flap sutured into defect, (**g**) Donar site sutured, (**h**) Base of flap sutured, (**i**) Lesion pinna, (**j**) Excision defect, (**k**) Flap markings with bridge outlined, (**l**) Flap outlined, (**m**) Flap raised with broad pedicle, (**n**) Flap tunneled into defect, (**o**) Flap inset into defect, (**p**) Donar site closure

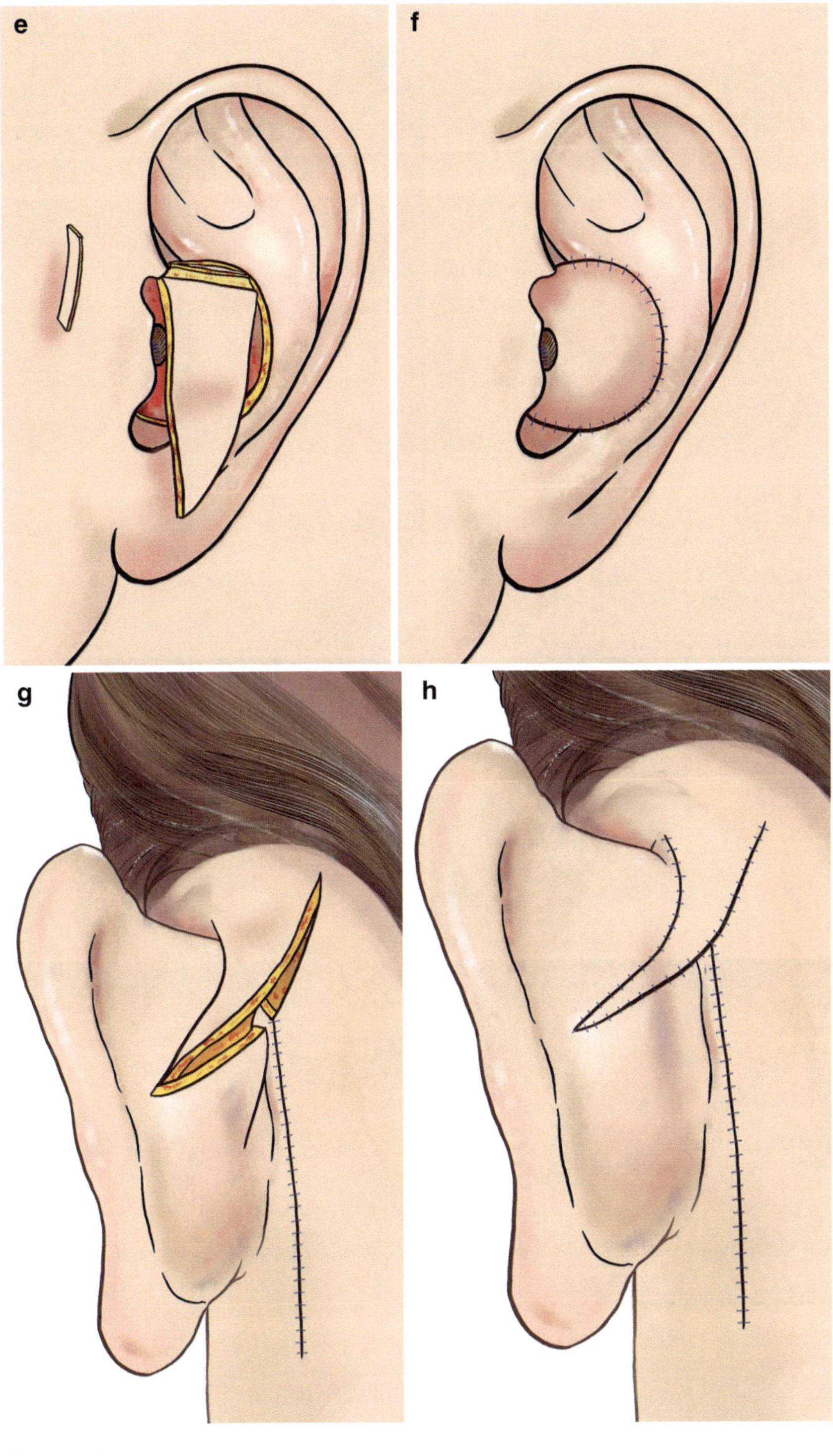

Fig. 9.5 (continued)

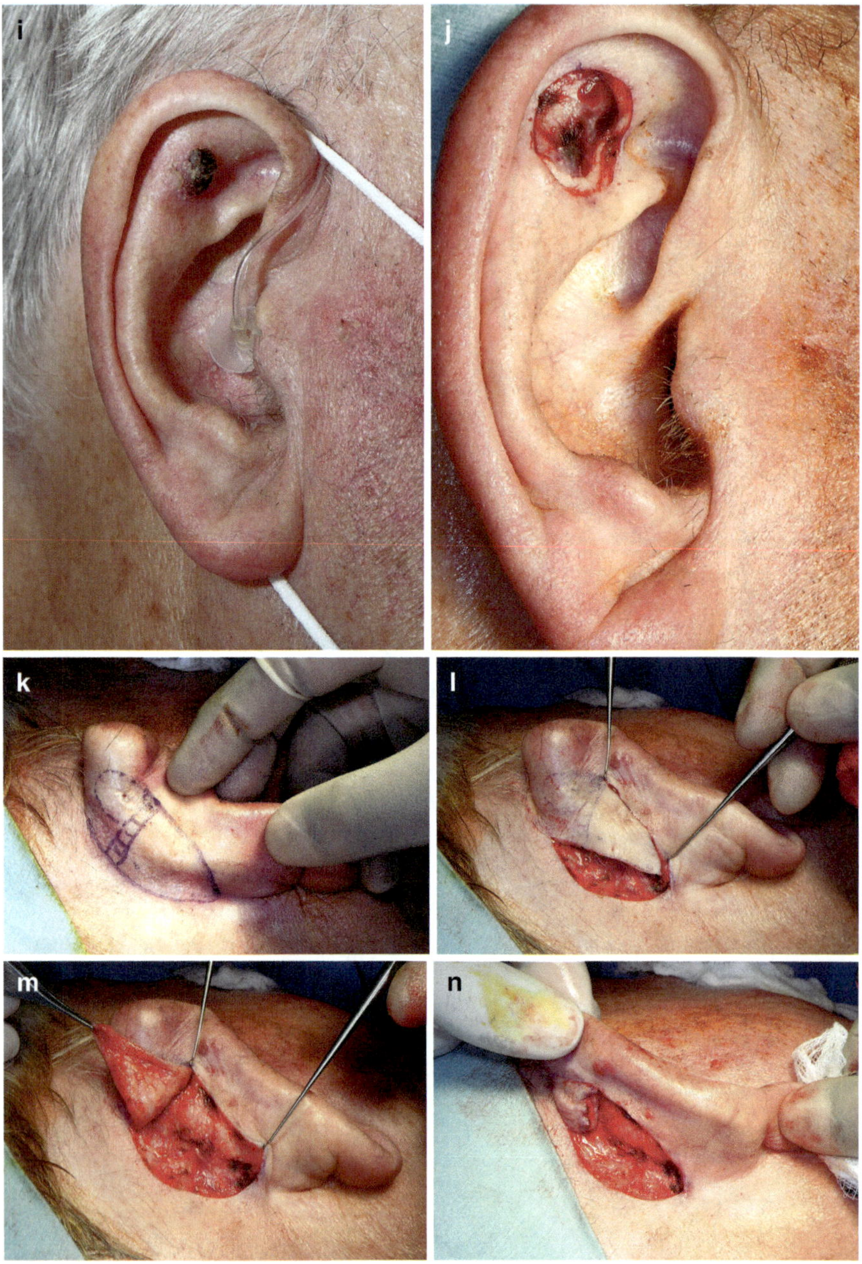

Fig. 9.5 (continued)

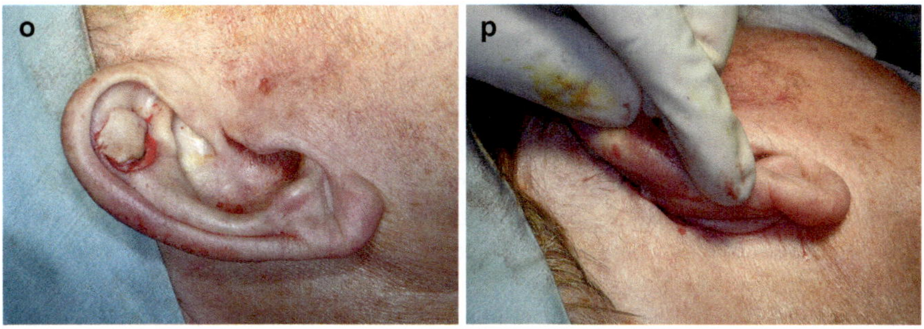

Fig. 9.5 (continued)

Pre-auricular Transposition Flap

Indications: Partial thickness defects (skin only/skin + cartilage).

Technique: A template is made to accurately reflect the defect, and the dimensions marked out in the pre-auricular skin. The flap can be based on a superior or inferior pedicle and raised in the subcutaneous plane. A full-thickness incision is made along the temporal/facial attachment of the ascending helix in case of a superiorly based flap, to create a tunnel into the defect. The flap is tunnelled anteriorly through to the defect and sutured into place. The section of the flap passing through the tunnel can be de-epithelialised, in case of a one-stage reconstruction. Alternatively, the flap pedicle is left intact can be divided after 3 weeks as a two-stage procedure and inset into the defect. The secondary defect can be closed primarily by undermining the surrounding tissues (See Fig. 9.12a–d).

An inferiorly based flap is more often considered when the conchal defect extends more inferiorly and laterally to include the intertragic notch, antitragus and antihelix. The remaining attachment of the lobule can be detached to aid inset of the flap and reattached (Fig. 9.6a–d). The flap can be thinned as a second staged procedure.

Tips: The tunnel should be of adequate dimension to prevent compression of the pedicle and vascular compromise. The hair distribution in the area should be taken into account, when designing the flap to prevent its inclusion into the reconstructed defect. Dog ears often have to be corrected and are best done inside the hairline and along the auriculocephalic sulcus.

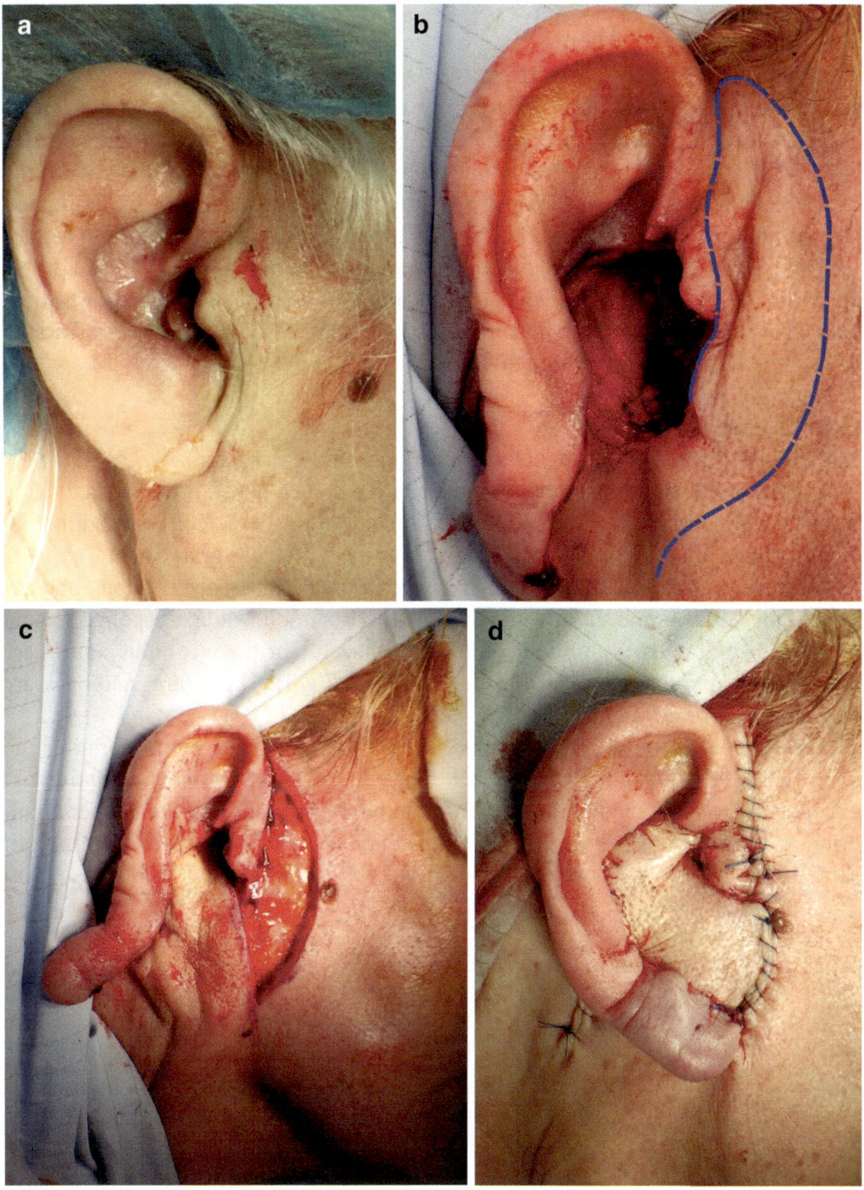

Fig. 9.6 Pre-auricular transposition flap. (**a**) Lesion conchal bowl, (**b**) Excision defect and markings for flap, (**c**) Flap transposed into defect, (**d**) Final closure

Antihelix

Healing by Secondary Intention

Indications: Partial thickness defects (skin only/skin + cartilage).

Technique: The partial thickness defect is left to heal by secondary intention. In case of skin only defects consideration can be given for perforating the underlying cartilage with a small punch biopsy core, to encourage granulation tissue ingress from the medial tissues. This can be useful, especially when perichondrium is lost.

Tips: A good wound care regimen is essential. The obvious disadvantage of this approach is the prolonged healing period and reliance on patient/career co-operation. Distortion due to scarring can be minimised by careful case selection and restricting its use to small- and medium-sized defects.

Skin Grafts

Indications: Partial thickness defects (skin only/skin + cartilage).

Technique: A suitable template is made of the defect, which is transferred to the donar site to harvest the graft. The graft is sutured to the defect, with additional "long" sutures that can be used for "tying" over the bolus. The graft can be "quilted" to the base, to decrease the risk of haematoma and dead space. A non-adherent dressing is laid over the sutured graft, over which a cotton wool ball/sponge soaked in proflavin or a suitable antibiotic ointment is placed. The tie-over bolus sutures are now used to hold the dressing in place (Fig. 9.7a–f, g–i). The sutures and pack are removed in 7–10 days time.

Tips: For skin only defects, consideration can be given for perforating the underlying cartilage with a small punch biopsy core, to encourage granulation tissue ingress from the medial tissues. This can be useful, especially when perichondrium is lost (See also Fig. 9.14e–i). Full-thickness grafts are preferred to split skin grafts.

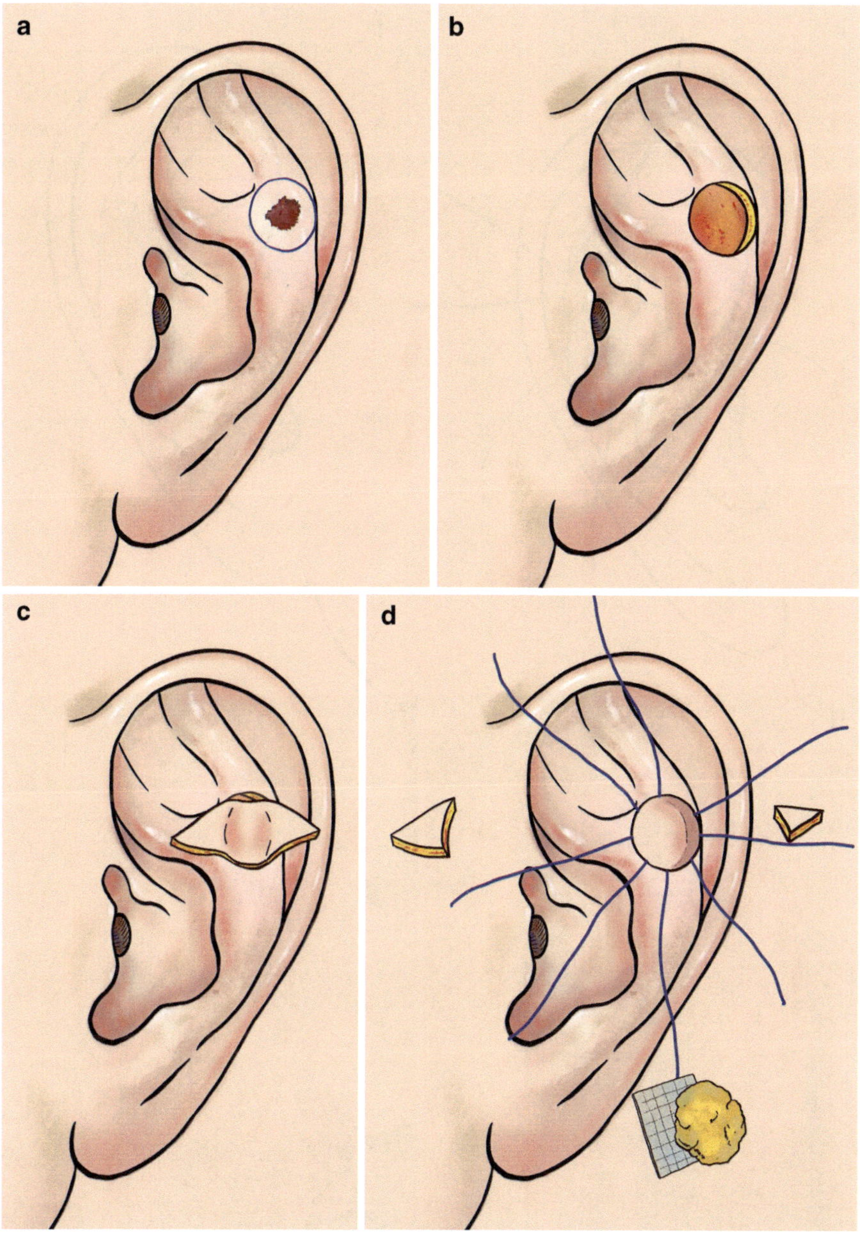

Fig. 9.7 Excision and skin graft. (**a**) Markings for excision, (**b**) Excision defect, (**c**) Skin graft insitu, (**d**) Skin graft sutured and tie over bolus sutures in place, (**e**) Non adherent and bolus dressing in situ, (**f**) Dressing sutured in place, (**g**) Excision defect, (**h**) Skin graft sutured in place, (**i**) Post operative result

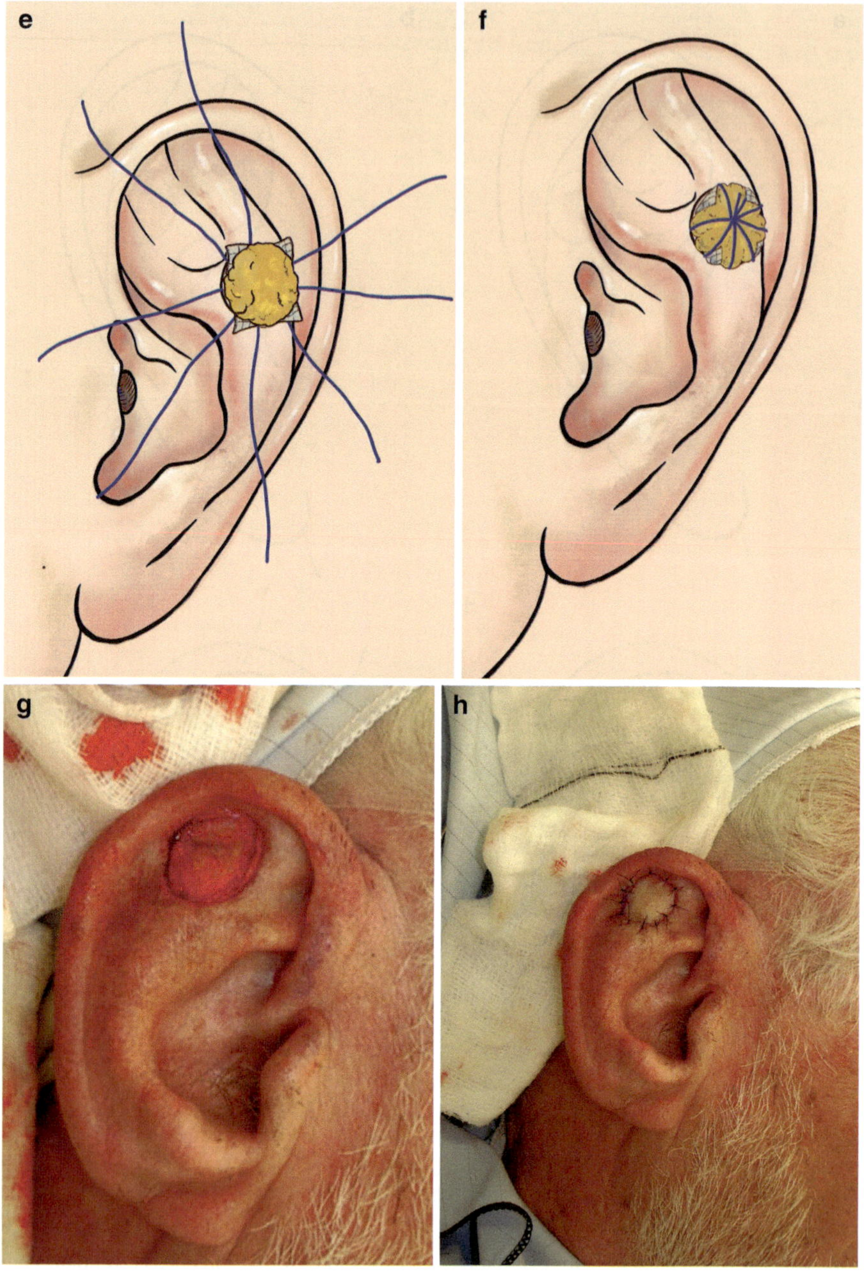

Fig. 9.7 (continued)

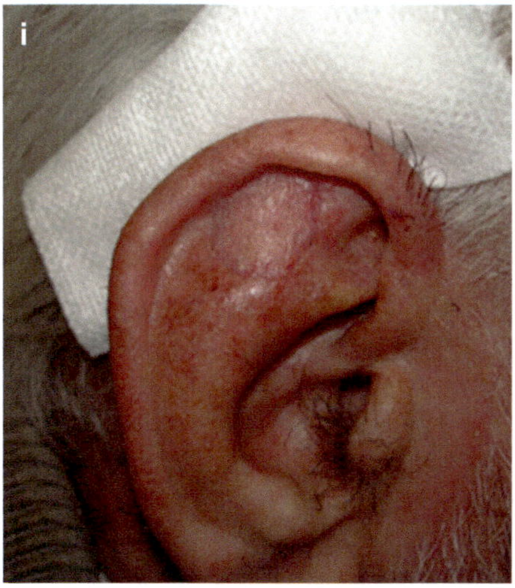

Fig. 9.7 (continued)

Helical Rim/Antihelix Extending to Helical Rim

Wedge Excision

Indications: Small/medium full-thickness defects.

Technique: The lesion is excised with adequate margins and the defect modified to a triangle, with the base along the helical rim and the apex extending medially across the antihelix. The wound is closed in three layers (anterior skin, cartilage and posterior skin (Fig. 9.8a–c, d–j).

Tips: Accurate approximation of the helical rim is essential to prevent notching. It is a simple technique for small defect and can be an acceptable technique for larger defects in patients, in whom more involved surgery is not indicated. The larger the wedge, the greater the "cupping" of the pinna. For larger defects, the medial extension of the wedge can be extended up to the concha. The cupping can be minimised by excising Burrows triangles along the scapha or junction of the antihelix and concha.

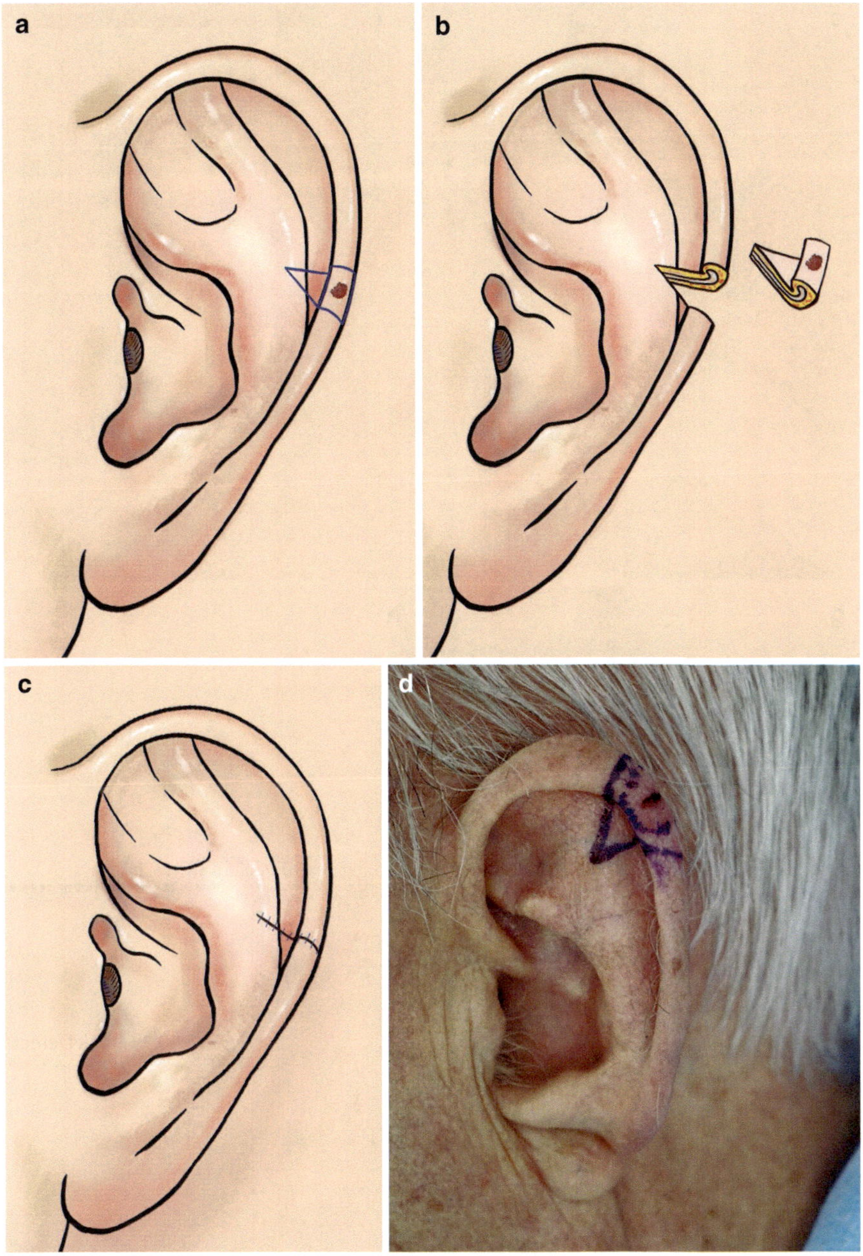

Fig. 9.8 Wedge excision and primary closure. (**a**) Markings for excision, (**b**) Excision defect, (**c**) Final closure, (**d**) Markings for excision - anterior view, (**e**) Markings for excision - posterior view, (**f**) Excision defect - anterior view, (**g**) Excision defect - posterior view, (**h**) Final closure - anterior view, (**i**) Final closure - posterior view, (**j**) Early post operative result

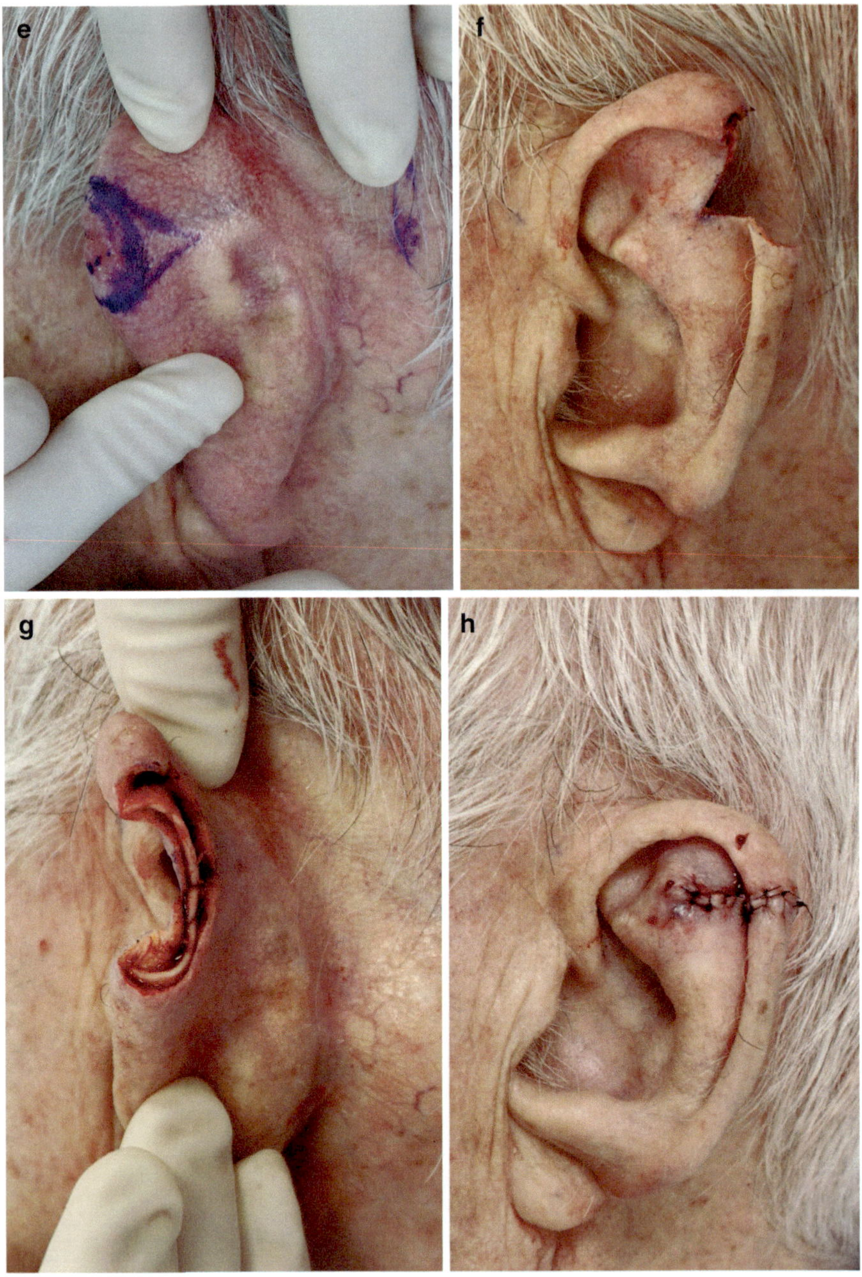

Fig. 9.8 (continued)

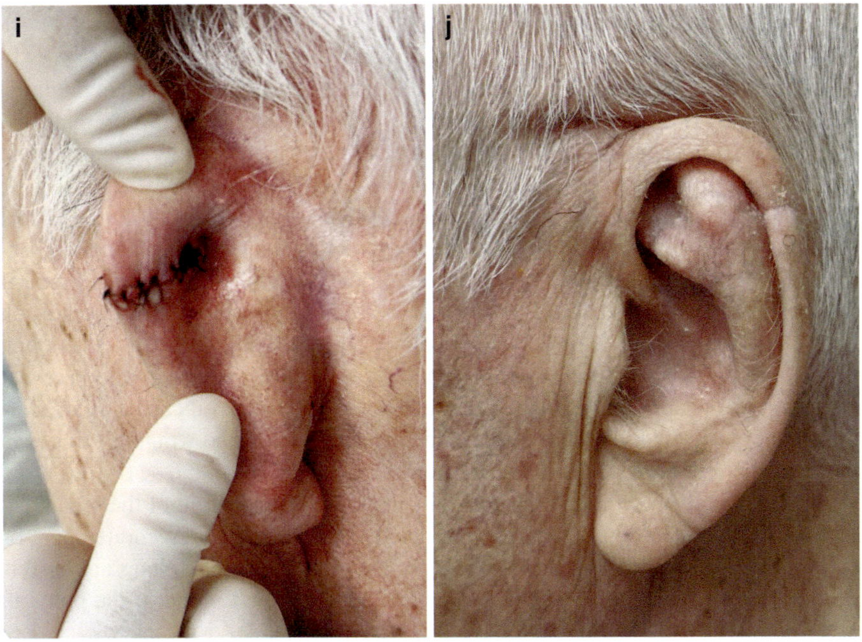

Fig. 9.8 (continued)

Rim Advancement (Posterior Pedicle)

Indications: Medium-sized full-thickness defects.

Technique: The lesion is excised with adequate margins and the defect modified to a rectangle. The skin in the anterior surface of the pinna is raised (minimally) to expose the underlying cartilage. An incision is made from the inferior base of the defect, through cartilage only up to the mid-lobule. (In the lobule, where cartilage is absent, the incision is deepened to the subcutaneous tissue.) The posterior skin is dissected of the cartilage from the medial margin of the flap, till adequate mobilisation is achieved. The resultant rim, pedicled on the posterior skin is rotated superiorly to close the defect. A similar flap can be raised superiorly, with the incision extending from the superior base of the defect, up to the helical crus. It is often necessary to remove additional cartilage and skin from the medial aspect to prevent distortion and "cupping" during flap inset. The cartilage removal can be as an additional rim along the medial margin, wedge or star shaped. The wound is closed in three layers (anterior skin, cartilage, posterior skin) (Fig. 9.9a–g, h–s, t–z, aa–ag).

Tips: Rim advancement flap results in a decrease in the height of the pinna, but prevents cupping and makes the reconstructed ear less obvious. Accurate approximation of the helical rim and cartilage is essential to prevent notching and distortion. Dog ears often have to be corrected on the posterior surface of the pinna to accommodate the flap.

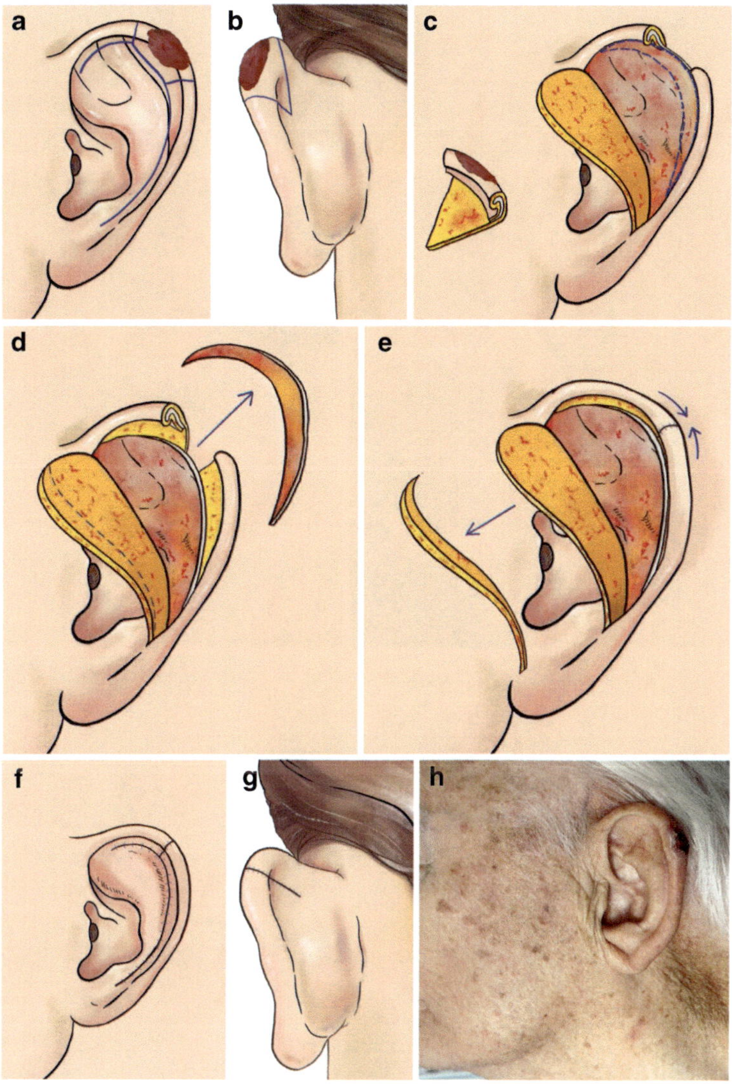

Fig. 9.9 Rim advancement flap. (**a**) Markings for excision and flap - anterior view, (**b**) Markings for excision - posterior view, (**c**) Excision defect and markings for additional cartliage excision, (**d**) Rim advancement flaps mobilised, additional cartilage excised and markings for additional skin excision, (**e**) Rim advancement flaps sutured into position and additional skin excised, (**f**) Final closure - anterior view, (**g**) Final closure - posterior view, (**h**) Lesion helical rim, (**i**) Markings for excision and flap - anterior view, (**j**) Markings for excision - posterior view, (**k**) Post excision defect - anterior view, (**l**) Post excision defect - Posterior view, (**m**) Inferior rim advancement flap delineated, (**n**) Posterior pedicle highlighted, (**o**) Flap advanced into defect; anterior cartilage overlap highlighted, (**p**) Anterior skin minimally elevated to delineate excess cartilage, (**q**) Wedge excison of additional cartilage, (**r**) Final closure - anterior view, (**s**) Final closure - posterior view, (**t**) Markings for excision, (**u**) Excision defect, (**v**) Markings for inferior rim advancement flap, (**w**) Incisions for flap, (**x**) Flap advanced into defect, (**y**) Final closure, (**z**) Post operative result, (**aa**) Markings for excision and flap, (**ab**) Excision defect - anterior view, (**ac**) Excision defect - posterior view, (**ad**) superior and inferior rim advancement flaps with Burrows triangle excised, (**ae**) Flaps advanced into defect, (**af**) Final closure, (**ag**) Post operative appearance

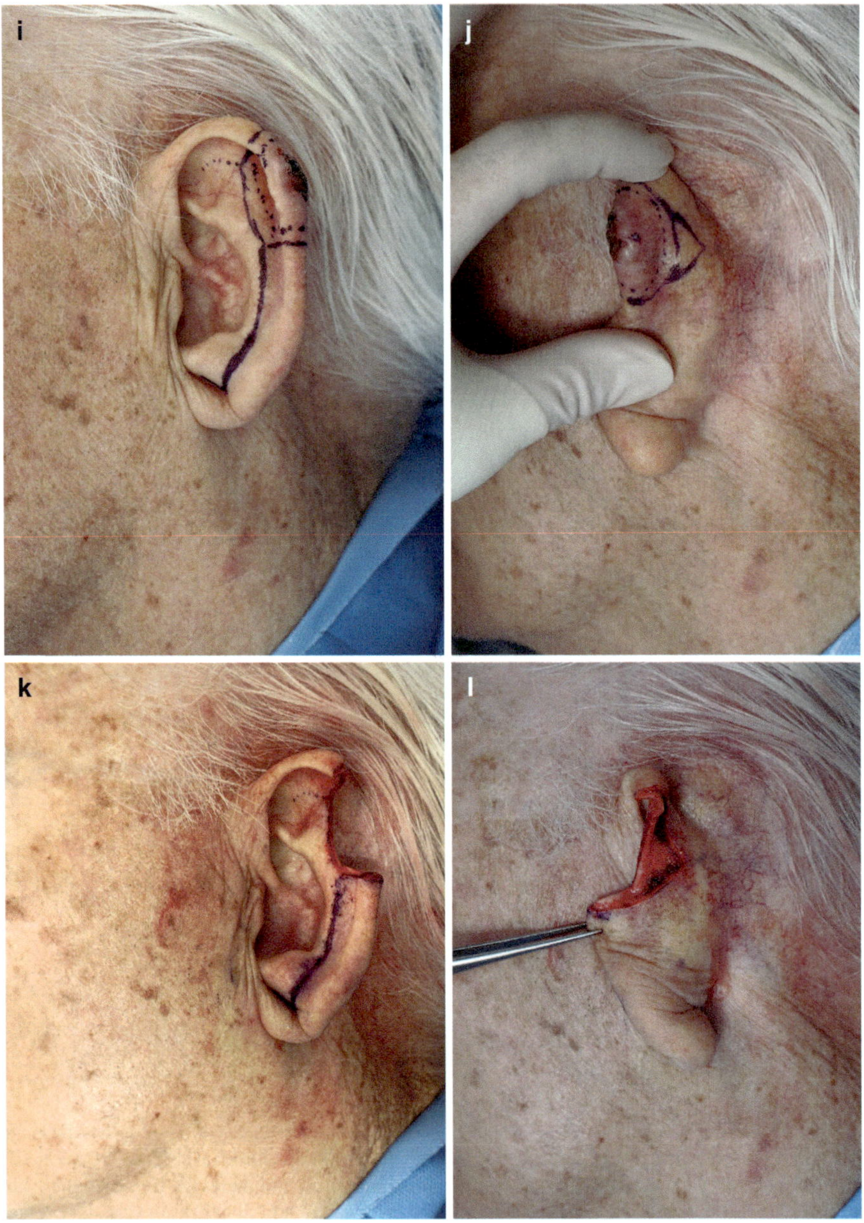

Fig. 9.9 (continued)

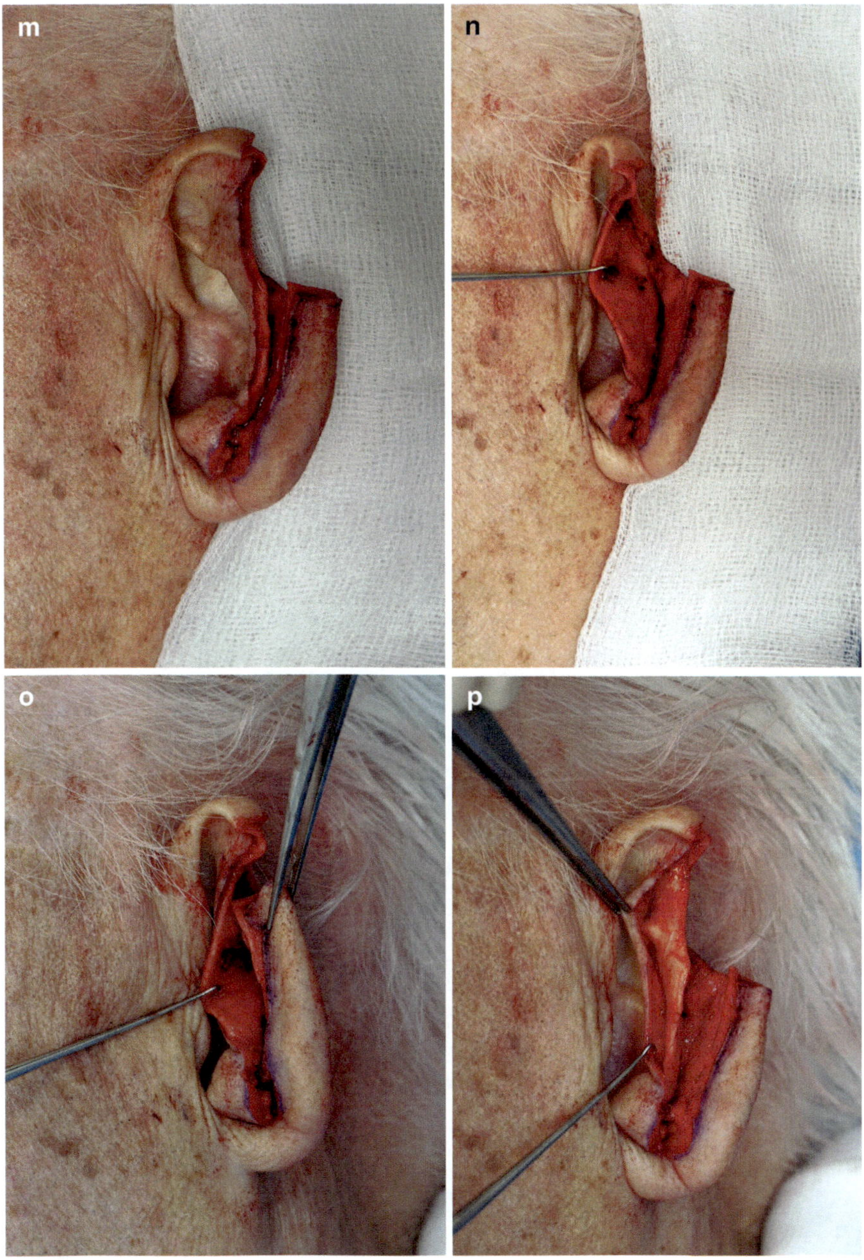

Fig. 9.9 (continued)

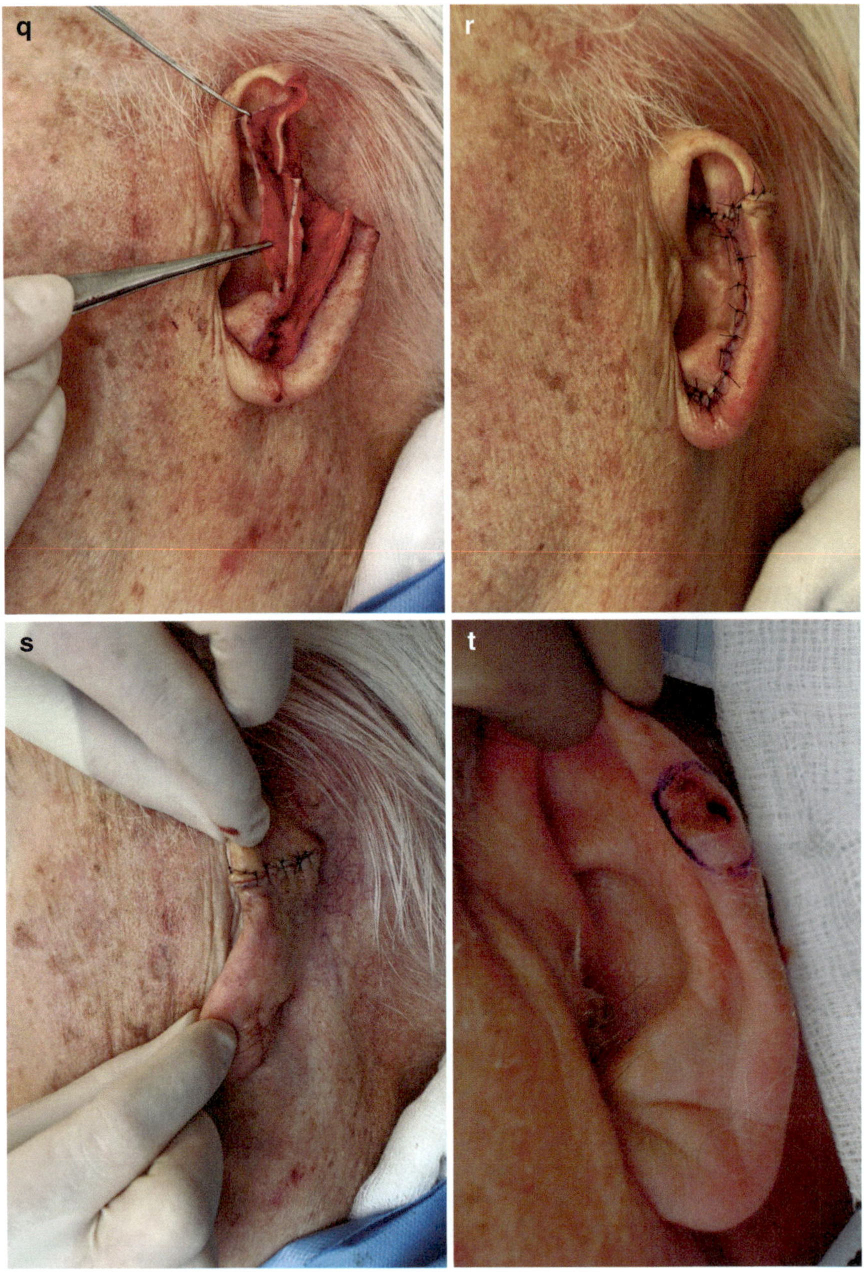

Fig. 9.9 (continued)

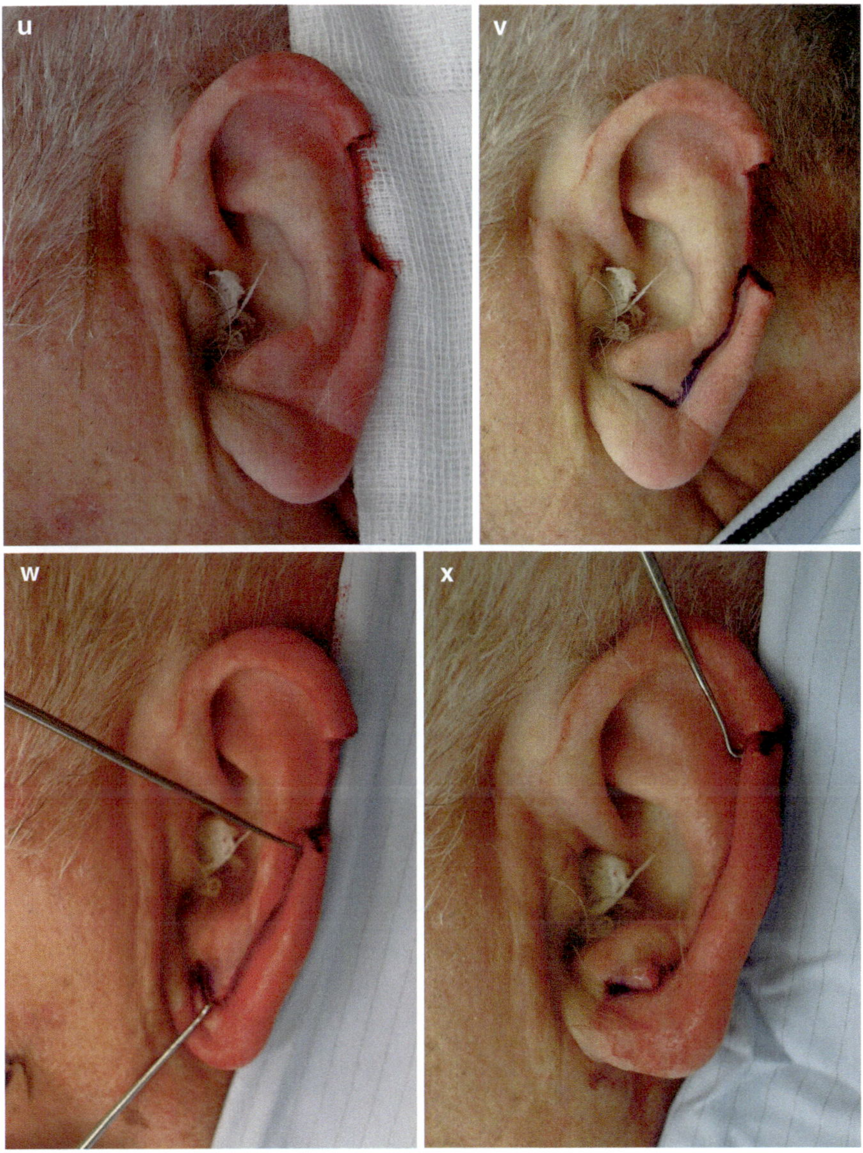

Fig. 9.9 (continued)

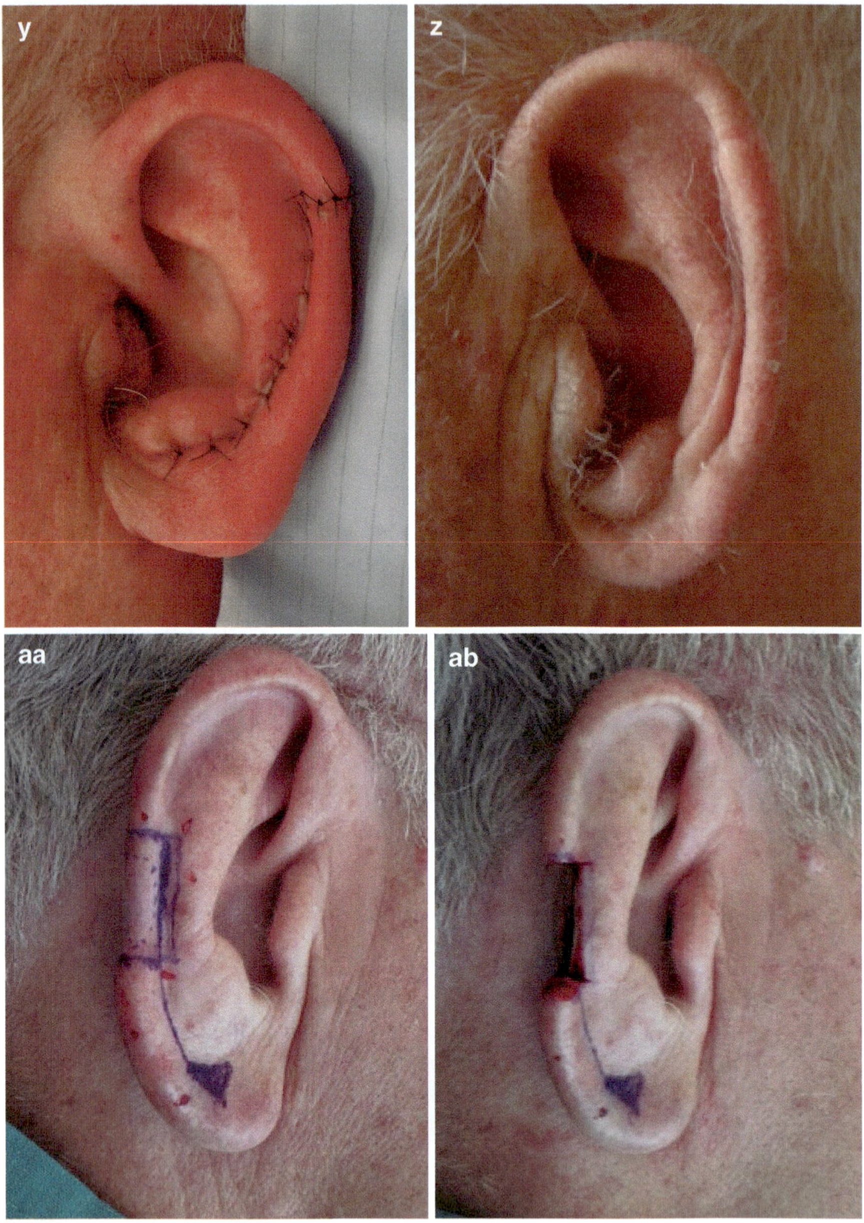

Fig. 9.9 (continued)

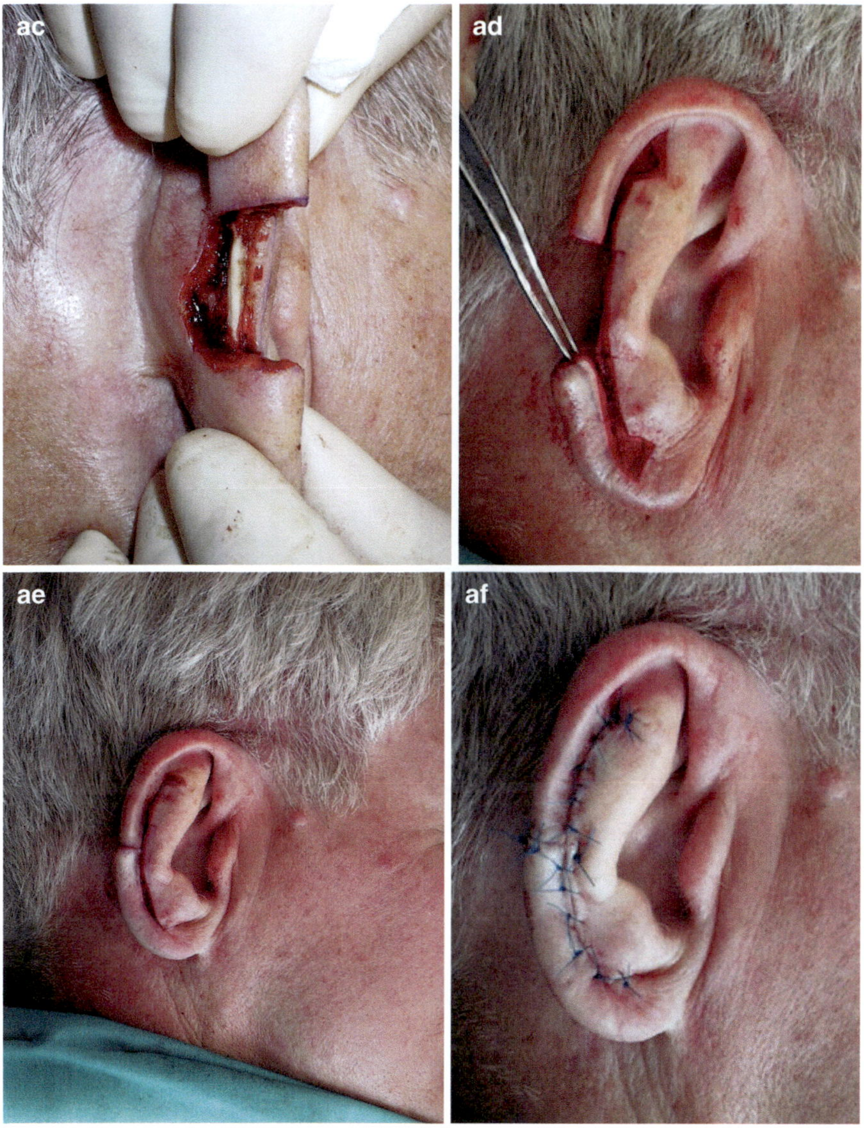

Fig. 9.9 (continued)

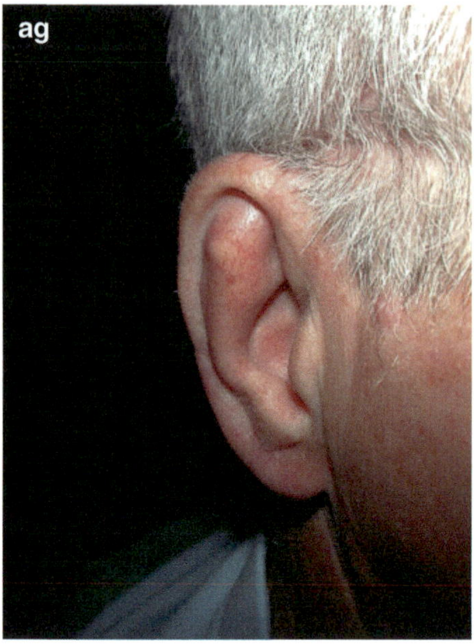

Fig. 9.9 (continued)

Modified Rim Advancement Flap

Indications: Medium-sized full-thickness defects, helix, antihelix, scapha.

Technique: The lesion is excised with adequate margins and the defect modified to a rectangle. An incision is from the base of the defect superiorly and inferiorly through the anterior skin and cartilage, taking care not to damage the posterior skin. Back cuts are made along the superior end to cross the triangular fossa and inferiorly extended to the antitragus. The posterior skin is dissected of the cartilage from the medial margin of the flap, till adequate mobilisation is achieved. The resultant rim, pedicled on the posterior skin is rotated superiorly to close the defect. It is often necessary to remove additional cartilage and skin from the medial aspect to prevent distortion and "cupping" during flap inset. The cartilage removal can be as an additional rim along the medial margin, The wound is closed in three layers (anterior skin, cartilage, posterior skin) (Fig. 9.10a–f, g–j).

Tips: Rim advancement flap results in a decrease in the height of the pinna, but prevents cupping and makes the reconstructed ear less obvious. Accurate approximation of the helical rim and cartilage is essential to prevent notching and distortion. Dog ears often have to be corrected on the posterior surface of the pinna to accommodate the flap.

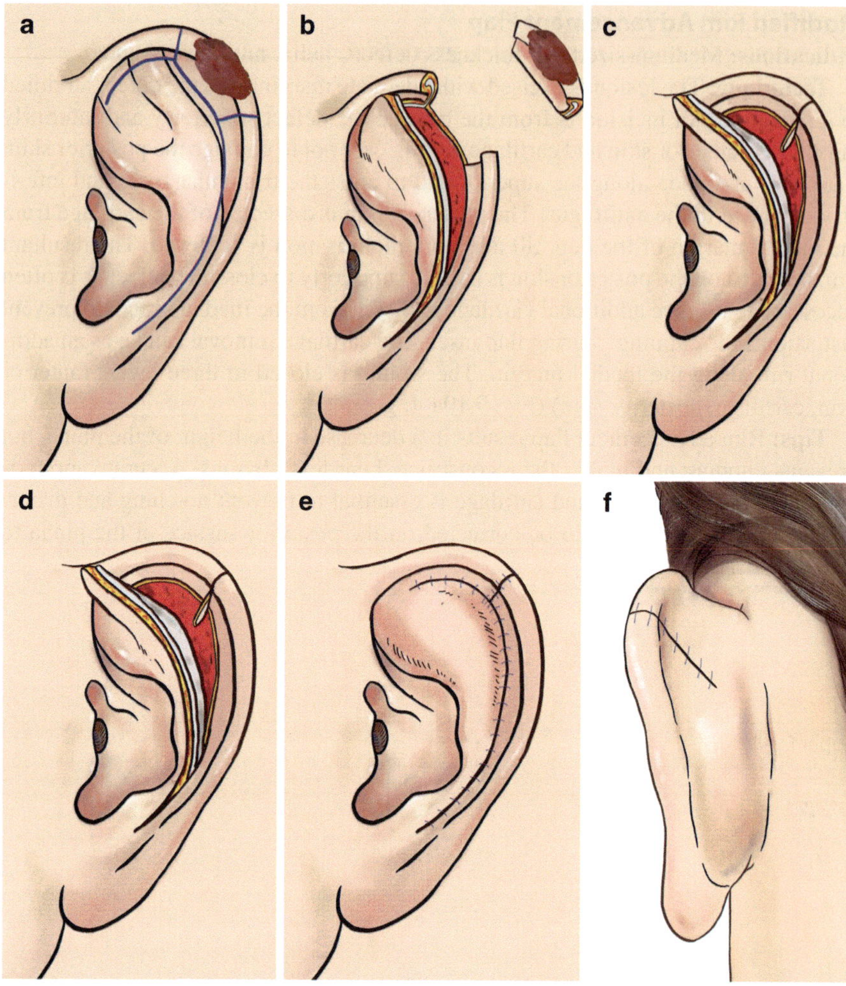

Fig. 9.10 Modified rim advancement flap. (**a**) Markings for excision and flap, (**b**) Excision defect and flap raised, (**c**) Rim advancement and closure of original defect; excess medial skin and cartilage to be excised highlighted, (**d**) Final closure - anterior view, (**e**) Final closure - posterior view, (**f**) Markings for excision and flap, (**g**) Excision defect and flap raised, (**i**) Closure of rim defect; excess skin cartilage highlighted, (**j**) Final closure

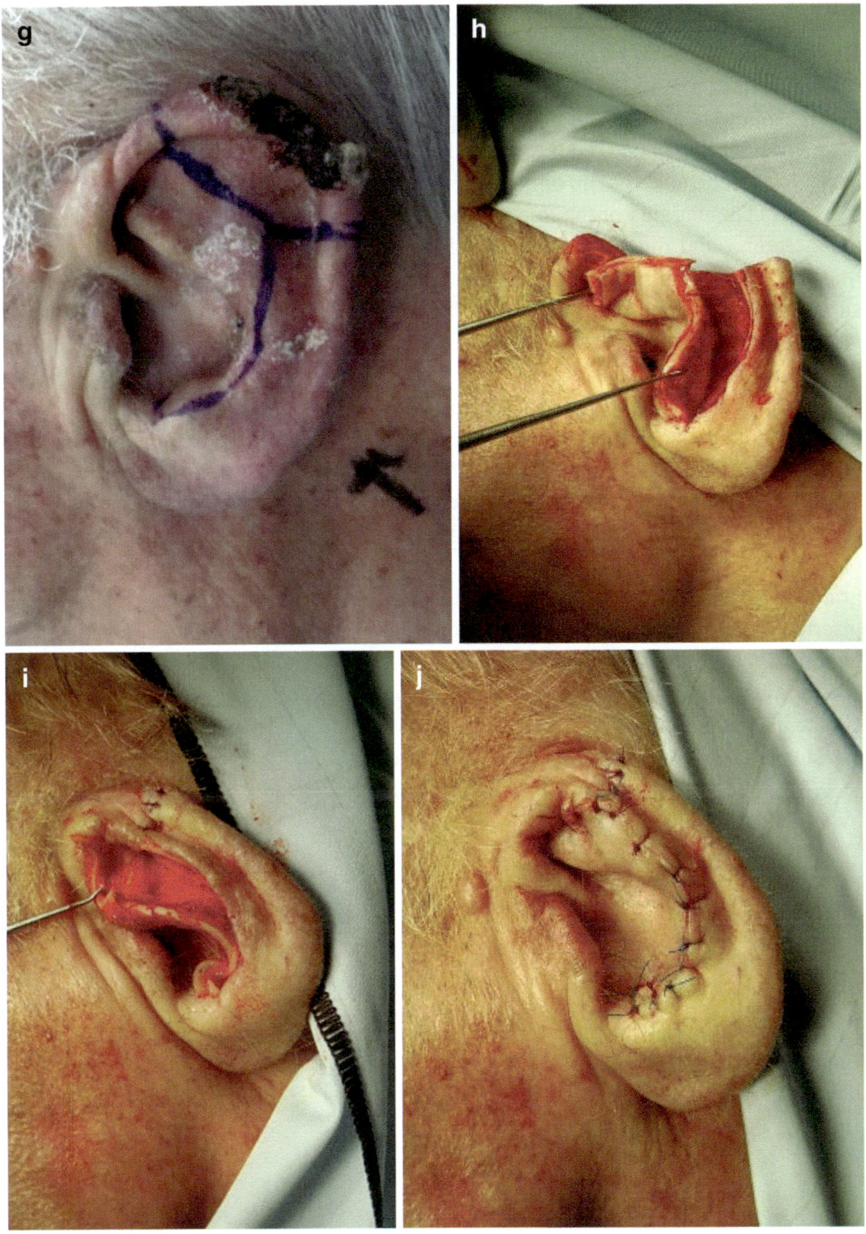

Fig. 9.10 (continued)

Two-stage Post-auricular Flap (Superiorly Based)

Indications: Medium-sized helical rim, helical rim + antihelix defects.

Technique: The lesion is excised with adequate margins and the defect modified to a rectangle or square with parallel superior and inferior edges. A superiorly based post-auricular flap is marked overlying the mastoid skin, at least 1 cm away from the auriculocephalic sulcus. The dimensions and reach of the flap are tested prior to any incisions. The margins of the flap are incised and the flap elevated on the surface of the sternomastoid muscle inferiorly and in the supra-periosteal plane overlying the mastoid. The mobilised flap is sutured into the defect on the anterior, inferior and superior margins. The pedicle will traverse over the intact skin in the auriculocephalic sulcus and is covered by Vaseline gauze. The donor defect is closed by undermining the wound margins (Fig. 9.11a–f).

The second stage is carried out 4 weeks later. The bridge is excised, and the distal end inset into the posterior margin of the pinna defect. The base of the flap is excised and inset into the remaining donor site (Fig. 9.11g).

Tips: The flap is useful for long defects, where a rim advancement flap is likely to result in significant shortening of the height of the ear. The flap can be inset across or along the defect, depending on the length of the defect. Interpositional cartilage grafts are beneficial in large defects to provide additional support. This can be inserted during the first or second stage. Additional contouring, if required can be undertaken as a third-stage procedure.

An inferiorly based post-auricular flap can also be used for similar defects. The choice between an inferiorly or superiorly based flap will depend on the position of the superior and inferior margins of the defect. A "low" inferior margin is better reconstructed with a superiorly based flap and vice versa, a "high" superior margin by an inferiorly based flap.

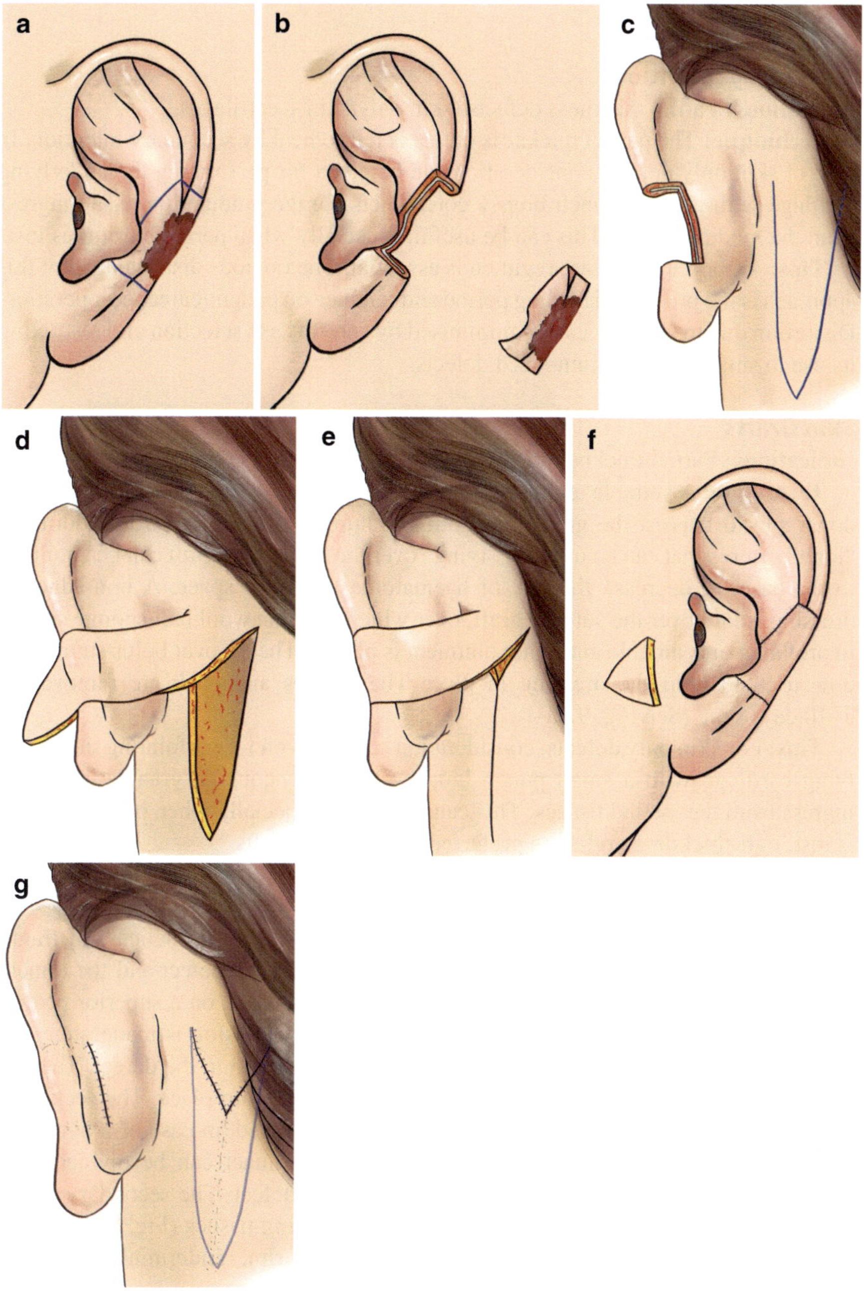

Fig. 9.11 Two stage post auricular flap (superiorly based). (**a**) Markings for excision, (**b**) Excision defect, (**c**) Markings for flap, (**d**) Flap raised and transposed into defect, (**e**) Closure of donar site, (**f**) Flap sutured into defect, (**g**) Second stage division and inset of pedicle

Triangular Fossa

Secondary Intention

Indications: Partial thickness defects (skin only/skin + cartilage).

Technique: The partial thickness defect is left to heal by secondary intention. In case of skin only defects consideration can be given for perforating the underlying cartilage with a small punch biopsy core, to encourage granulation tissue ingress from the medial tissues. This can be useful, especially when perichondrium is lost.

Tips: A good wound care regimen is essential. The obvious disadvantage of this approach is the prolonged healing period and reliance on patient/career co-operation. Distortion due to scarring can be minimised by careful case selection and restricting its use to small- and medium-sized defects.

Skin Grafts

Indications: Partial thickness defects (skin only/skin + cartilage).

Technique: A suitable template is made of the defect, which is transferred to the donar site to harvest the graft. The graft is sutured to the defect, with additional "long" sutures that can be used for "tying" over the bolus. The graft can be "quilted" to the base, to decrease the risk of haematoma and dead space. A non-adherent dressing is laid over the sutured graft, over which a cotton wool ball/sponge soaked in proflavin or a suitable antibiotic ointment is placed. The tie-over bolus sutures are now used to hold the dressing in place The sutures and pack are removed in 7–10 days time (See Fig. 9.6a–i).

Tips: For skin only defects, consideration can be given for perforating the underlying cartilage with a small punch biopsy core, to encourage granulation tissue ingress from the medial tissues. This can be useful, especially when perichondrium is lost. Full-thickness grafts are preferred to split skin grafts.

Superiorly Based Pre-auricular Flap

Indications: Partial thickness defects (skin only, skin + cartilage), helical rim, tragus

Technique: A template is made to accurately reflect the defect and the dimensions marked out in the pre-auricular skin. The flap is based on a superior pedicle and raised in the subcutaneous plane. A full-thickness incision is made along the facial attachment of the ascending helix to create a tunnel into the defect. The flap is tunnelled anteriorly through to the defect and sutured into place. The section of the flap passing through the tunnel can be de-epithelialised, in case of a one-stage reconstruction. Alternatively, the flap pedicle is left intact can be divided after 3 weeks as a two-stage procedure and inset into the defect. The secondary defect can be closed primarily by undermining the surrounding tissues (Fig. 9.12a–d). In patients in whom the defect includes the helical rim, undermining and de-epithelialisation are not necessary (Fig. 9.12e–m).

Tips: The tunnel should be of adequate dimension to prevent compression of the pedicle and vascular compromise. The hair distribution in the area should be taken into account, when designing the flap to prevent its inclusion into the reconstructed defect. Dog ears often have to be corrected and are best done inside the hairline and along the auriculocephalic sulcus.

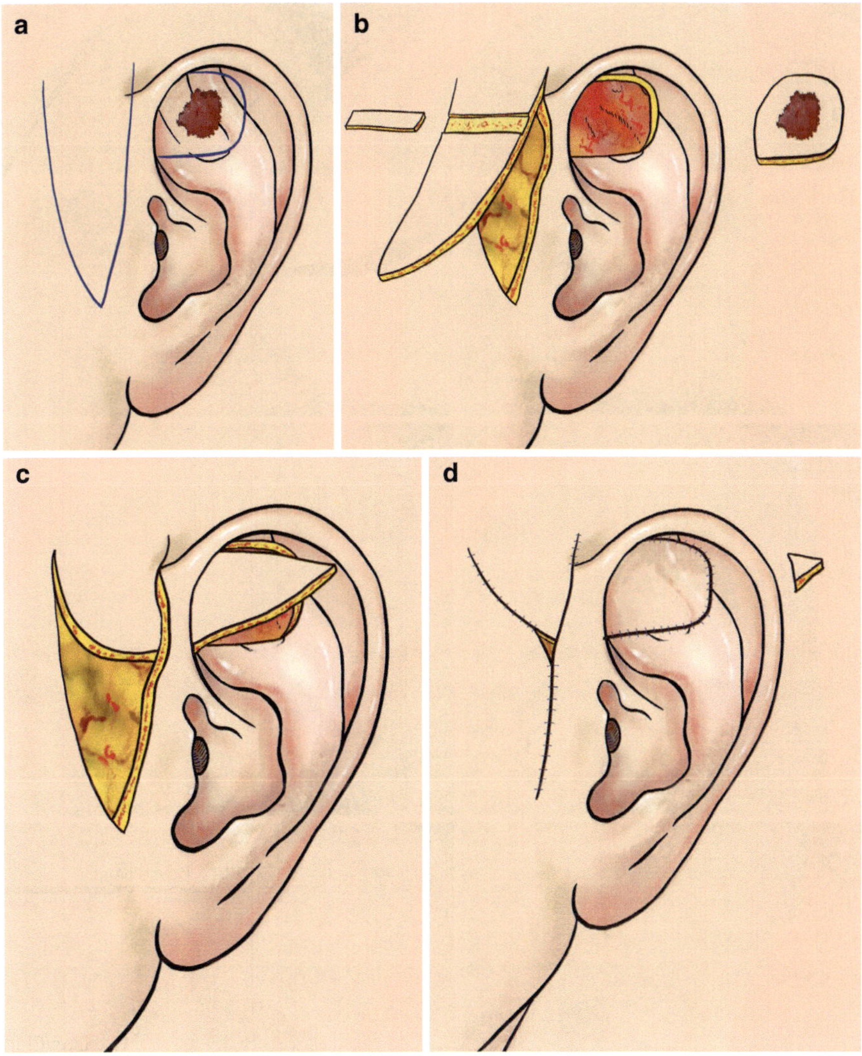

Fig. 9.12 Superiorly based pre-auricular flap. (**a**) Markings for excision and flap, (**b**) Excision defect and flap raised with bridge de-epithelialised, (**c**) Flap tunnled into defect, (**d**) Flap sutured in place, (**e**) Markings for excision, (**f**) Markings for excision - posterior view, (**g**) Markings for flap, (**h**) Excision defect, (**i**) Flap incision, (**j**) Trial transfer into defect, (**k**) Final closure - anterior view, (**l**) Final closure - posterior view, (**m**) Post operative appearance

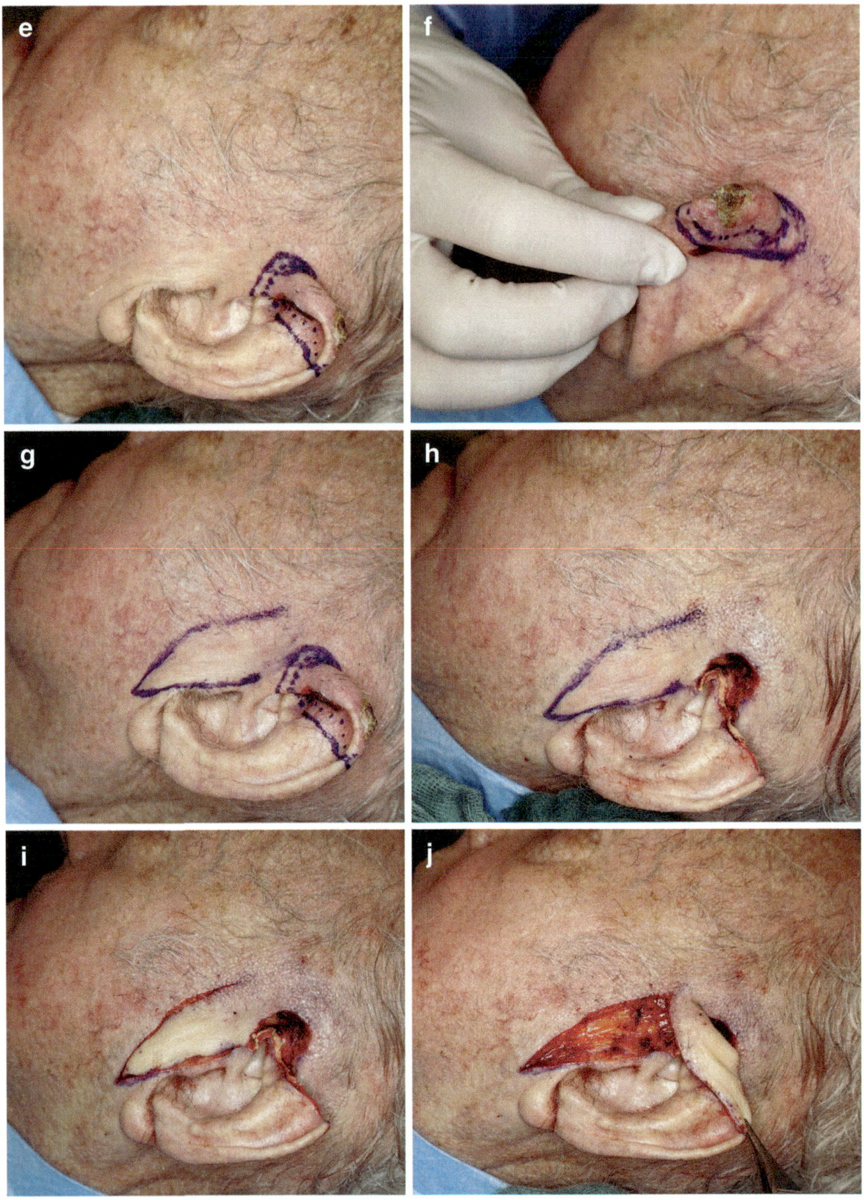

Fig. 9.12 (continued)

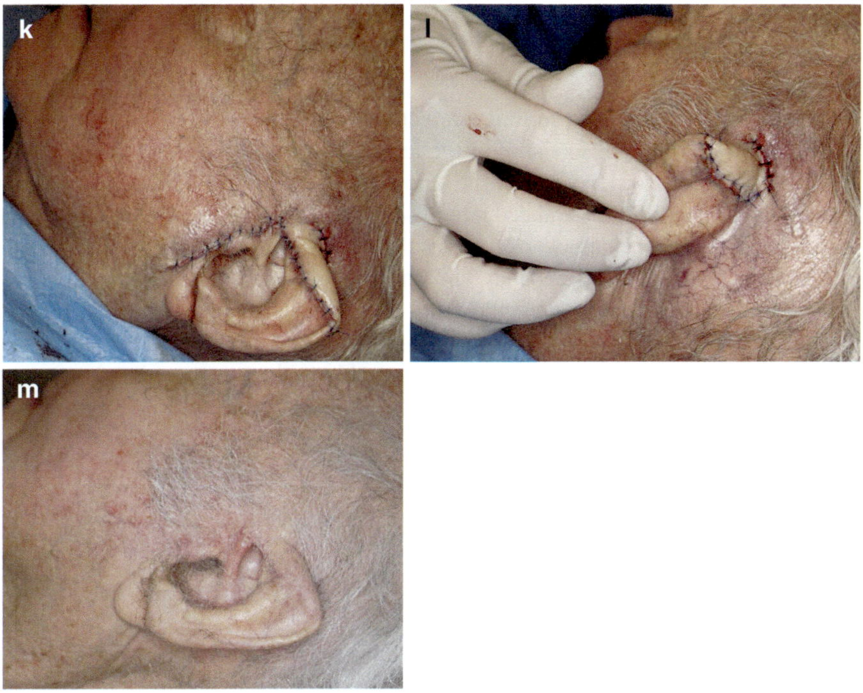

Fig. 9.12 (continued)

Tragus

Advancement Flap

Indications: Skin only, skin cartilage defects.

Technique: Following excision of the lesion, two parallel or slightly diverging incisions are made from the base of the defect and the skin flap is raised in a subcutaneous plane. The skin is advanced into the defect and the leading edge sutured into the meatal aspect of the defect, to start with. The rest of the wound is sutured, taking into account the length discrepancy and any dog ears appropriately managed. In case of a skin and cartilage defect, the distal end of the flap can be "folded" to create a neo tragus (Fig. 9.13a–c, d–g).

Tips: Raise the flap of adequate length to enable folding to accommodate suturing into the meatal surface of the defect.

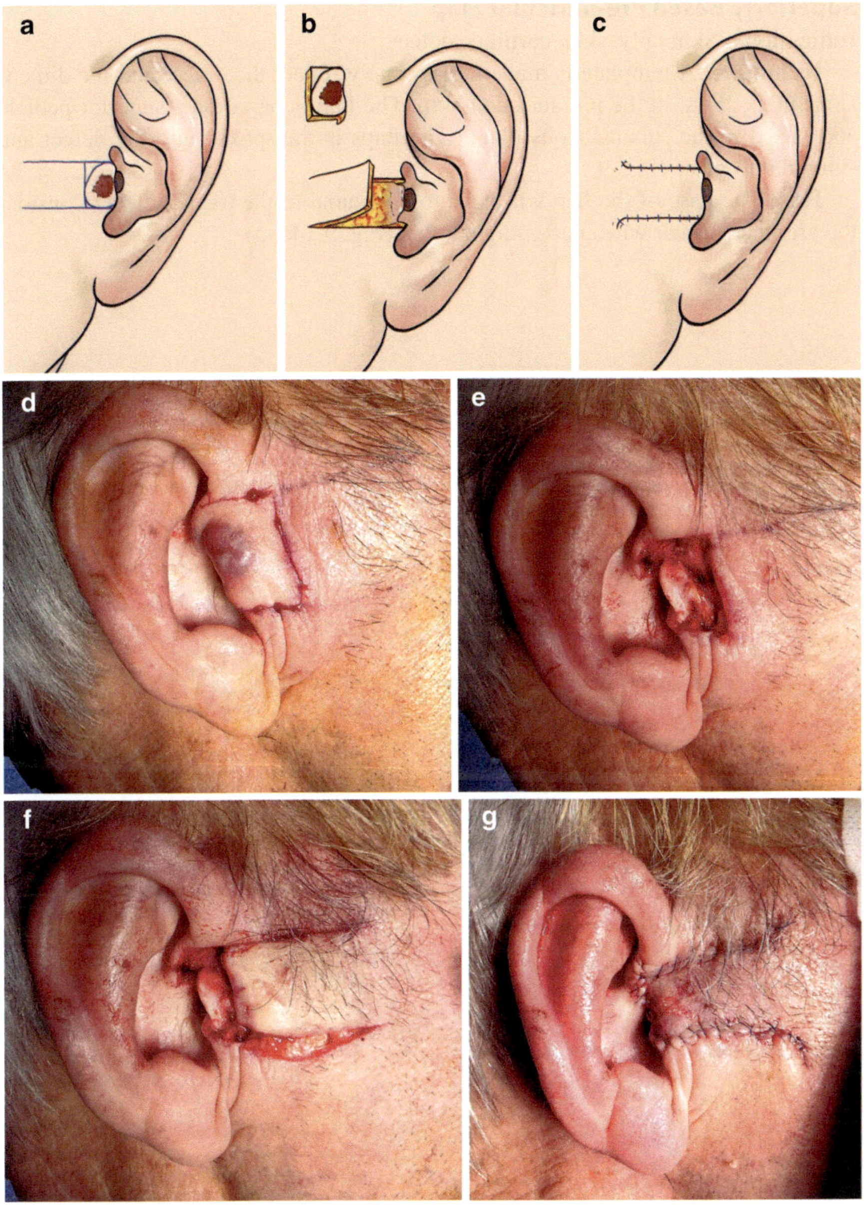

Fig. 9.13 Advancement flap. (**a**) Markings for excision and flap, (**b**) Excision defect and flap raised, (**c**) Final closure, (**d**) Outline of excision, (**e**) Excision defect, (**f**) Flap raised, (**g**) Final closure

Superiorly Based Pre-auricular Flap

Indications: Skin only, skin/ cartilage defects

Technique: A template is made to accurately reflect the defect and the dimensions marked out in the pre-auricular skin. The flap is based on a superior pedicle and raised in the subcutaneous plane. The flaps is transposed into the defect and sutured into place (Fig. 9.14a–g).

Tips: The base of the flap will have to be cranial to the tragal defect. Consider the presence of hair when designing the flap (Fig. 9.14a–g).

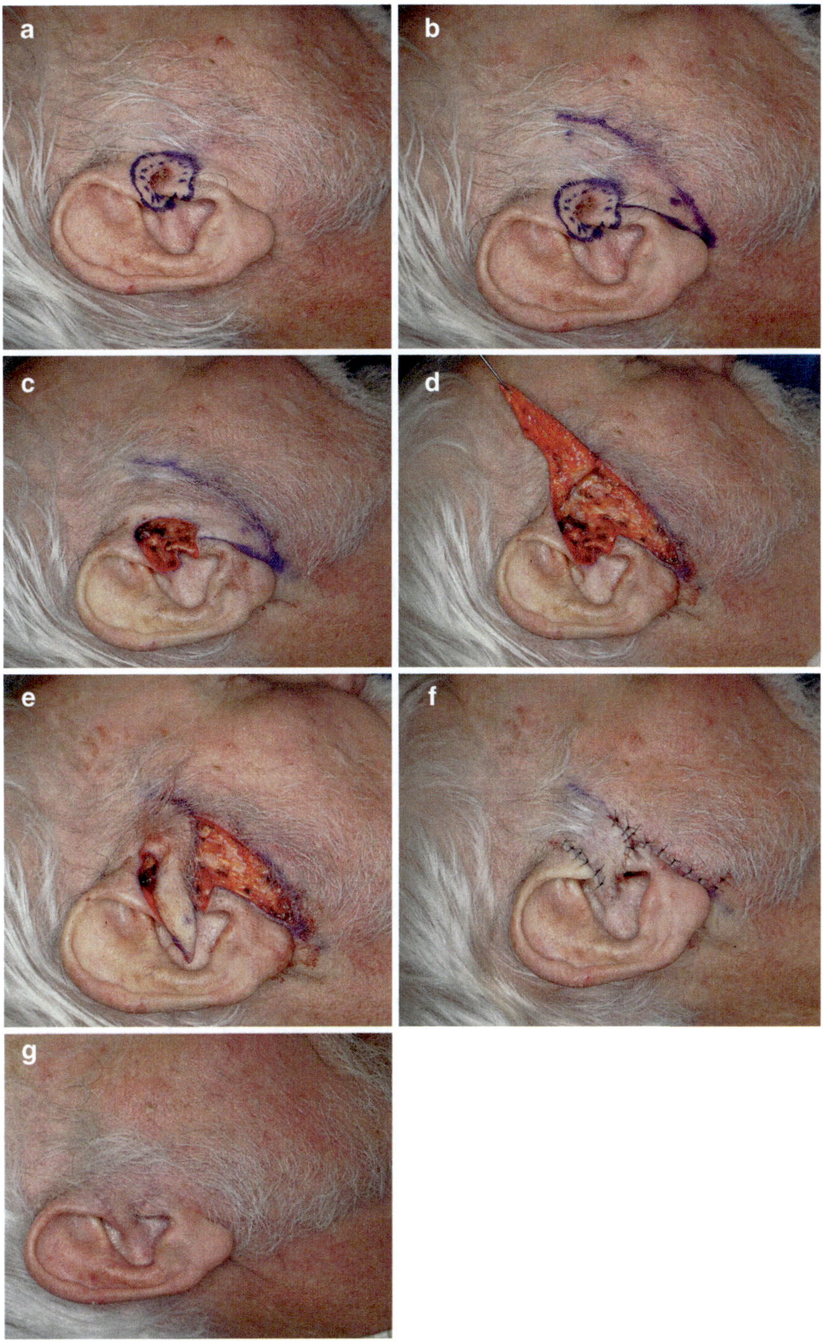

Fig. 914 (**a**) Markings for excision, (**b**) markings for flap, (**c**) excision defect, (**d**) Flap raised (**e**) Flap transposed into defect (**f**) final closure (**g**) early appearance with no revisions

Posterior Surface of Pinna

Healing by Secondary Intention

Indications: Partial thickness defects (skin only/skin + cartilage).

Technique: The partial thickness defect is left to heal by secondary intention. In case of skin only defects consideration can be given for perforating the underlying cartilage with a small punch biopsy core, to encourage granulation tissue ingress from the medial tissues. This can be useful, especially when perichondrium is lost.

Tips: A good wound care regimen is essential. The obvious disadvantage of this approach is the prolonged healing period and reliance on patient/career co-operation. Distortion due to scarring can be minimised by careful case selection and restricting its use to small- and medium-sized defects.

Primary Closure

Indications: Partial thickness defects (skin only/skin + cartilage).

Technique: The defect is converted into an ellipse. The adjacent skin is mobilised in the plane above the perichondrium, and the wound is closed in layers. For larger defects that extend across the auriculocephalic sulcus onto the mastoid skin, the wound edge of the posterior surface of the pinna can be sutured to the mastoid wound edge, with a resultant "pinning" back of the pinna.

Tips: Pinning back can interfere with the fit of the hearing aid and would have to be discussed with the patient.

Skin Graft

Indications: Partial thickness defects (skin only/skin + cartilage).

Technique: A suitable template is made of the defect, which is transferred to the donar site to harvest the graft. The graft is sutured to the defect, with additional "long" sutures that can be used for "tying" over the bolus. The graft can be "quilted" to the base, to decrease the risk of haematoma and dead space. A non-adherent dressing is laid over the sutured graft, over which a cotton wool ball/sponge soaked in proflavin or a suitable antibiotic ointment is placed. The tie-over bolus sutures are now used to hold the dressing in place The sutures and pack are removed in 7–10 days time (Fig. 9.15a–d).

Tips: For skin only defects, consideration can be given for perforating the underlying cartilage with a small punch biopsy core, to encourage granulation tissue ingress from the medial tissues. This can be useful, especially when perichondrium is lost (Fig. 9.15e–i). Full-thickness grafts are preferred to split skin grafts.

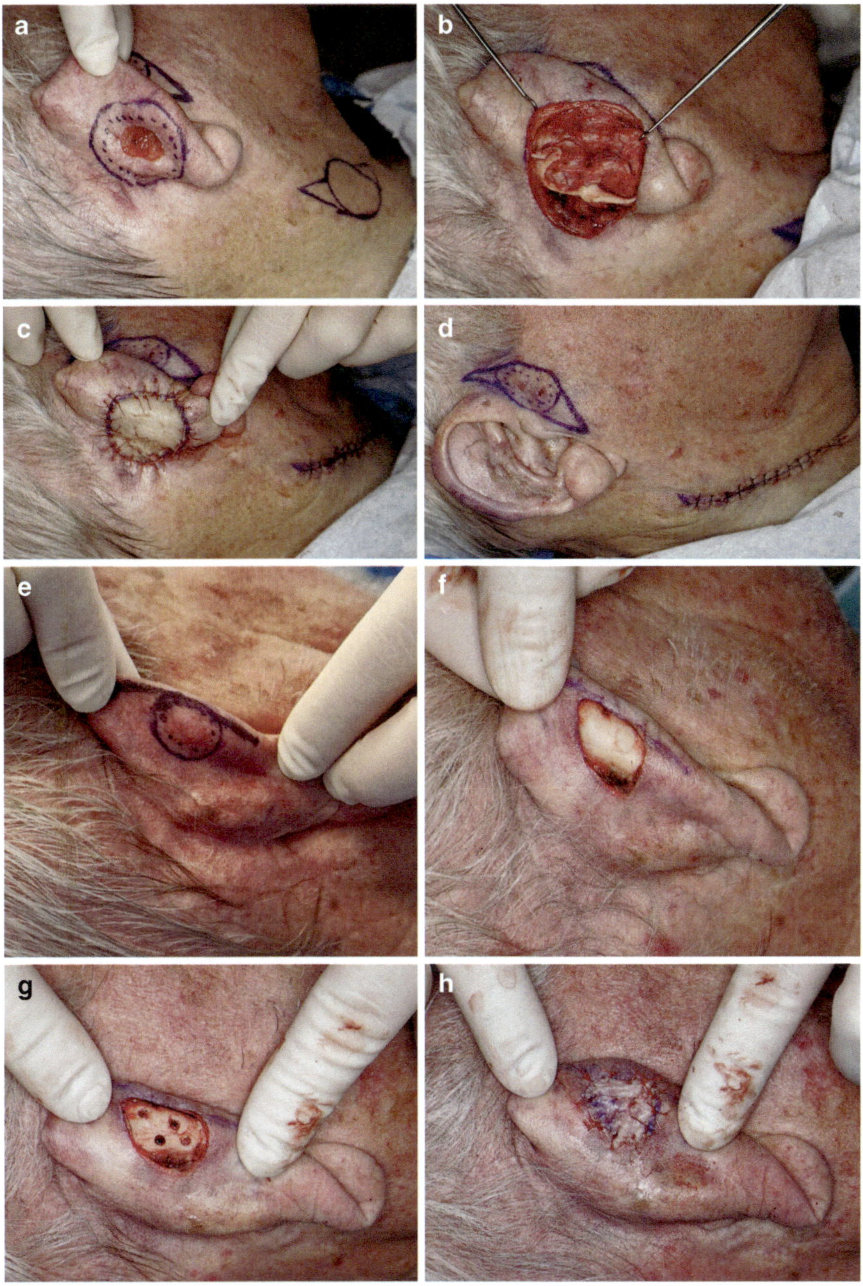

Fig. 9.15 Skin graft reconstruction. (**a**) Markings for excision and neck skin graft, (**b**) Excision defect, (**c**) Skin graft sutured and quilted in place, (**d**) Quilting sutures anterior surface and donar site closure, (**e**) Markings for excision, (**f**) Excision defect over bare cartilage, (**g**) Cartilage perforations with smal punch, (**h**) Skin graft quilted and sutured in place, (**i**) Appearance quilting from anterior surface

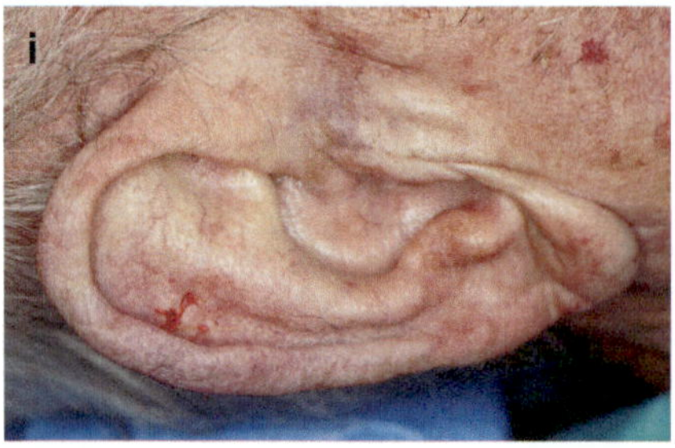

Fig. 9.15 (continued)

Advancement Flap

Indications: Medium/large defects.

Technique: Two parallel incisions are made from the superior and inferior margins of the defect and extended across the auriculocephalic sulcus onto the mastoid skin. The flap is initially raised above the perichondrium in the pinna and above the periosteum overlying the mastoid. The mobilised flap is suture into the defect in layers (Fig. 9.16a–c, d–g).

Tips: The difference in length of the flaps will have to be accommodated by differential suturing and any dog ears that results will have to be corrected. Additional subcutaneous sutures along the auriculocephalic sulcus will help prevent "tenting" of the flap. The reconstruction can interfere with the fit of a hearing aid and would have to be discussed with the patient.

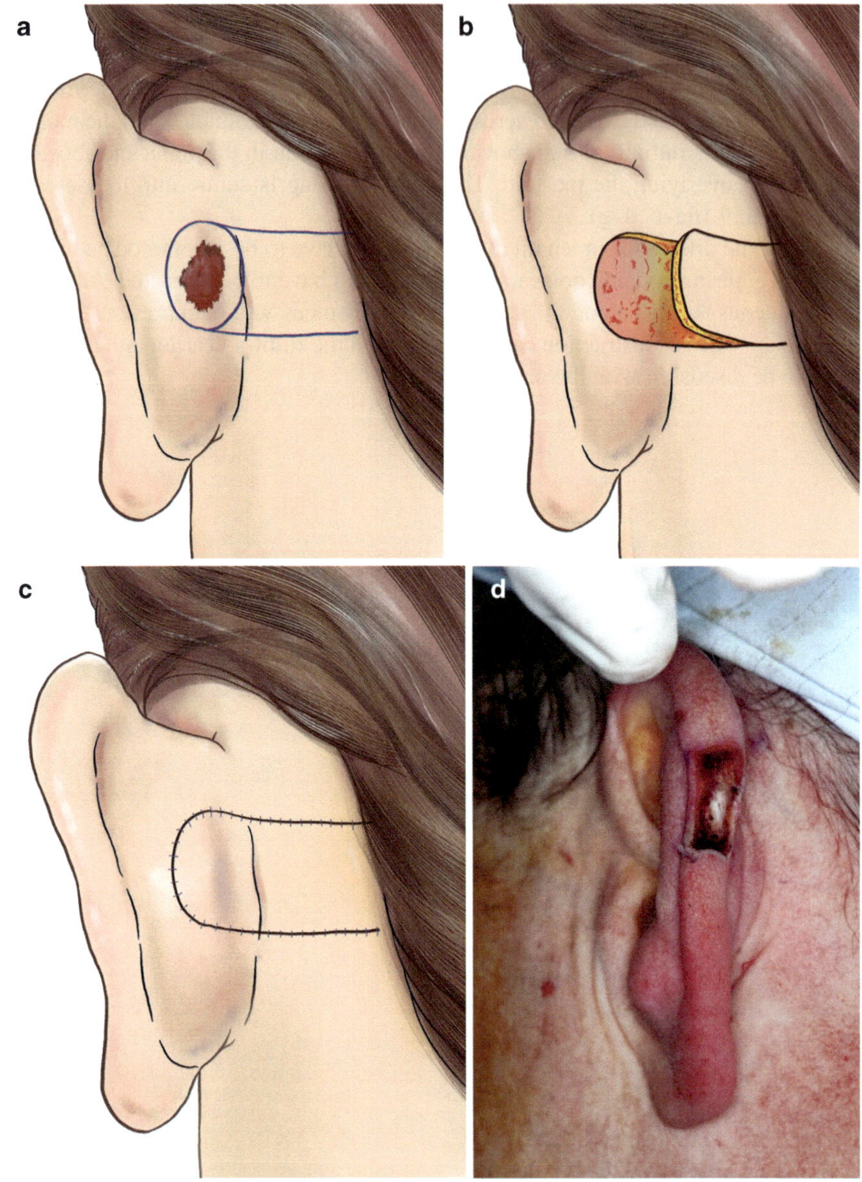

Fig. 9.16 Advancement flap. (**a**) Markings for excision and flap, (**b**) Excision defect and flap raised, (**c**) Final closure, (**d**) Excision defect, (**e**) Flap raised, (**f**) Final closure - posterior view, (**g**) Final closure - anterior view

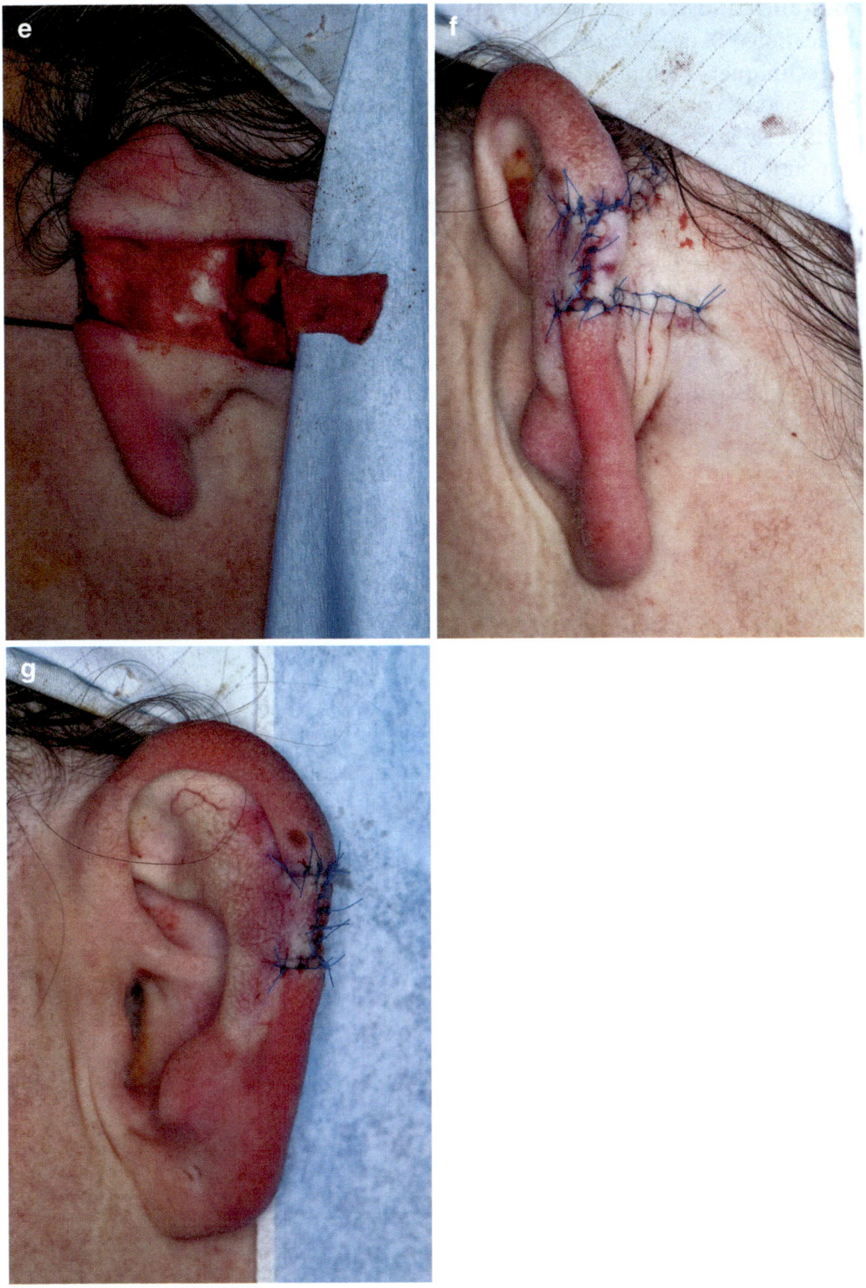

Fig. 9.16 (continued)

Post-auricular Transposition Flaps

Indications: Skin +/– cartilage defect.

Technique: A template is made to accurately reflect the defect and the dimensions marked out in the posterior auricular/mastoid skin. The flap can be raised on a superior or inferiorly based pedicle, consisting of skin, subcutaneous tissue and post-auricular muscle. The margins of the flap are incised down to periosteum, and the flap raised in the supra-periosteal plane. The secondary defect can be closed primarily by undermining the surrounding tissues. The transfer can be carried out as a single-stage or two-stage procedure, depending on the location and size of the defect (Fig. 9.17a–f, See also Fig. 9.11a–g).

Tips: The pinna might be "pinned" back when the secondary defect extends across the auriculocephalic sulcus. This can interfere with the fit of an existing hearing aid and would have to be discussed with the patient.

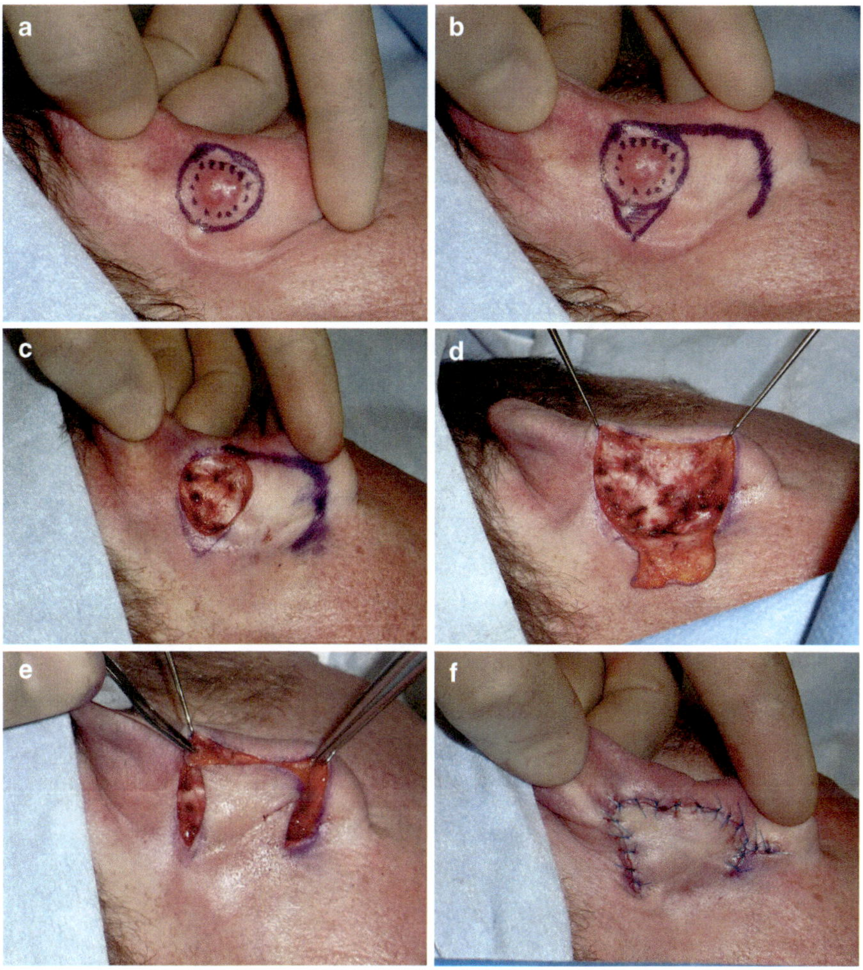

Fig. 9.17 Post auricular transposition flap. (**a**) Markings for excision, (**b**) Markings for excision and flap, (**c**) Excision defect, (**d**) Flap raised, (**e**) Flap transposed into defect, (**f**) Final closure

Rhombic Flap

Indications: Medium defects. For defects that are rhomboid or can be converted into a rhombus, the Limberg flap offers the advantage of utilising the skin laxity in the inferior aspect of the pinna.

Technique: Though technically four flaps can be raised for any given defect, it is often based inferiorly, determined by the tissue laxity and the orientation of the eventual scars. An incision is made by extending the short diagonal by a length equal to one side of the defect and a further incision is made from its extremity parallel to the adjacent side of the defect, again of equal length. The wound is closed in layers (Fig. 9.18a–d).

Tips: The amount of skin available in the adjacent area can be assessed using the "pinch test". With a rhomboid flap, some but not all the scars can be placed along the skin creases. It is often easier to close the secondary defect first followed by the primary defect. In the case of circular defects, it is not always necessary to remove additional tissue to convert the defect into a rhomboid.

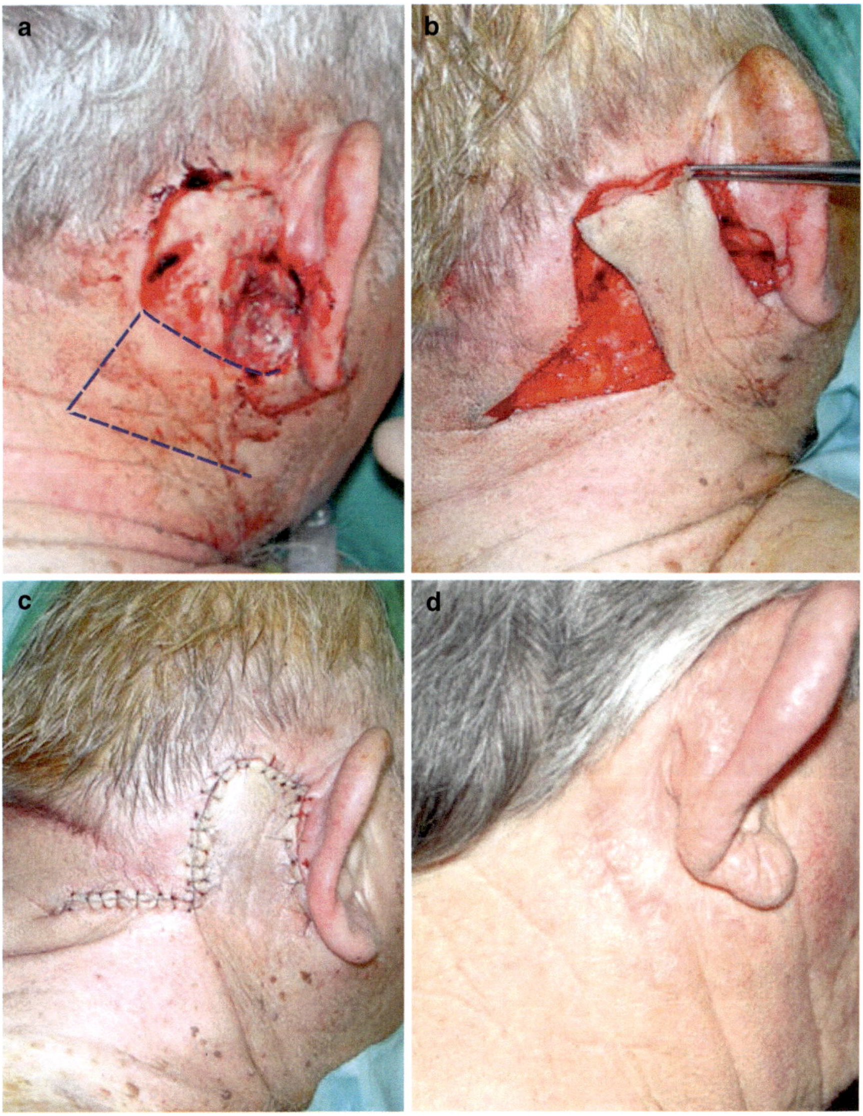

Fig. 9.18 Rhombic flap. (**a**) Excision defect and flap markings, (**b**) Flap transfered into defect, (**c**) Final closure, (**d**) Post operative appearance

Lobule

Primary Closure

Indications: Small/medium defects.

Technique: The lesion is excised with adequate margins and the defect modified into a triangle. Sufficient mobility is often present in the lobule, and the wound is closed in layers (Fig. 9.19a–c).

Tips: There is often a reduction in height and width of the lobule.

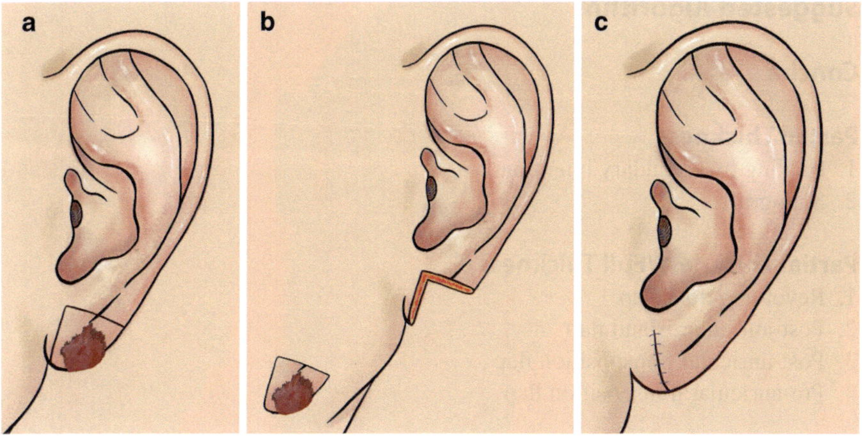

Fig. 9.19 Wedge excision and primary closure. (**a**) Markings for excision, (**b**) Excision defect, (**c**) Final closure

Suggested Algorithm

Concha

Partial Thickness

1. Healing by secondary intention
2. Skin graft

Partial Thickness/Full Thickness

1. Revolving door flap
2. Post-auricular island flap
3. Post-auricular transposition flap
4. Pre-auricular transposition flap

Antihelix/Helix

Partial Thickness

1. Healing by secondary intention (antihelix)
2. Skin graft (antihelix)

Full Thickness

1. Wedge excision
2. Helical rim advancement
3. Superiorly based pre-auricular flap
4. Two-stage post-auricular flap

Triangular Fossa

1. Healing by secondary intention
2. Skin graft
3. Superiorly based pre-auricular flap

Tragus

1. Superiorly based pre-auricular flap
2. Advancement flap

Posterior Surface of Pinna

1. Healing by secondary intention
2. Primary closure
3. Skin graft
4. Post-auricular advancement/transposition flap
5. Rhombic flap

Lobule

1. Primary closure

Cheek Defects

10

Subunits and Anatomical Considerations

The cheek is the largest aesthetic unit in the face. It has an undulating contour and is defined by the nasofacial, melolabial and mentolabial folds medially, infra-orbital rim and zygomatic arch superiorly, pinna and angle of the mandible posteriorly and the lower border of the mandible inferiorly. It can be divided into medial, buccal, infra-orbital, zygomatic, lateral and mandibular subunits (Fig. 10.1).

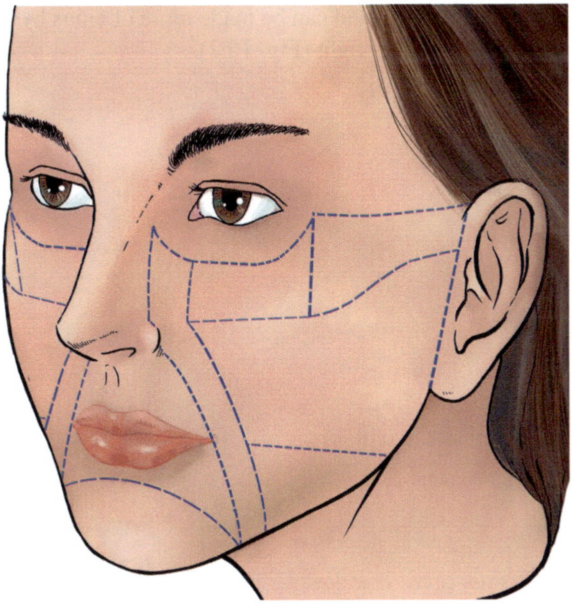

Fig. 10.1 Subunits of the cheek

V. Ilankovan et al., *Local Flaps in Facial Reconstruction*,
https://doi.org/10.1007/978-3-031-49464-2_10

The medial subunit consists of skin adjacent to the nasofacial, melolabial and mentolabial folds. The buccal subunit encompasses the central cheek area lateral to the medial unit. The infra-orbital unit represents the area below the lower eyelid. The lateral subunit is the area adjacent to the pinna and angle of the mandible. The zygomatic subunit is between the buccal, infra-orbital unit and temple and overlies the zygomatic prominence. The mandibular subunit encompasses the area overlying the body of the mandible.

The facial artery and vein course the cheek unit obliquely from the lower border of the mandible, just anterior to the insertion of the masseter muscle up to the medial canthus region. They lie deep to the muscles of facial expression. The branches of the facial nerve emerge from the anterior border of the parotid gland and supply the muscles of facial expression and lie on their deep surface. The nerve is relatively unprotected in the cheek and mandibular subunits. The infra-orbital nerve provides sensory supply to most of the cheek and emerges from the infra-orbital foramen, deep to the orbicularis oculi and levator labii superioris.

The skin in the subunits of the cheek varies in their characteristics. Reconstructive options should take into account adjacent tissue laxity and the likelihood of distorting the surrounding landmarks (eyelids, nose, lips and pinna).

Scars are best placed along the aesthetic borders, and consideration should be given to extending the defect, especially in the medial and lateral subunits. When this is inappropriate, scars are best designed to be parallel to the RSTL. The RSTLs in the cheeks are curvilinear or radially fan out from the lateral canthus area (crow's foot) and offer excellent camouflage for the scars. The skin creases are more prominent in the elderly and can be made more obvious by requesting the patient to smile and shut their eyes tight (Fig. 10.2).

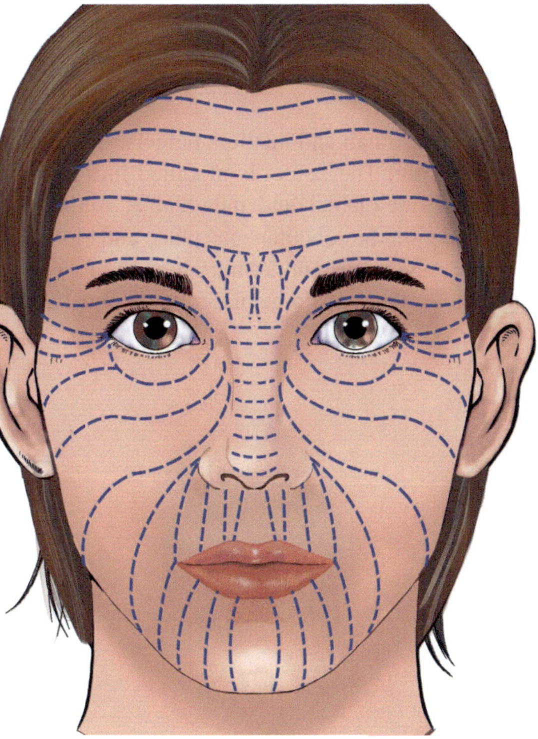

Fig. 10.2 Orientation of RSTL's in the cheek

Medial Subunit

Primary Closure

Indications: Small and medium defects.

Technique: The defect is modified into an ellipse to lie along the axis of the nasofacial, melolabial and mentolabial folds. The adjacent wound margins are undermined in the subcutaneous plane and closed in layers (Fig. 10.3a–c, d–f, g–i).

Tips: Asymmetric undermining, with greater undermining in the lateral aspect often allows the scars to be placed in the most advantageous position.

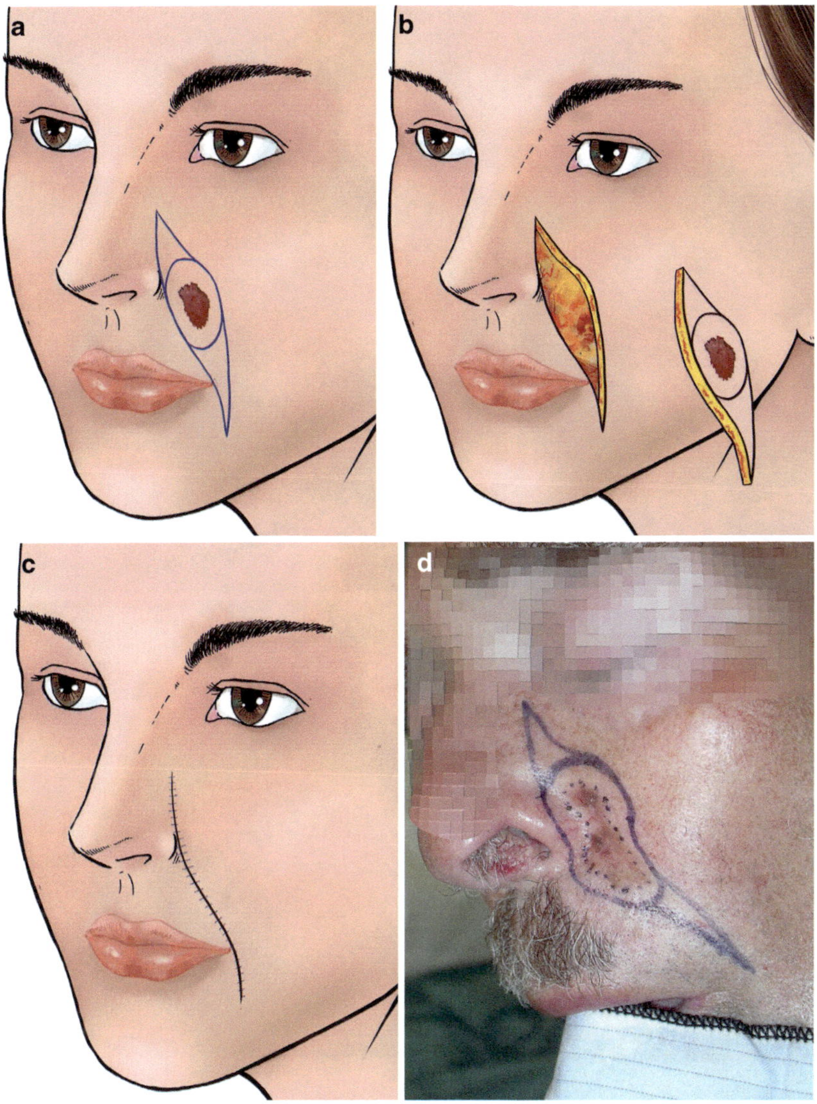

Fig. 10.3 Excision and primary closure. (**a**) Markings for excision, (**b**) Excision defect, (**c**) Final closure, (**d**) Markings for excision, (**e**) Excision defect, (**f**) Final closure, (**g**) Markings for excision, (**h**) Excision defect, (**i**) Final closure

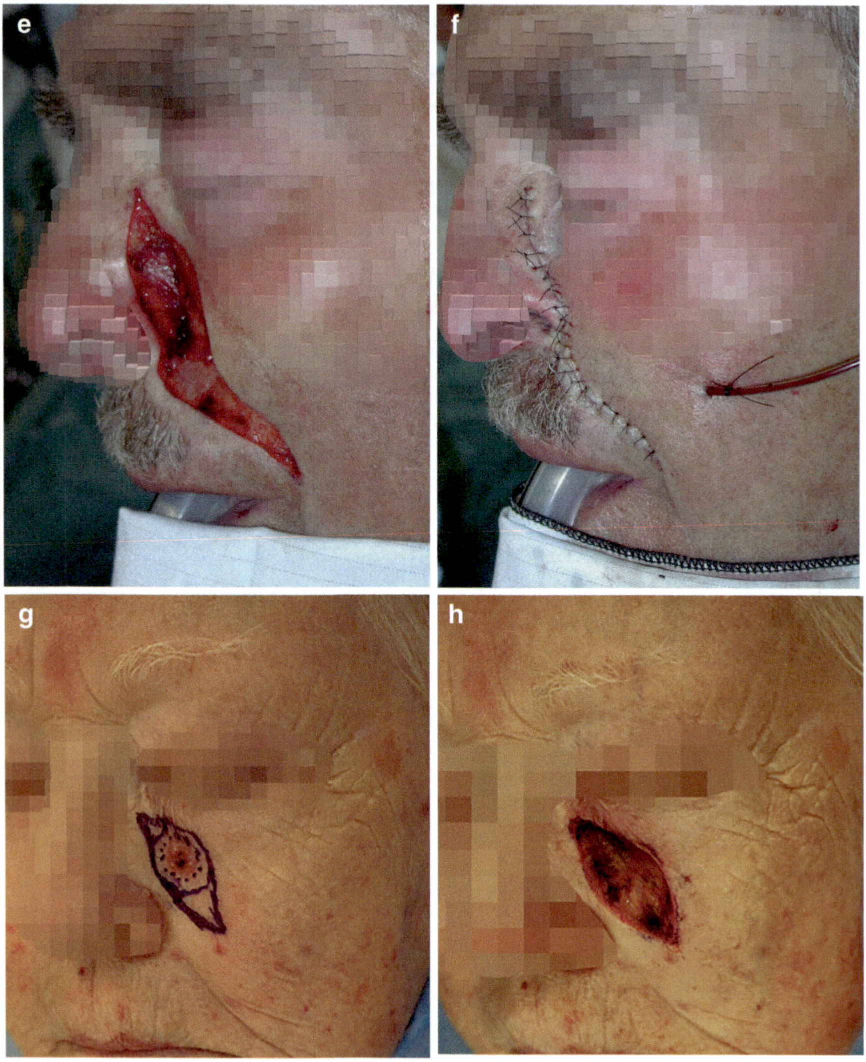

Fig. 10.3 (continued)

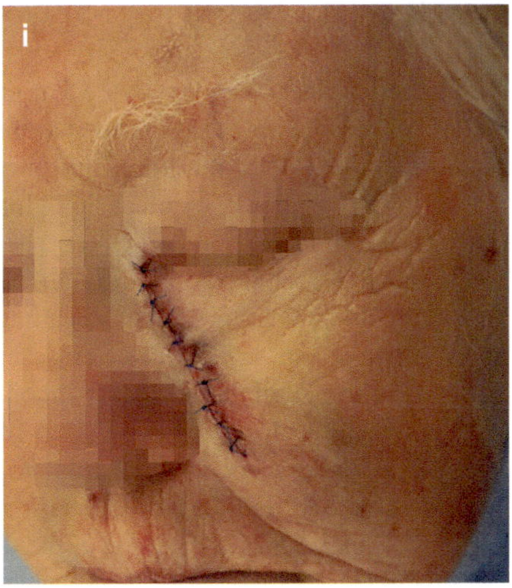

Fig. 10.3 (continued)

Island Advancement Flap

Indications: Small and medium defects adjacent to the alar facial, nasofacial folds.

Technique: The defect is modified to place the medial margins along the alar-facial/nasofacial fold and a parallel lateral margin. Curvilinear incisions are made from the superior and inferior margins of the defect, to delineate a triangular skin island, at least two to three times the length of the defect. The flap is oriented along the melolabial fold. The incision is deepened only through the skin along the entire outline of the flap. The central subcutaneous tissue, beneath the flap is preserved to provide the vascularity. The flap subcutaneous tissue closest and furthest from the defect is released incrementally to obtain the necessary mobility. The flap is mobilised into the defect, and the wound is closed in layers (Fig. 10.4a–c, d–i, j–o).

Tips: The defect can be enlarged to place the base along the alar-facial and nasofacial folds for best scar camouflage. For larger defects, the curvilinear incision should be made parallel to the cheek RSTLs. The size of the skin pedicle will determine the extent of safe subcutaneous dissection. It is mandatory to retain an adequate subcutaneous island pedicle, the size of which needs to take into account additional tissue release that might be required to obtain the necessary mobility.

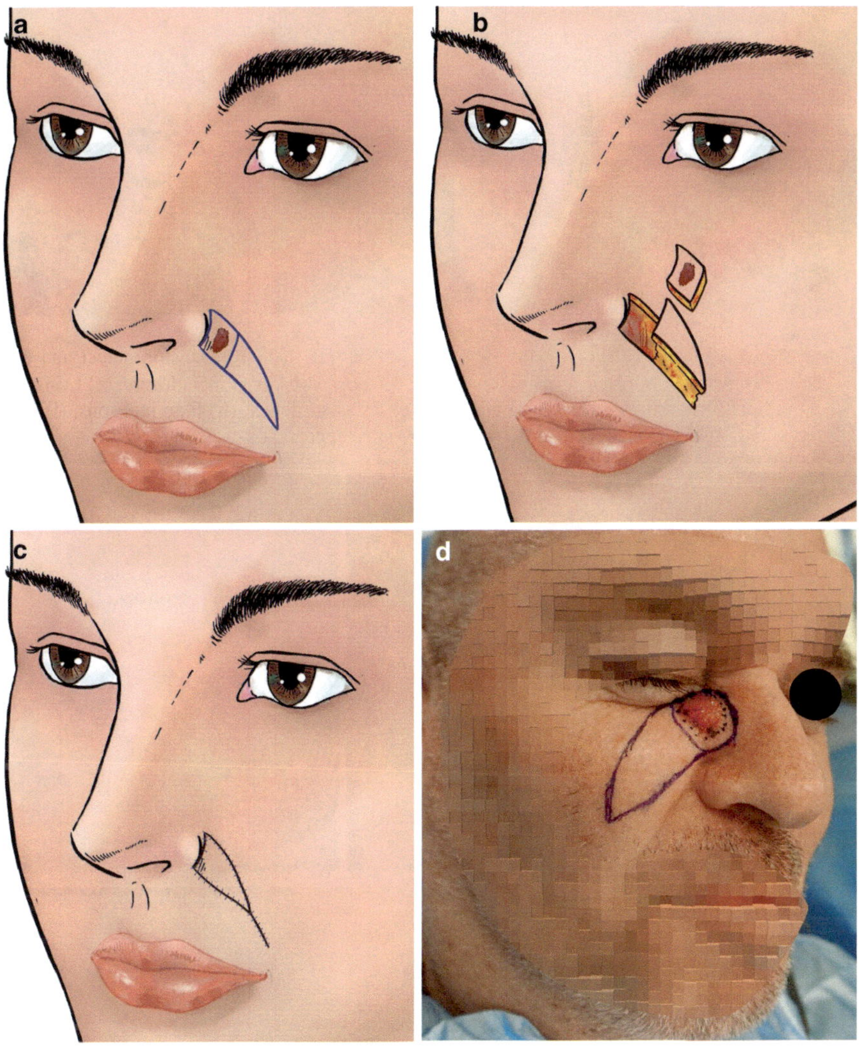

Fig. 10.4 Island advancement flap. (**a**) Markings for excision and flap, (**b**) Excision defect and flap raised, (**c**) Final closure, (**d**) Markings for excision and flap, (**e**) Excision defect, (**f**) Flap incision (**g**) Subcutaneous pedicle, (**h**) Final closure, (**i**) Post operative appearance, (**j**) Markings for excision and flap, (**k**) Excision defect and flap raised, (**l**) Flap mobilised into defect, (**m**) Final closure, (**n**) markings for excision and flap, (**o**) Final closure

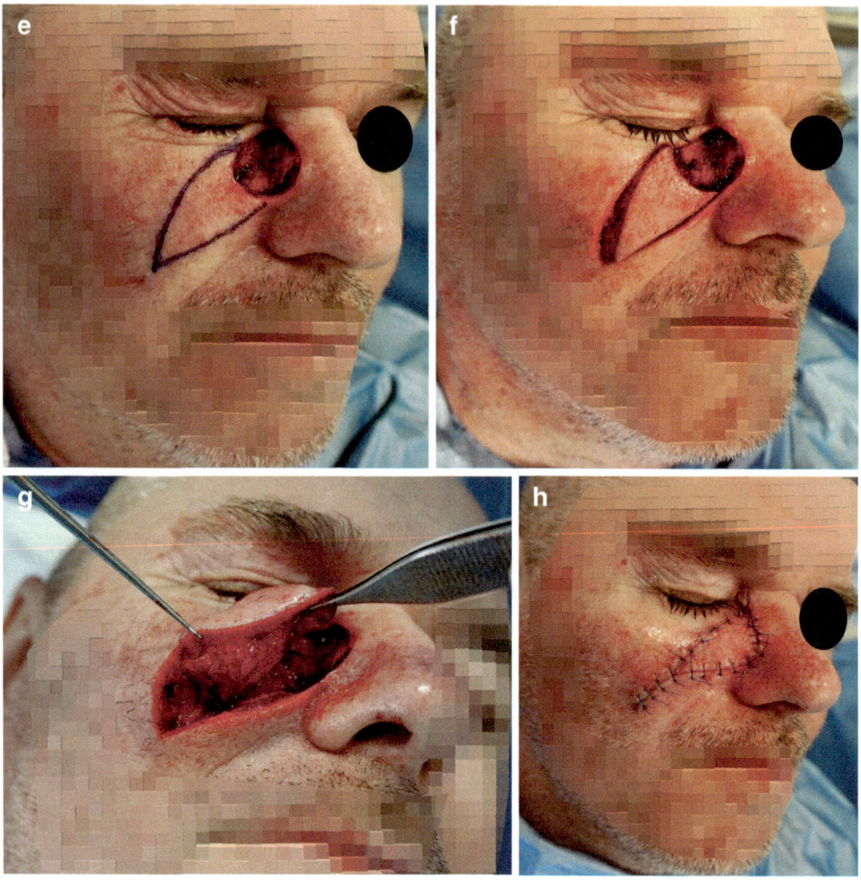

Fig. 10.4 (continued)

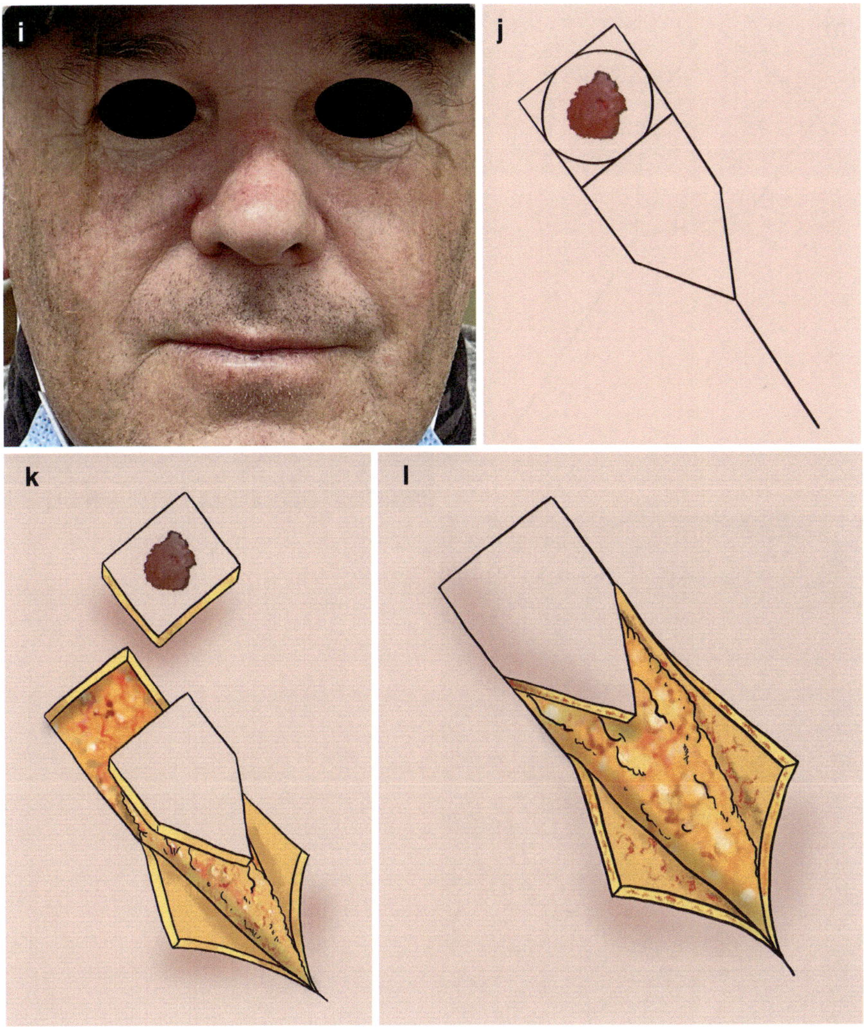

Fig. 10.4 (continued)

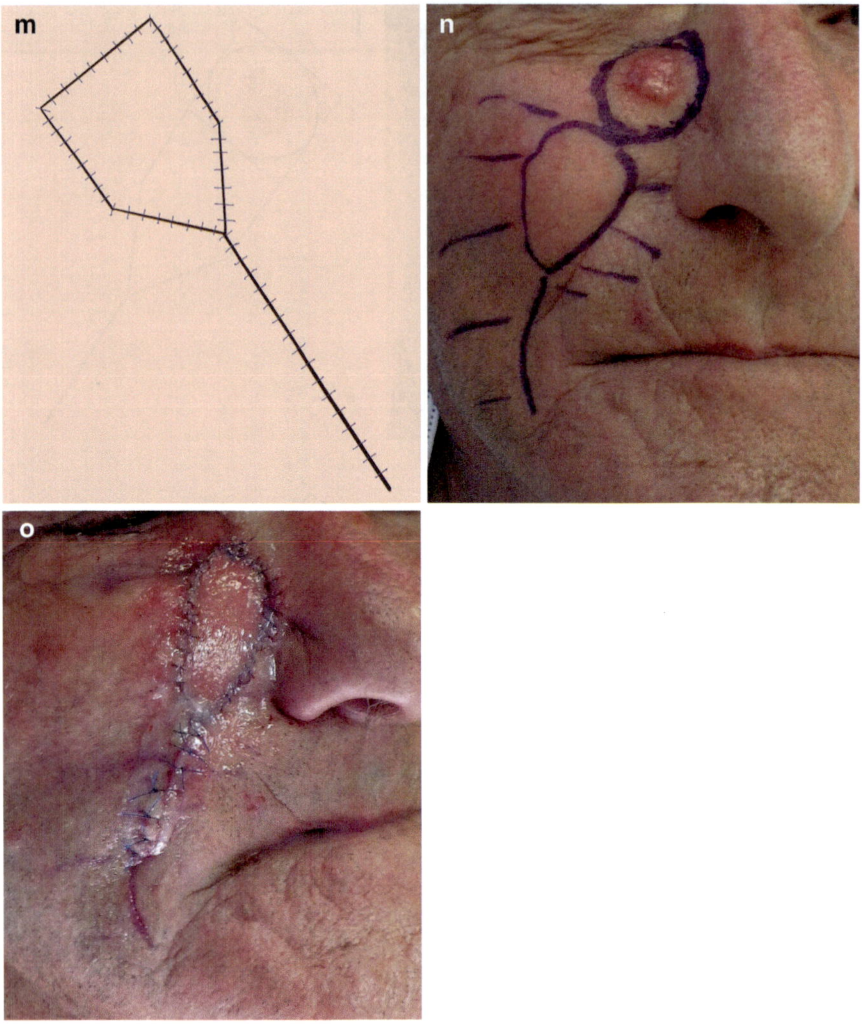

Fig. 10.4 (continued)

Buccal Subunit

Primary Closure

Indications: Small and medium defects.

Technique: The defect is modified into an ellipse to lie along the axis of the cheek RSTLs (Fig. 2). The adjacent wound margins are undermined in the subcutaneous plane and closed in layers (Fig. 10.5a–c).

Tips: Fairly large defects can be closed primarily, especially in the elderly with skin laxity. Care should be taken to avoid damage to the facial nerve.

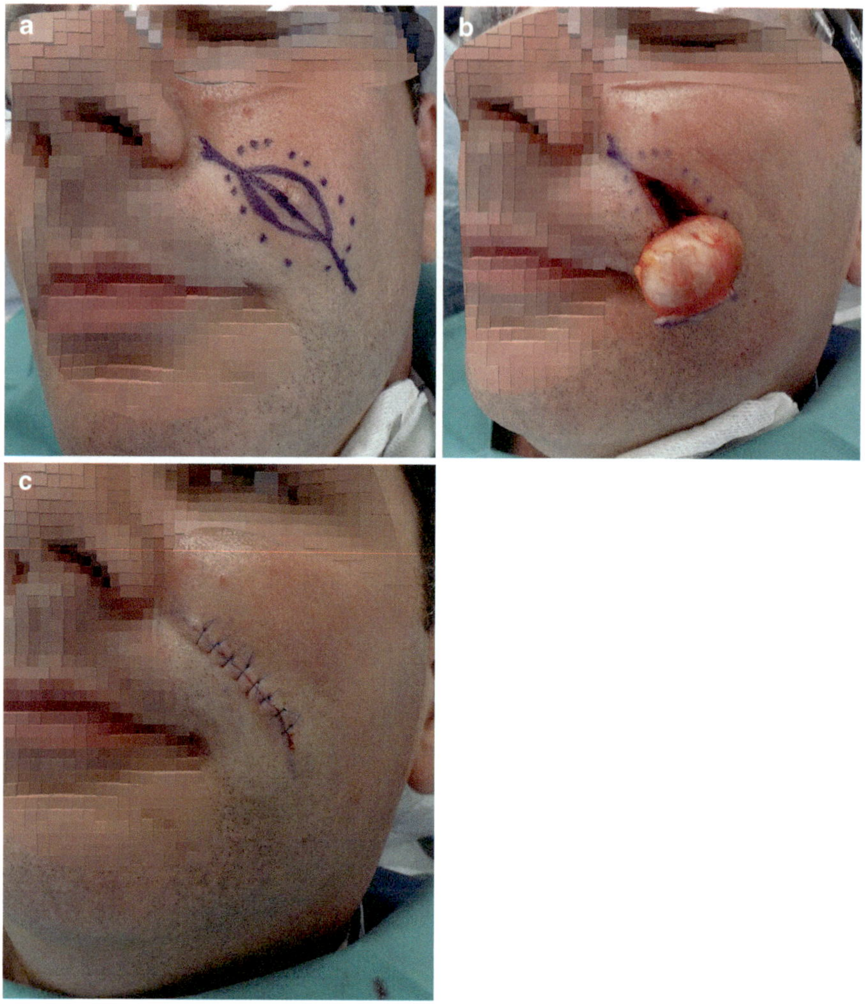

Fig. 10.5 Excision and primary closure. (**a**) Markings for excision, (**b**) Excision defect, (**c**) Final closure

Rhombic Flap

Indications: Medium-sized defects.

Technique: The defect is modified into a rhombus with 60° and 120° internal angles. A rhomboid flap is designed by extending the short diagonal to a distance equal to one of the sides, and a further line is drawn from its extremity, parallel to the adjacent side of the defect. The flap is raised in the subcutaneous plane and mobilised into the defect. The wound is closed in layers (Fig. 10.6a–c).

Tips: Given the design of the rhombic flaps, it will not be possible to align all the scars along the RSTL. Four flaps can be designed for any given defect, and the ideal one is chosen based on tissue laxity, best orientation of scars and avoiding distortion of adjacent landmarks.

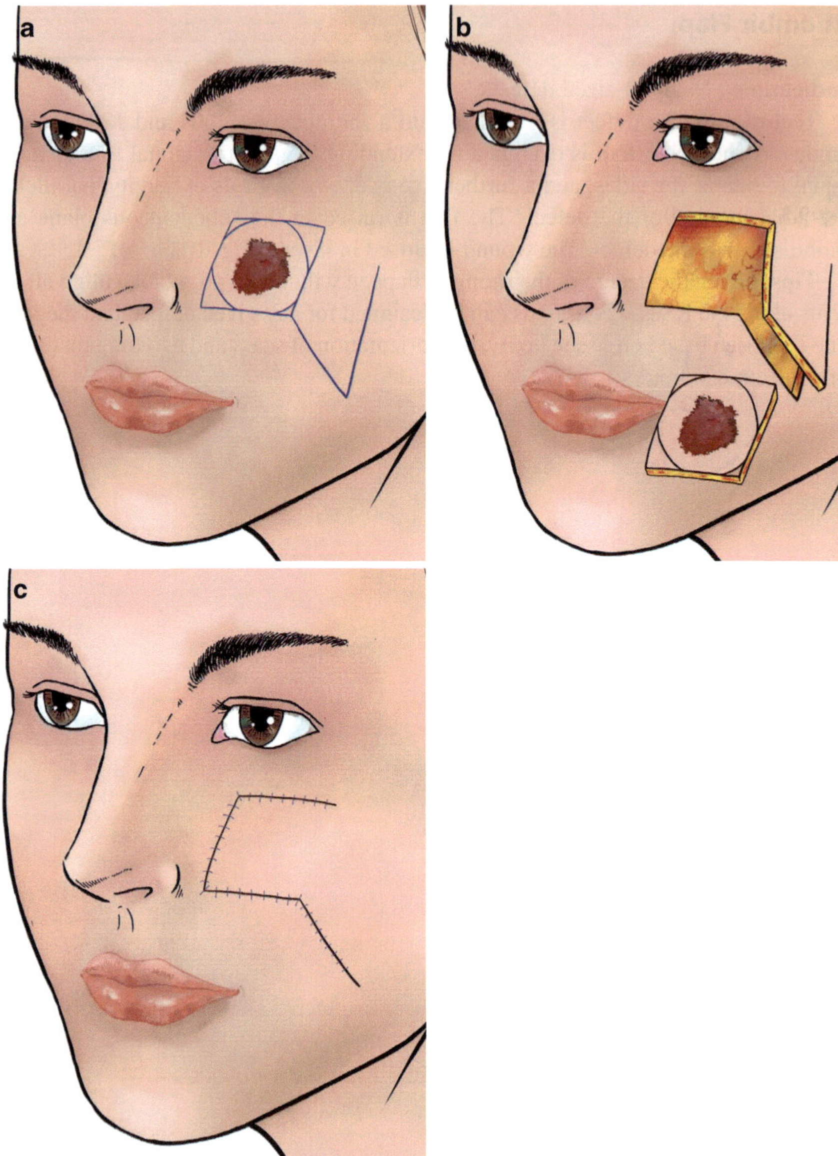

Fig. 10.6 Rhombic flap. (**a**) Markings for excision and flap, (**b**) Excision defect and flap raised, (**c**) Final closure

Laterally Based Rotation/Transposition Flap

Indications: Medium/large defects medial, buccal, infra-orbital subunits.

Technique: The defect is modified into a triangle, with the medial border along the nasofacial/melolabial fold and the base superiorly. A curvilinear incision is made from the base of the defect laterally, along the infra-orbital/crow's feet skin creases, with an "exaggerated" superior extension. The lateral/inferior extension is dictated by the size of the required flap and follows the pre-auricular skin crease. The flap is raised in the subcutaneous plane and mobilised into the defect. Any dog ears that develop are corrected along the melolabial fold. The wound is sutured in layers and a drain inserted as required (Fig. 10.7a–d, e–h).

Tips: The exaggerated superior extension is necessary to decrease the risk of ectropion. If a large flap is raised, additional "anchoring/suspension" sutures should be placed from the deep surface of the flap to the periosteum overlying the zygoma/zygomatic arch, to prevent flap decent and ectropion. A McGregor type "Z" plasty can also be incorporated to reduce the risk of ectropion (Fig. 10.7i–l). The flap can be extended inferiorly into a neck skin crease (cervicofacial) or even past the clavicle (thoraco-cervicofacial) if required (See Fig. 6.18). The cervical extension can be placed behind the lobule of the ear and close to the hairline to camouflage the scars.

When extending into the neck, the plane of dissection is in the supra-platysmal plane. If dissection is undertaken deep to the platysma, care should be taken to avoid damage to the mandibular branch of the facial nerve.

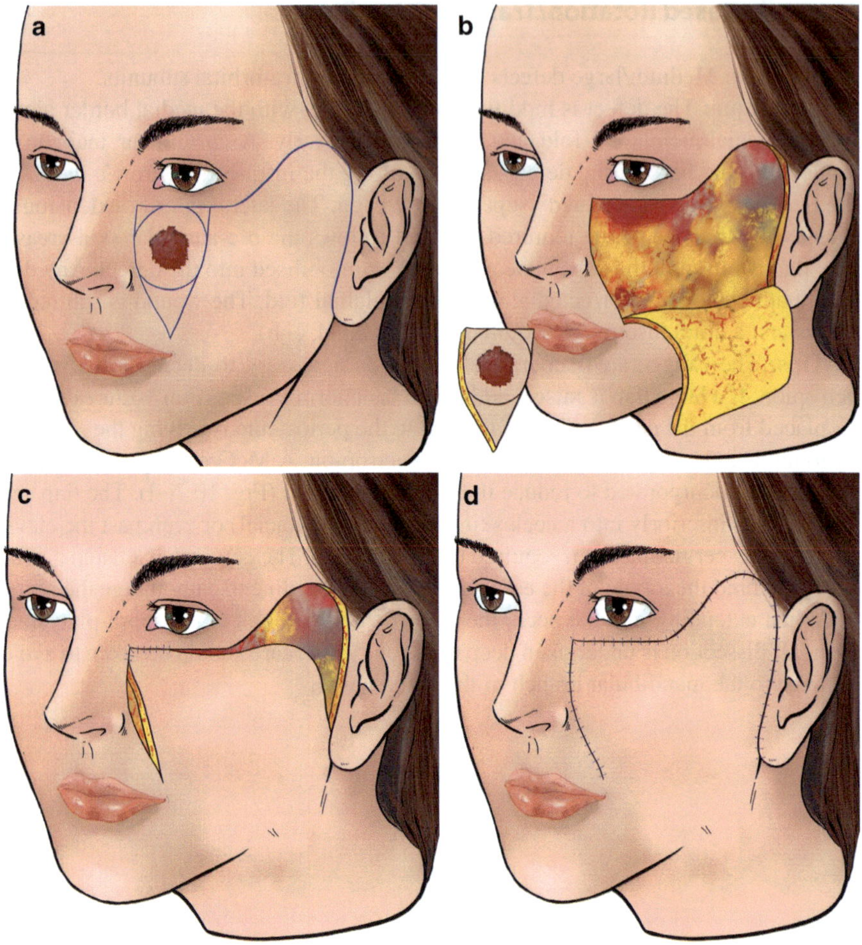

Fig. 10.7 Laterally based rotation/transposition flap. (**a**) Markings for excision and flap, (**b**) Excision defect and flap raised, (**c**) Flap mobilised into defect, (**d**) Final closure, (**e**) Markings for excision and flap, (**f**) Markings for excision and flap (lateral view), (**g**) Final closure, (**h**) Final closure (lateral view), (**i**) Lesion cheek, (**j**) Markings for excision and flap, (**k**) Excision defect, (**l**) Final closure

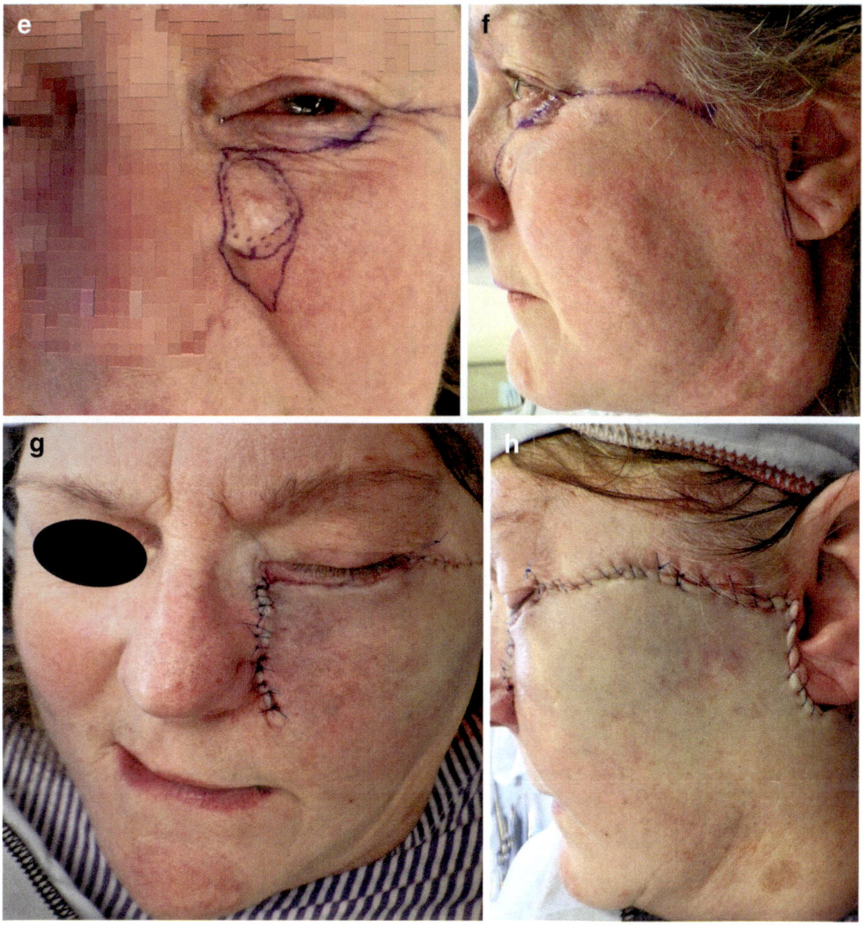

Fig. 10.7 (continued)

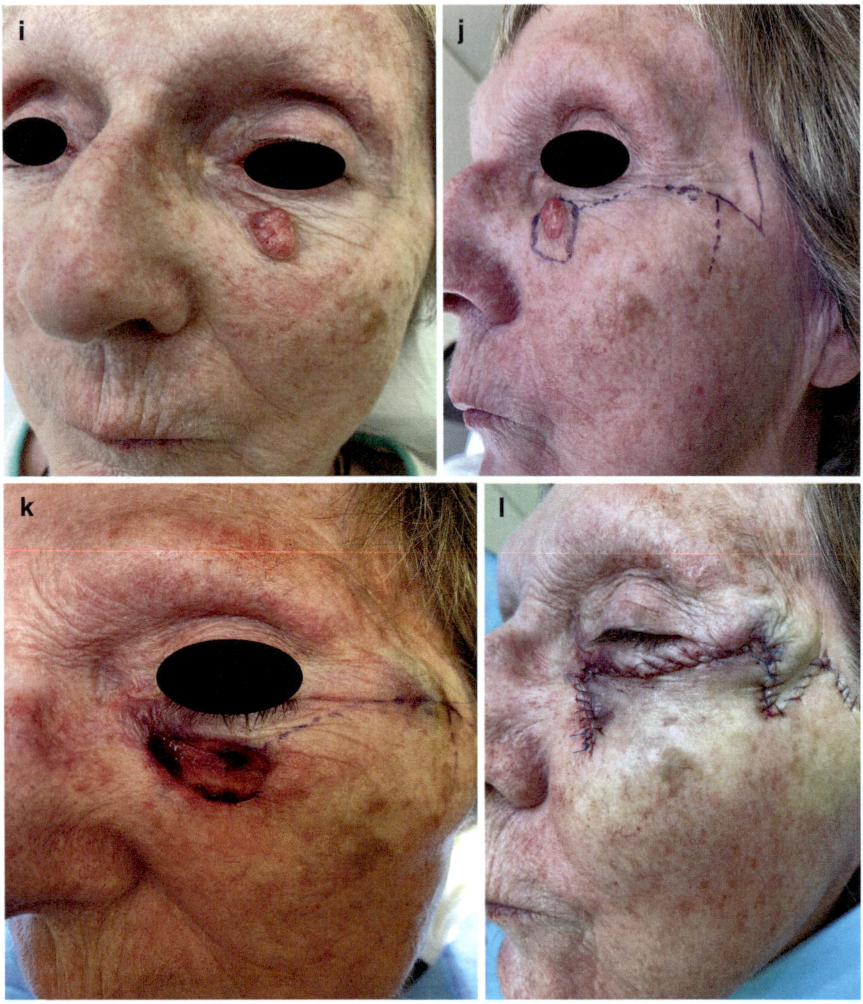

Fig. 10.7 (continued)

Inferiorly Based Rotation Advancement Flap

Indications: Medium-sized defects, medial cheek, superior buccal.

Technique: The defect is converted into a triangle, with the base along the nasofacial sulcus. An incision is made inferiorly from the base of the defect along the nasofacial, melolabial and mentolabial folds. The skin flap is raised in the subcutaneous plane, till the required mobility is obtained. Meticulous haemostasis is obtained, the flap moved into the defect, and the wound is closed in layers. A drain is inserted as required. Any dog ear is excised along the infra-orbital skin crease and the mentolabial fold (Fig. 10.8a–c, d–h).

Tips: Additional tissue can be excised medially to place the suture line along the nasofacial folds. Anchoring sutures in the region of the zygomatic prominence are placed, when a large flap is raised. Care must be taken to avoid tension in the lower eyelid, to prevent ectropion. The flap can be extended into the neck if required. The extent of inferior extension is determined by the size of the defect and tissue laxity in the "jowl" area. This can be assessed by the "pinch" test. "Z" plasties can be incorporated in the neck extension to prevent bowstringing across the cervicofacial junction.

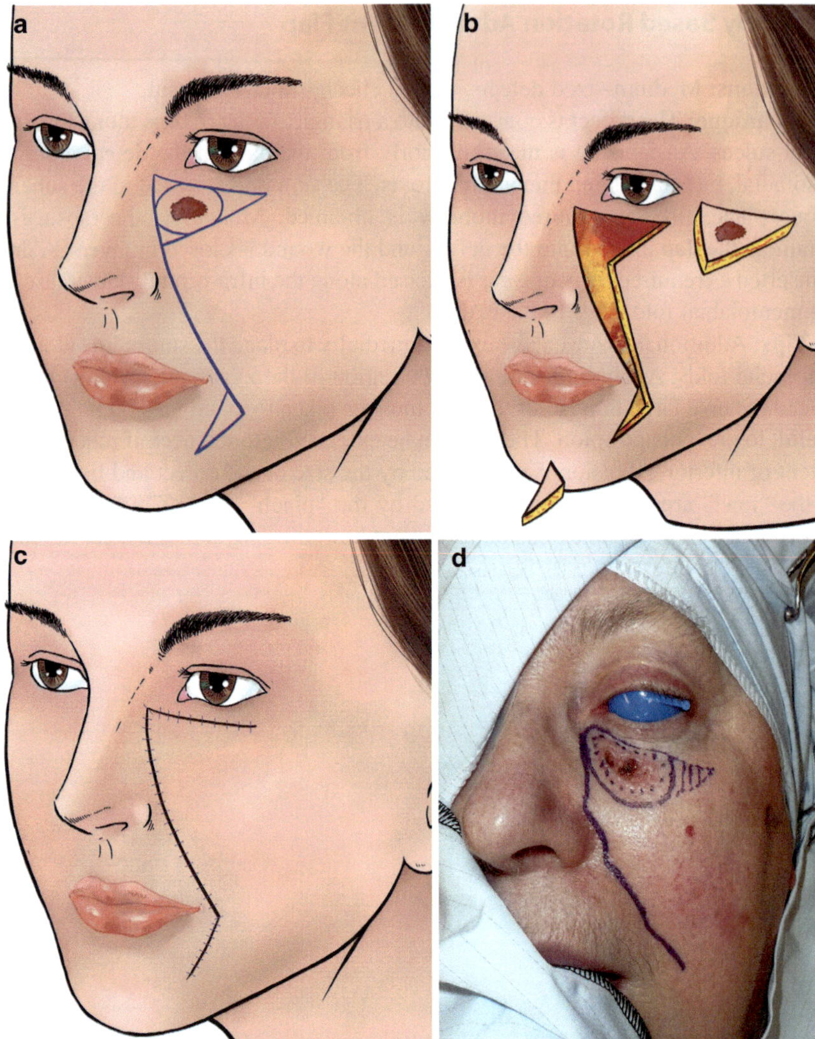

Fig. 10.8 Inferiorly based rotation/advancement flap. (**a**) Markings for excision and flap, (**b**) Excision defect and flap raised, (**c**) Final closure, (**d**) Markings for excision and flap, (**e**) Excision defect, (**f**) Flap raised, (**g**) Flap mobilised into defect, (**h**) Final closure

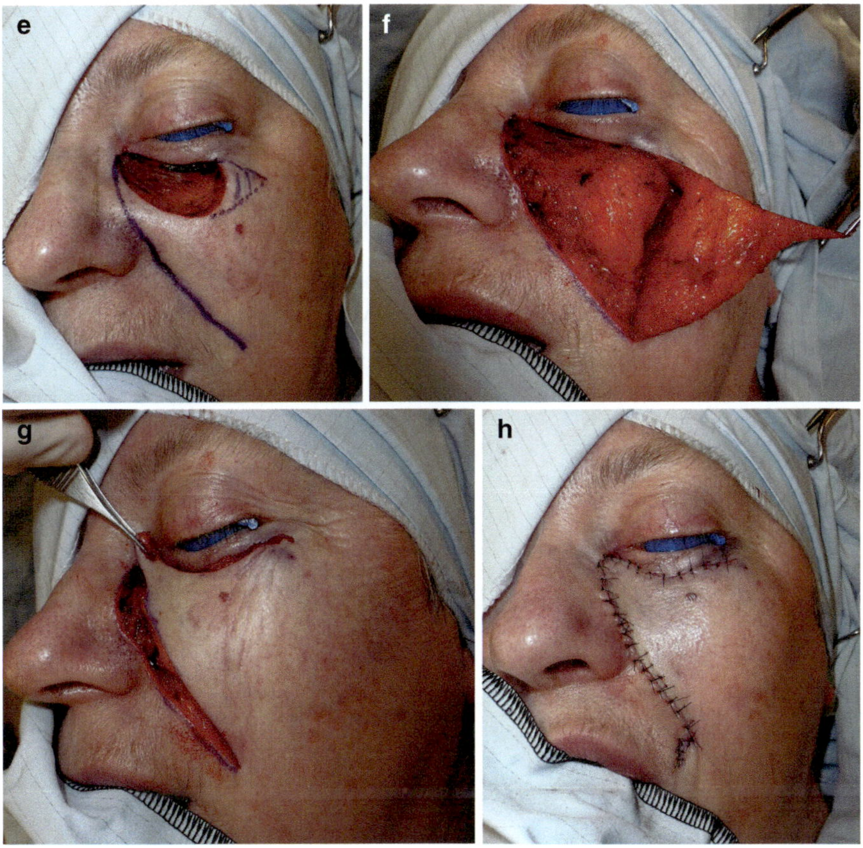

Fig. 10.8 (continued)

Zygomatic Subunit

Primary Closure

Indications: Small defect.

Technique: The defect is modified into an ellipse to lie along the axis of RSTLs (Fig. 10.2). The adjacent wound margins are undermined in the subcutaneous plane and closed in layers (Fig. 10.9a–c).

Tips: The patient can be requested to shut their eye tight and give a smile to identify skin creases. Care should be taken to avoid damage to the facial nerve.

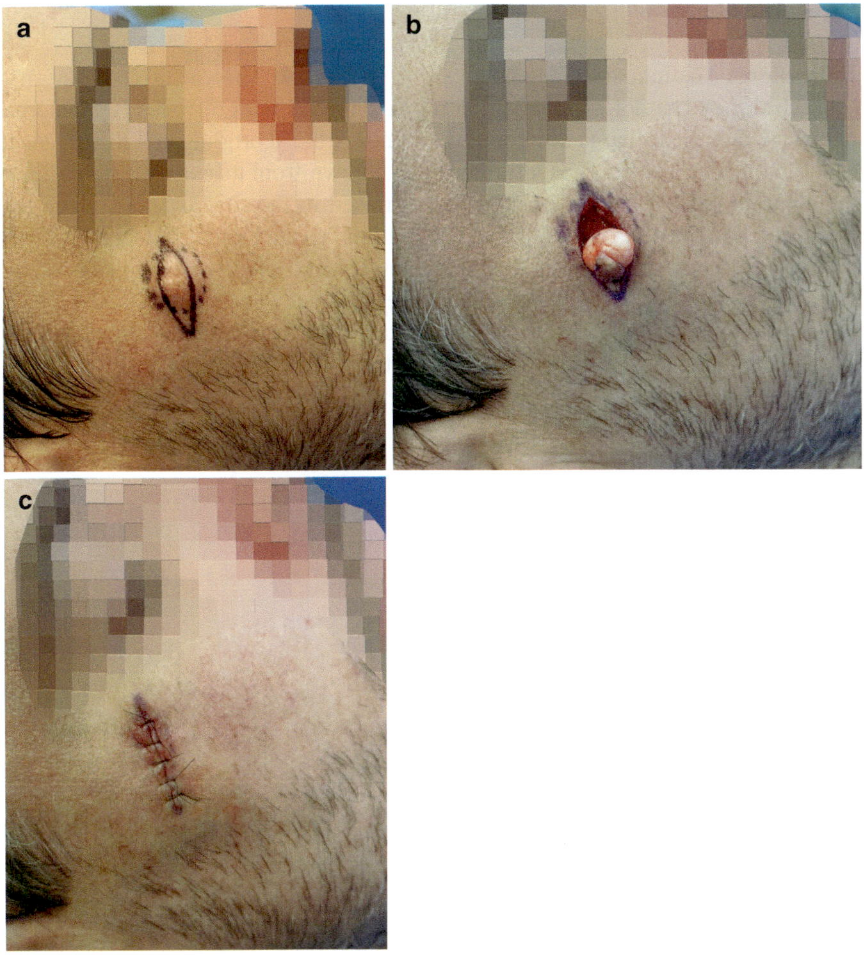

Fig. 10.9 Excision and primary closure. (**a**) Markings for excision, (**b**) Excision defect, (**c**) Final closure

Rhombic Flap

Indications: Medium-sized defects.

Technique: The defect is modified into a rhombus with 60° and 120° internal angles. A rhomboid flap is designed by extending the short diagonal to a distance equal to one of the sides, and a further line is drawn from its extremity, parallel to the adjacent side of the defect. The flap is raised in the subcutaneous plane and mobilised into the defect. The wound is closed in layers (Fig. 10.10a–c, d–f).

Tips: Given the design of the rhombic flaps, it will not be possible to align all the scars along the RSTL. Four flaps can be designed for any given defect, and the ideal one is chosen based on tissue laxity, best orientation of scars and avoiding distortion of adjacent landmarks. A superiorly based lateral flap often works best for a zygomatic defect.

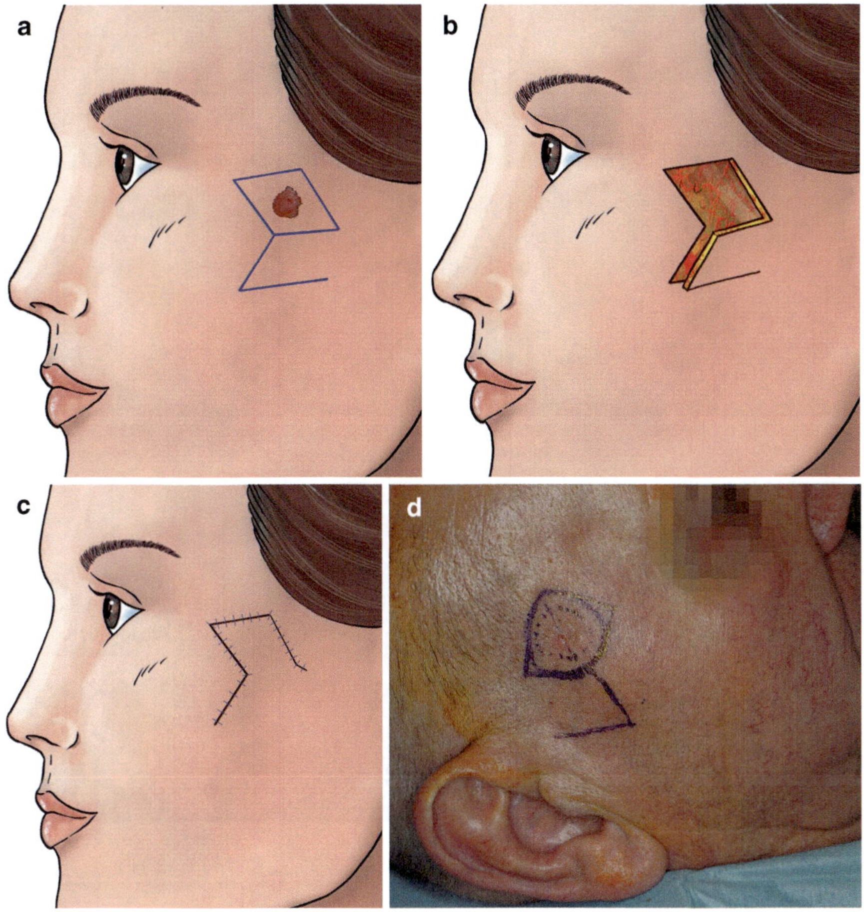

Fig. 10.10 Rhombic flap. (**a**) Markings for excision and flap, (**b**) Excision defect and flap raised, (**c**) Final closure, (**d**) Markings for excision and flap, (**e**) Excision defect and flap incision, (**f**) Flaps raised, (**g**) Flap transposed and closure od secondary defect, (**h**) Final closure

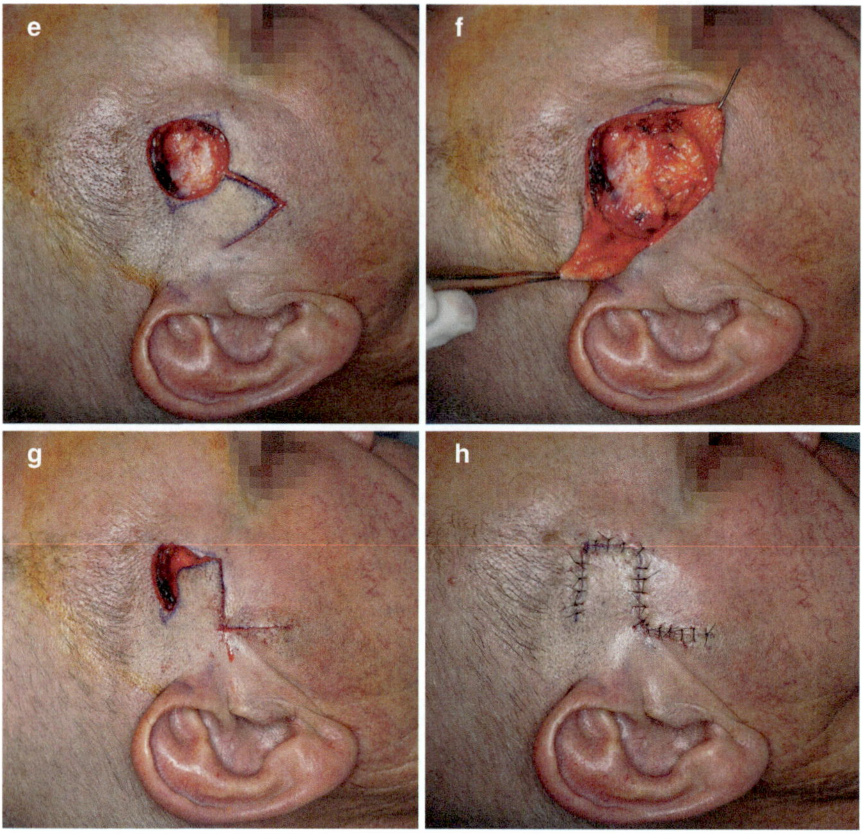

Fig. 10.10 (continued)

Rotation/Transposition Flap

Indications: Medium and large defects.

Technique: The defect is modified into a triangle, with the base superiorly. A curvilinear incision is made from the base of the defect laterally up to the pre-auricular skin crease and extended inferiorly along it. The flap is raised in the sub-cutaneous plane and mobilised into the defect. Any dog ears that develop are corrected along the cheek RSTLs. The wound is sutured in layers, and a drain inserted as required (Fig. 10.11a–g).

Tips: The exaggerated superior extension of the lateral limb and additional "anchoring/suspension" sutures placed from the deep surface of the flap to the periosteum overlying the zygoma/zygomatic arch are helpful to prevent flap decent and ectropion. The flap can be extended inferiorly into a neck skin crease (cervicofacial) or even past the clavicle (thoraco-cervicofacial) if required. The cervical extension can be placed behind the lobule of the ear and close to the hairline to camouflage the scars.

When extending into the neck, the plane of dissection is in the supra-platysmal plane. If dissection is undertaken deep to the platysma, care should be taken to avoid damage to the mandibular branch of the facial nerve.

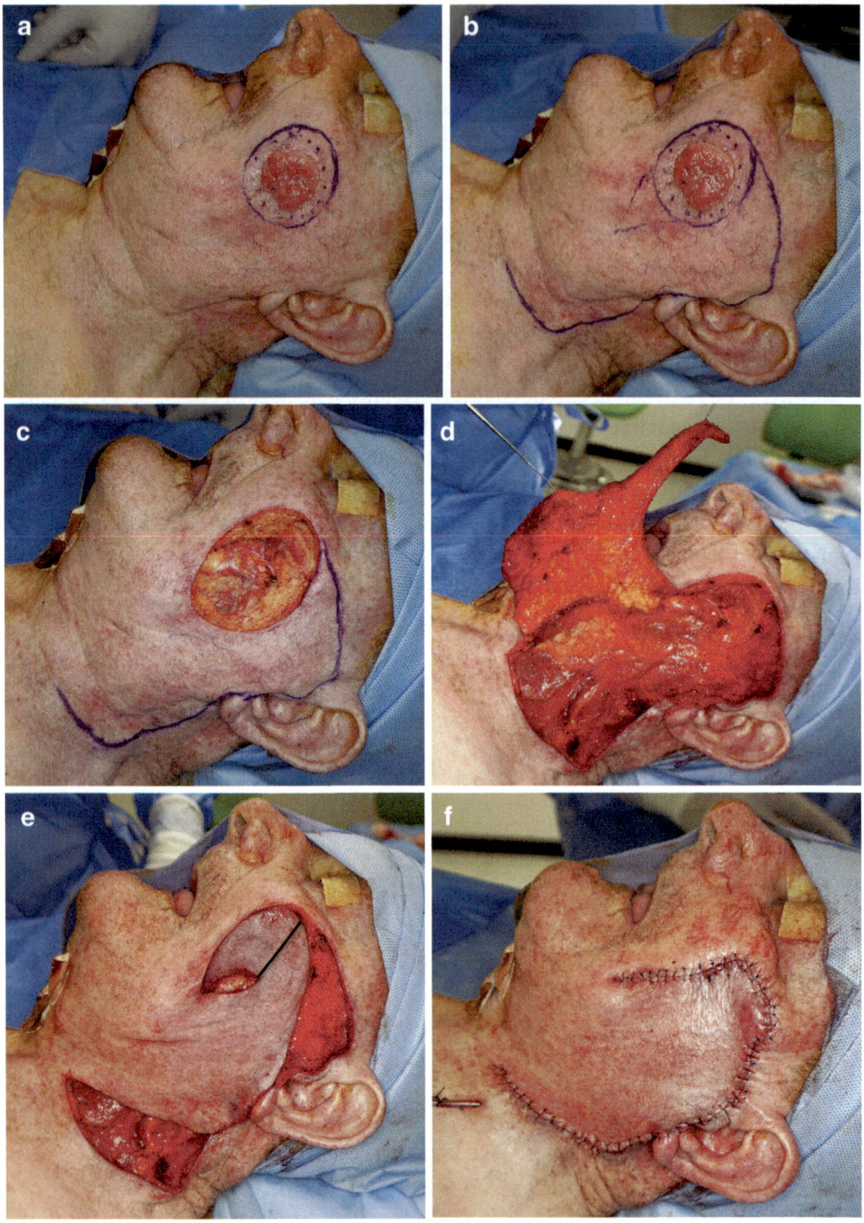

Fig. 10.11 Rotation/transposition flap. (**a**) Markings for excision, (**b**) Markings for excision and flap, (**c**) Excision defect, (**d**) Flap raised, (**e**) Flap transposed into defect/ excess tissue marked for trimming, (**f**) Final closure, (**g**) Post operative appearance

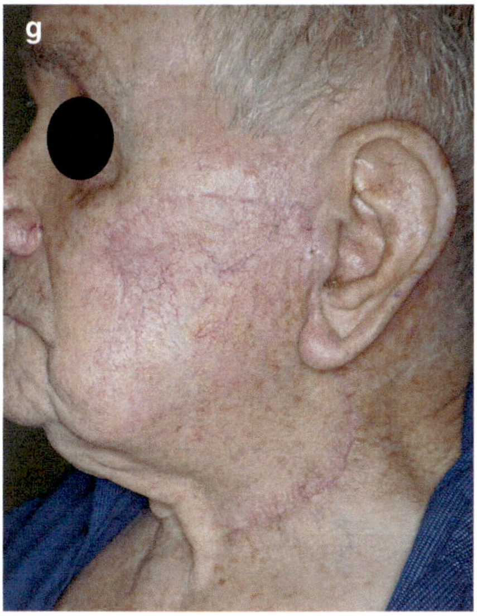

Fig. 10.11 (continued)

Island Advancement Flap

Indications: Small and medium defects.

Technique: The defect is modified to have a straight leading edge adjacent to the flap. Curvilinear incisions are made from the superior and inferior margins of the defect, to delineate a triangular skin island, at least two to three times the length of the defect. These incisions are oriented along the RSTL. The incision is deepened only through the skin along the entire outline of the flap. The central subcutaneous tissue, beneath the flap is preserved to provide the vascularity. The flap subcutaneous tissue closest and furthest from the defect is released incrementally to obtain the necessary mobility. The flap is mobilised into the defect, and the wound is closed in layers (Fig. 10.12a–f).

Tips: The curvilinear incision should be made parallel to the cheek RSTLs. The size of the skin pedicle will determine the extent of safe subcutaneous dissection. It is mandatory to retain an adequate subcutaneous island pedicle, the size of which needs to take into account additional tissue release that might be required to obtain the necessary mobility.

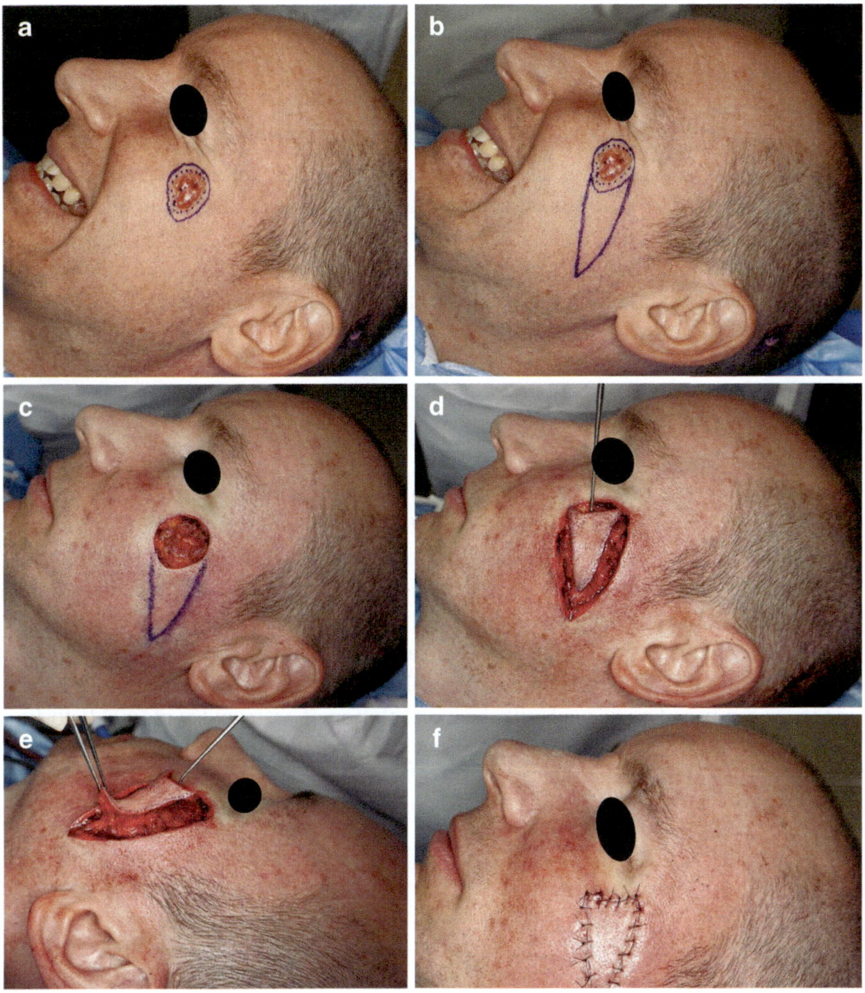

Fig. 10.12 Island advancement flap. (**a**) Markings for excision, (**b**) Markings for excision and flap, (**c**) Excision defect, (**d**) Flap mobilised into defect, (**e**) Sub cutaneous pedicle, (**f**) Final closure

Mandibular Subunit

Primary Closure

Indications: Small and medium defects.

Technique: The defect is modified into an ellipse to lie along the axis of the cheek RSTLs (Fig. 10.2). The adjacent wound margins are undermined in the subcutaneous plane and closed in layers.

Tips: Fairly large defects can be closed primarily, especially in the elderly with skin laxity. Care should be taken to avoid damage to the facial nerve.

Rhombic Flap

Indications: Medium-sized defects.

Technique: The defect is modified into a rhombus with 60° and 120° internal angles. A rhomboid flap is designed by extending the short diagonal to a distance equal to one of the sides and a further line is drawn from its extremity, parallel to the adjacent side of the defect. The flap is raised in the subcutaneous plane and mobilised into the defect. The wound is closed in layers (Fig. 10.13a–d, e–p).

Tips: Given the design of the rhombic flaps, it will not be possible to align all the scars along the RSTL. Four flaps can be designed for any given defect, and the ideal one is chosen based on tissue laxity, best orientation of scars and avoiding distortion of adjacent landmarks. An inferiorly based lateral flap often works best for a mandibular subunit defect.

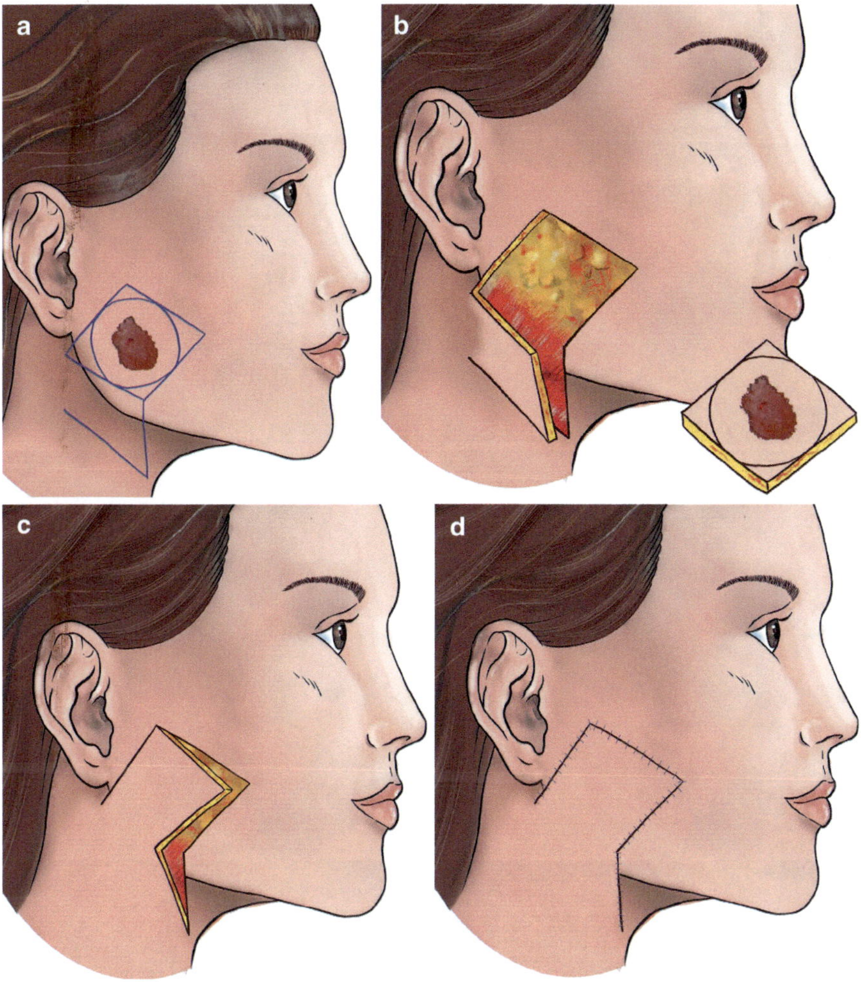

Fig. 10.13 Rhombic flap. (**a**) Markings for excision and flap, (**b**) Excision defect and flap raised, (**c**) Flap transposed into defect, (**d**) Final closure, (**e**) Lesion for excision, (**f**) Markings for excision and flap, (**g**) Excision defect and flap raised, (**h**) Trial transposition of flap, (**i**) Undermining of margins, (**j**) Initial closure of secondary defect, (**k**) Flap transposed into defect, (**l**) Adjustment of margins, (**m**) Delineation of dog ear, (**n**) Incision across base, (**o**) Excess tissue marked for excision, (**p**) Final closure

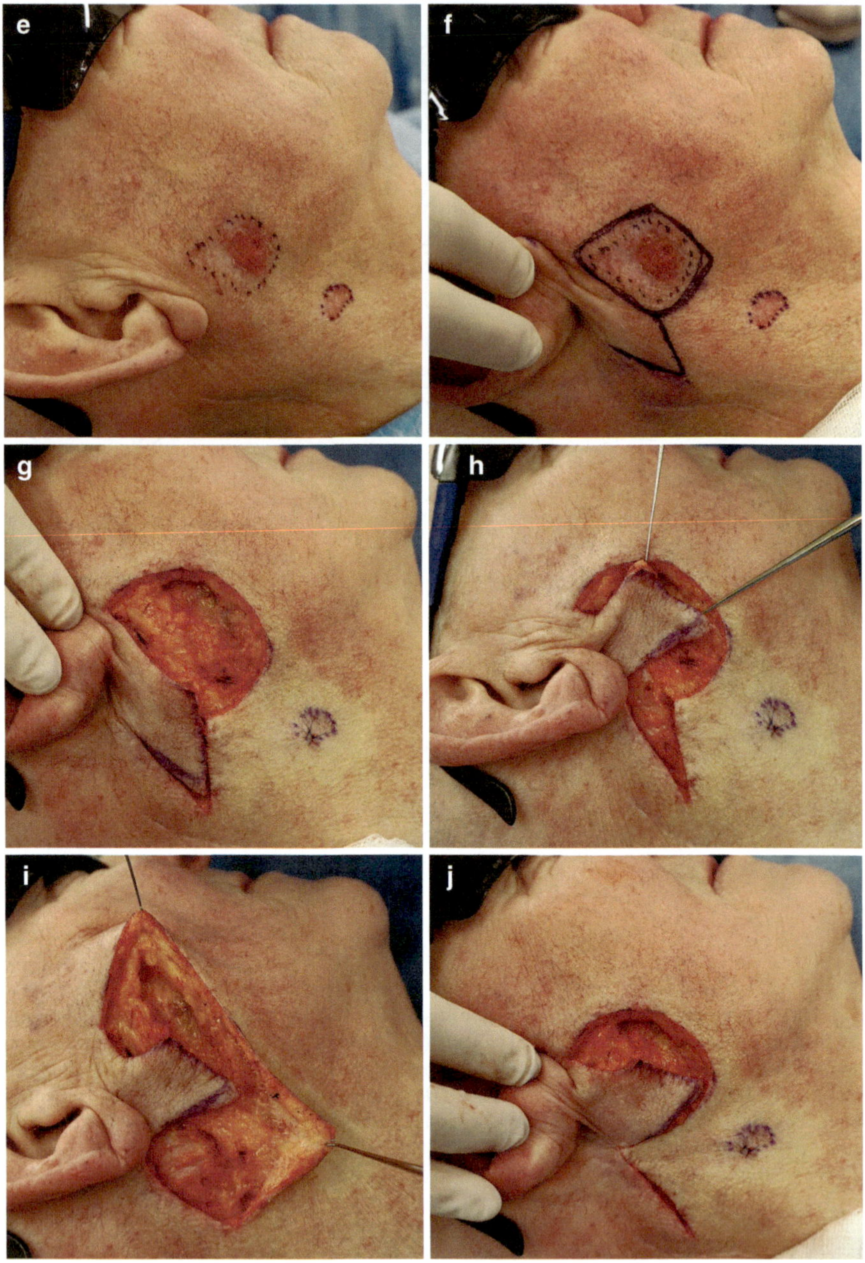

Fig. 10.13 (continued)

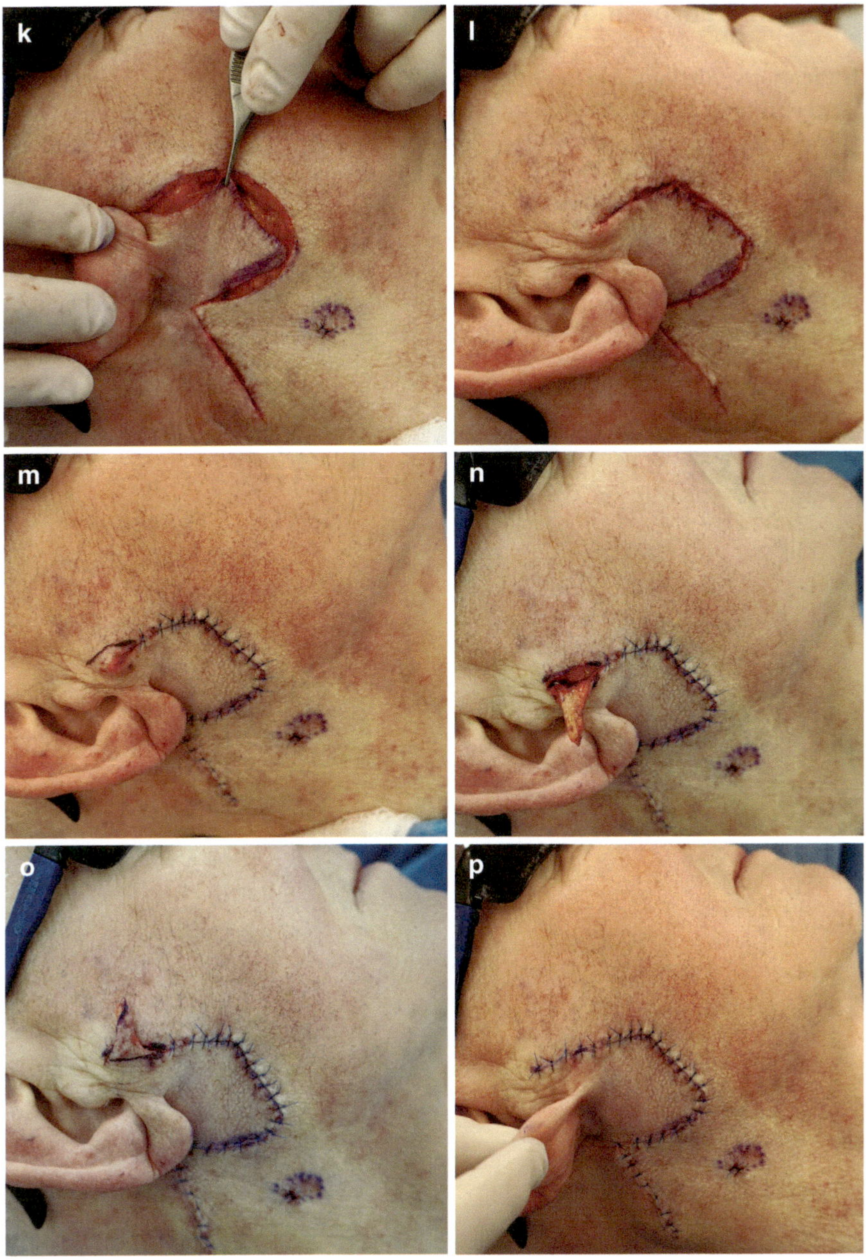

Fig. 10.13 (continued)

Rotation/Transposition Flap

Indications: Medium and large defects.

Technique: The defect is modified into a triangle, with the base superiorly/laterally. A curvilinear incision is made from the base of the defect laterally/inferiorly along the cheek RSTLs. The flap is raised in the subcutaneous plane and mobilised into the defect. Any dog ears that develop are corrected along the RSTLs. The wound is sutured in layers, and a drain inserted as required (Fig. 10.14a–c, d–h).

Tips: When extending into the neck, the plane of dissection is in the supra-platysmal plane. If dissection is undertaken deep to the platysma, care should be taken to avoid damage to the mandibular branch of the facial nerve.

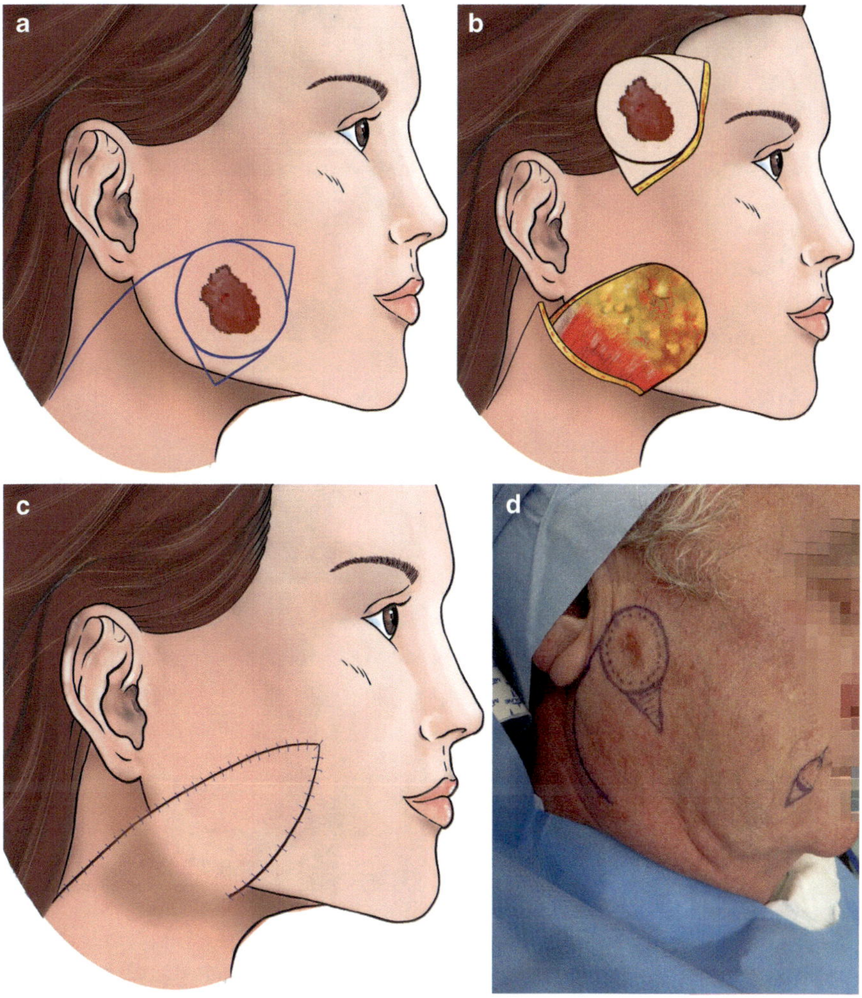

Fig. 10.14 Rotation/transposition flap. (**a**) Markings for excision and flap, (**b**) Excision defect and flap raised, (**c**) Final closure, (**d**) Markings for excision and flap, (**e**) Excision defect, (**f**) Flap raised, (**g**) Flap mobilised into defect, (**h**) Final closure

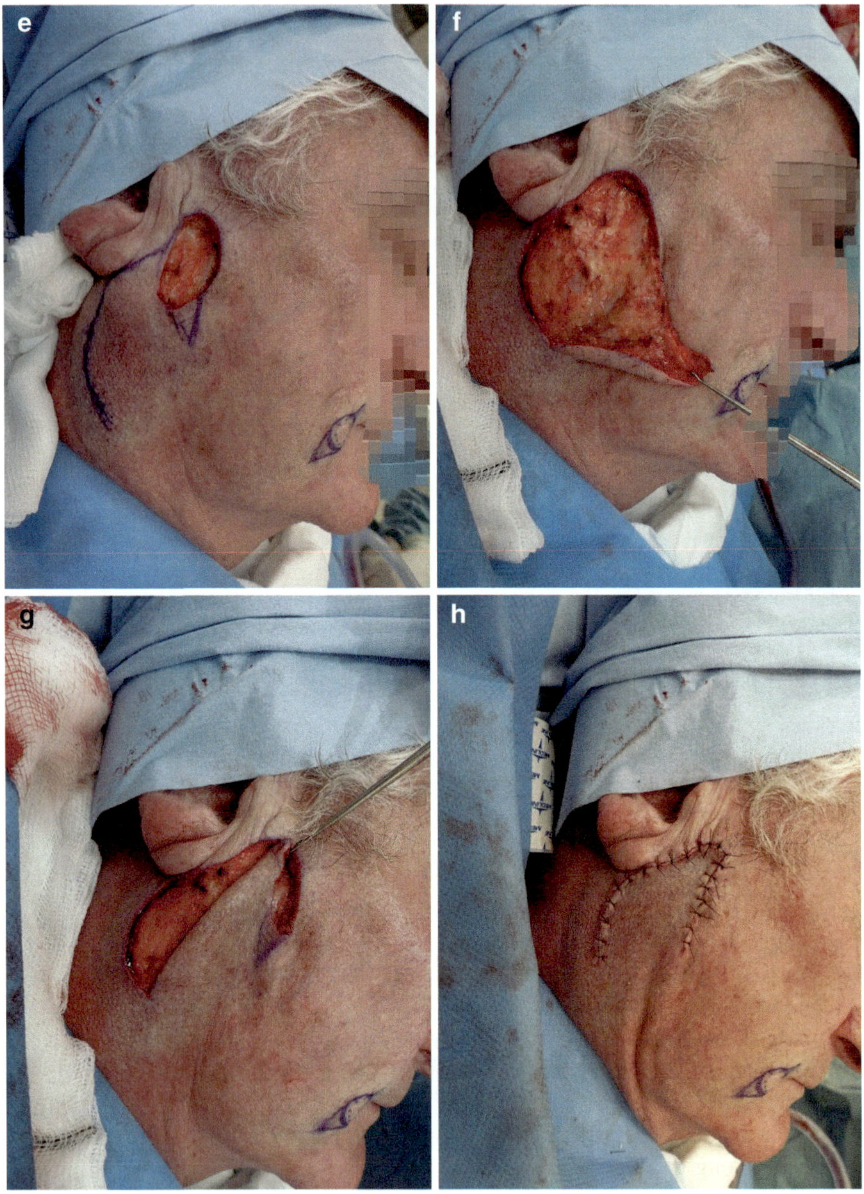

Fig. 10.14 (continued)

Lateral Subunit

Primary Closure

Indications: Small and medium defects.

Technique: The defect is modified into an ellipse to lie along the pre-auricular RSTLs. The adjacent wound margins are undermined in the subcutaneous plane and closed in layers.

Tips: Fairly large defects can be closed primarily, especially in the elderly with skin laxity. Care should be taken to avoid damage to the facial nerve. The superficial temporal vessels are present in the vicinity and if transected require appropriate haemostasis.

Asymmetric Primary Closure

Indications: Medium-sized pre-auricular defects.

Technique: The lesion is excised as an ellipse and the inferior pole extended inferior and posterior to the lobule, along the auriculocephalic sulcus. The anterior and inferior margins are widely undermined in the subcutaneous plane, to obtain the required mobility. The wound is closed in layers and any excess tissue removed to place the suture line along the pre-auricular skin fold and auriculocephalic sulcus (Fig. 10.15a–e, f, g).

Tips: Care should be taken when undermining the tissue to avoid damage to the facial and great auricular nerves. Any excess tissue is removed in segments, by overlapping it over the pre-auricular skin crease and auriculocephalic sulcus. The incisions along the lobule are best placed a few millimetres away to avoid distorting it.

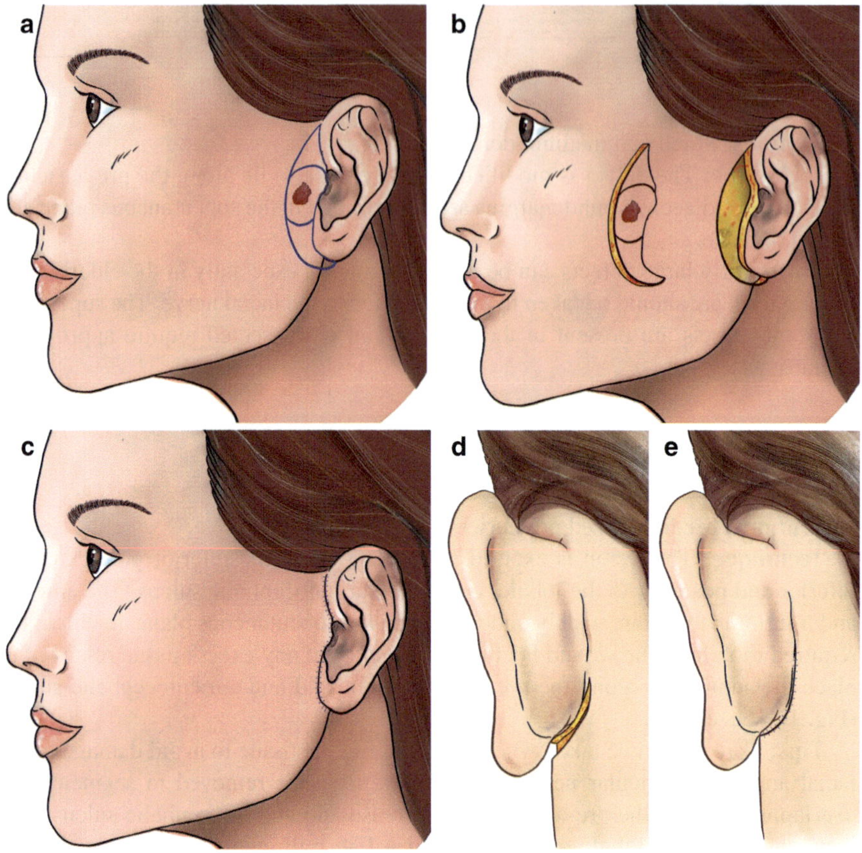

Fig. 10.15 Excision and asymmetric primary closure. (**a**) Markings for excision, (**b**) Excisiion defect, (**c**) Final closure, (**d**) post auricular extension, (**e**) Post auricular closure, (**f**) Markings for excision, (**g**) Final closure

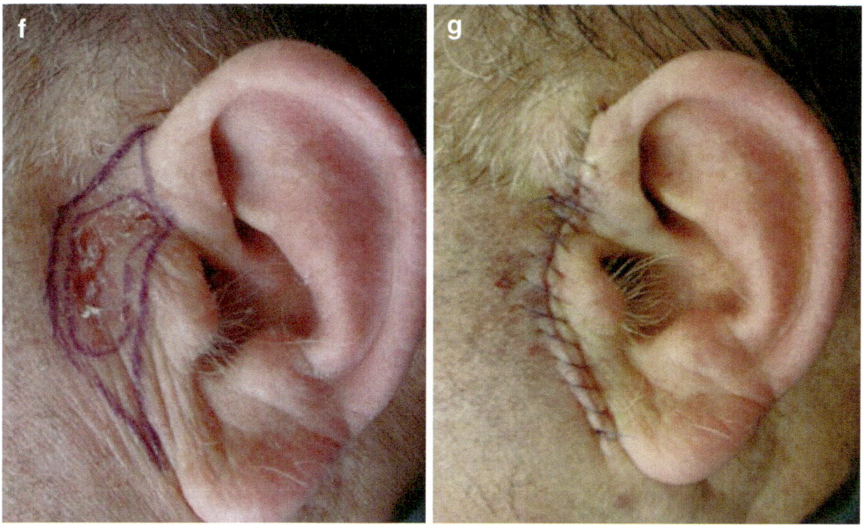

Fig. 10.15 (continued)

Rhombic Flap

Indications: Medium-sized defects.

Technique: The defect is modified into a rhombus with 60° and 120° internal angles. A rhomboid flap is designed by extending the short diagonal to a distance equal to one of the sides and a further line is drawn from its extremity, parallel to the adjacent side of the defect. The flap is raised in the subcutaneous plane and mobilised into the defect. The wound is closed in layers (See Fig. 10.12).

Tips: Given the design of the rhombic flaps, it will not be possible to align all the scars along the RSTL. Four flaps can be designed for any given defect and the ideal one is chosen based on tissue laxity, best orientation of scars and avoiding distortion of adjacent landmarks. An inferiorly based flap often works best for an inferior lateral subunit defect.

Bilobed Flap

Indications: Medium- and large-sized defects lateral, mandibular and buccal units.

Technique: It is best suited for circular defects. The first lobe is designed to be of similar dimensions to the defect, and the second lobe can be made slightly narrower, but longer to accommodate pointed ends on the summit, for primary closure. The flap is raised in the subcutaneous plane and mobilised into the defect. The wound margins are widely undermined and the defect closed in layers. Closure is best carried out in an orderly sequence; the tertiary defect is closed first, followed closure of the primary defect. The flap covering the secondary defect is appropriately trimmed and closed next, and the dog ear is addressed last (Fig. 10.16a–d, e–j, see also Fig. 3.5a–d).

Tips: The flap is designed to best utilise the tissue laxity, avoid distorting adjacent structures and placement of scars. Due to curvilinear incisions, it is not possible to accommodate all the scars along RSTLs and there is a tendency for "pin cushioning" of the flap. This can be partly mitigated by modifying the defect and flap margin to include right-angled corners and parallel wound margins. Care must be taken to avoid damage to the facial and great auricular nerves.

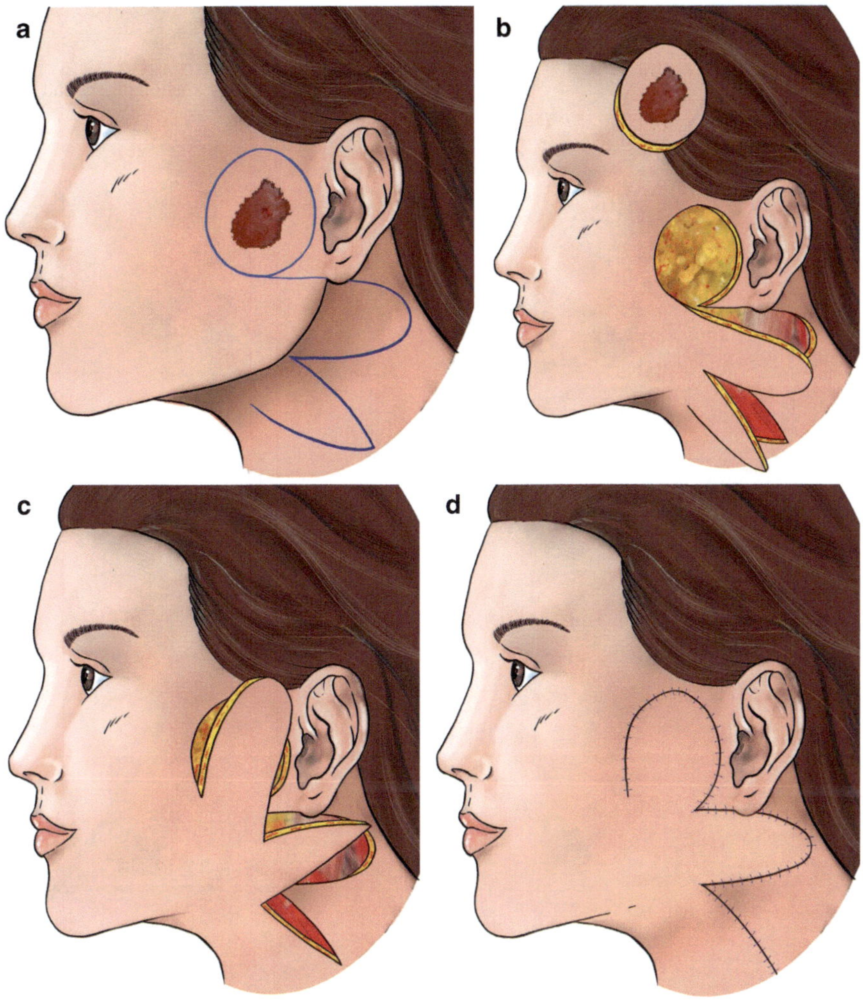

Fig. 10.16 Bilobed flap. (**a**) Markings for excision and flap, (**b**) Excision defect and flaps raised, (**c**) Flaps transposed into defect, (**d**) Final closure, (**e**) Markings for excision, (**f**) Markings for excision and flap, (**g**) Excision defect, (**h**) Flaps raised, (**i**) Flaps transposed into defects, (**j**) Final closure

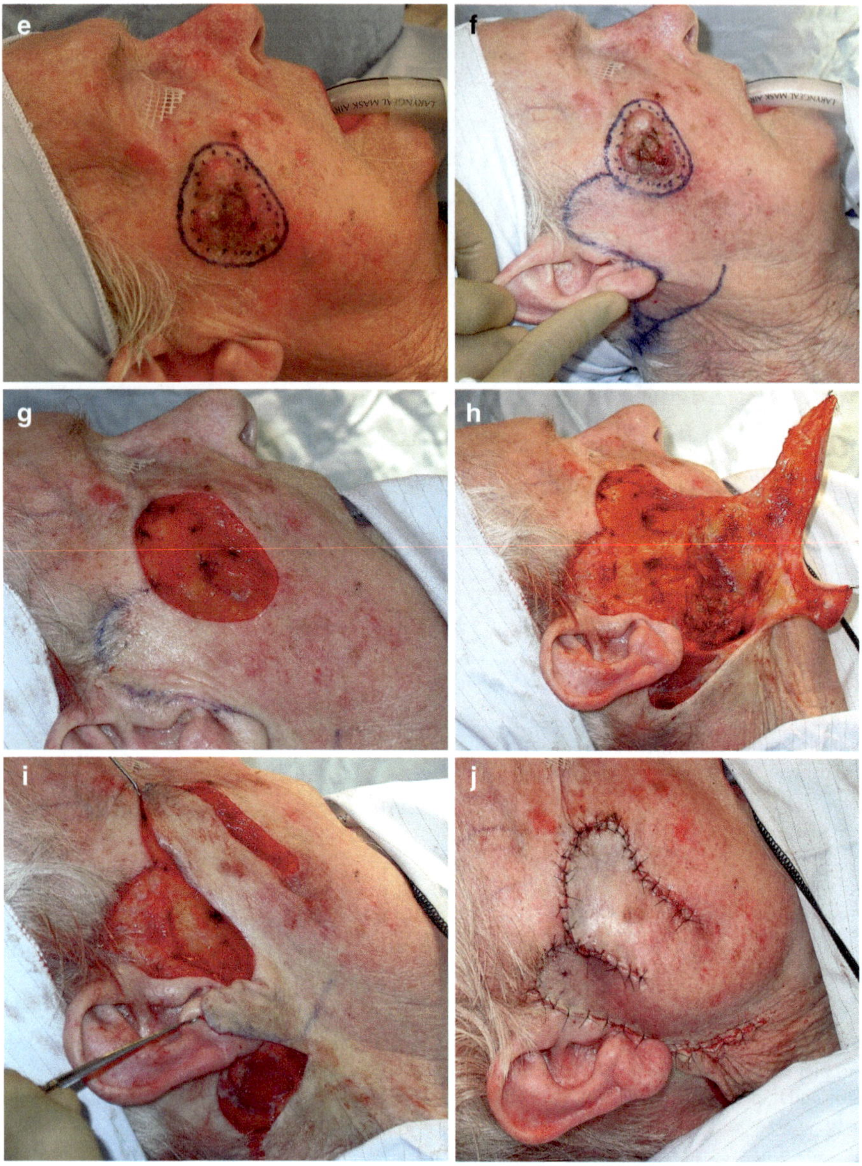

Fig. 10.16 (continued)

Suggested Algorithm

Medial

Small
1. Primary closure

Medium
1. Island advancement flap
2. Rotation/transposition flap (lateral)
3. Rotation/transposition flap (inferior)

Buccal

Small
1. Primary closure

Medium
1. Primary closure
2. Rhombic flap
3. Rotation/transposition flap (lateral)
4. Rotation/transposition flap (inferior)
5. Island advancement flap
6. Bilobed flap

Zygomatic Unit

Small
1. Primary closure

Medium
1. Rhombic flap
2. Rotation/transposition flap
3. Mustarde' flap
4. Island advancement flap

Mandibular

Small
1. Primary closure

Medium

1. Rhombic flap
2. Rotation/transposition flap
3. Bilobed flap

Lateral Unit

Small

1. Primary closure

Medium

1. Asymmetric primary closure
2. Rhombic flap
3. Rotation/transposition flap
4. Bilobed flap

Lips/Chin

11

Lips

Subunits and Anatomical Considerations

The upper and lower lips have prominent aesthetic and social connotations and form a distinct facial aesthetic unit. The lip unit is defined by the base of the nose superiorly, nasolabial fold laterally and mentolabial fold inferiorly. The lip aesthetic unit can be divided into the cutaneous upper lip, cutaneous lower lip and the vermillion subunits. The upper lip can be further divided into a philtrum and two lateral subunits (Fig. 11.1).

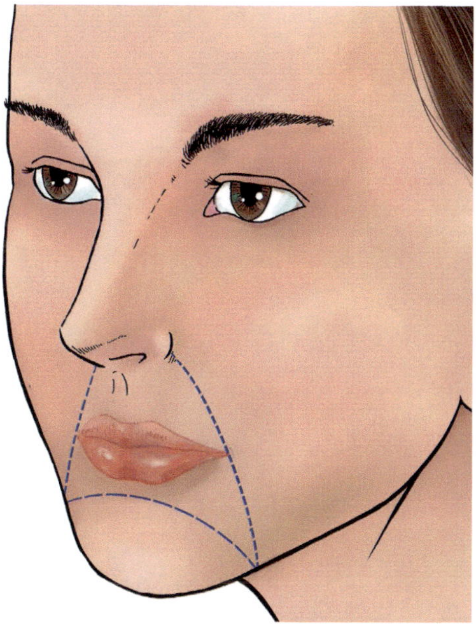

Fig. 11.1 Lip unit and subunits

V. Ilankovan et al., *Local Flaps in Facial Reconstruction*,
https://doi.org/10.1007/978-3-031-49464-2_11

The lip is a composite structure made up of skin, muscle and mucosa. The mucocutaneous junction is defined by the vermillion border and represents a very important facial landmark. The RSTLs are oriented radially around the oral stoma and are vertical in the central region and oblique in the lateral aspects (Fig. 11.2).

The labial arteries run in the submucosal plane, along the free lip margins. They lie on the posterior surface of the orbicularis oris, and its pulsation can often be felt in this region. The sensory (infra-orbital/mental) and motor (facial) nerve supply are arranged in a radial fashion around the oral stoma.

Lip reconstruction needs to address both aesthetics and function. Satisfactory function requires the presence of intact sensory and motor nerves and restoration of the orbicularis oris muscle sphincter.

Ideally tissue mobilised from within the lip complex provides the best match. Incisions should be placed parallel to the perioral rhytids for simple excisions. It is extremely important not to distort the vermillion border, and its precise approximation is mandatory. Flaps mobilised from the adjacent areas, should ideally have their incisions along the aesthetic borders (base of nose, vermillion, nasolabial and mentolabial folds). Consideration should be given to modifying the defect, so as to place the scar in the most advantageous position.

The specific reconstructive options will depend on a multitude of factors, including the presence of full and partial thickness defects.

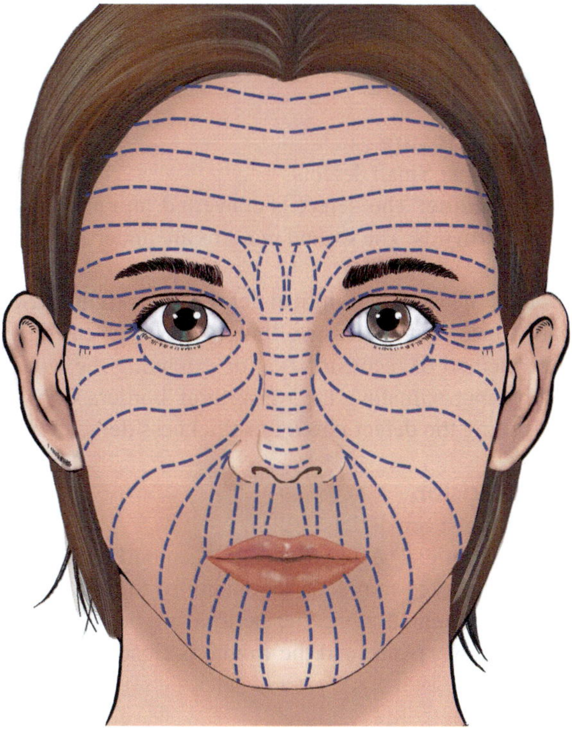

Fig. 11.2 Orientation of lip RSTL's

Lower Lip

Skin Only

Primary Closure

Indications: Small defects.

Technique: The defect is converted into an ellipse to orient the scar along the perioral rhytids. The wound margins are undermined in the sub-cuatneous plane and closed in layers.

Tips: Closure of elliptical defects leads to increase in length of the scar and can cause distortion of the vermillion border. This can be overcome by utilising an alternate method of reconstruction or extending the wound into the mucosa and accurately approximating the vermillion border. Consideration should be given to converting the defect into a full-thickness defect to aid closure.

M/W Excision

Indications: Small defects.

Technique: The excision defect is modified to include M/W extremities, instead of an ellipse, to minimise the length of the overall defect. The overall axis of the defect is oriented along the perioral rhytids. The margins are undermined in the subcutaneous plane, and the wound is closed in layers (Fig. 11.3a–c).

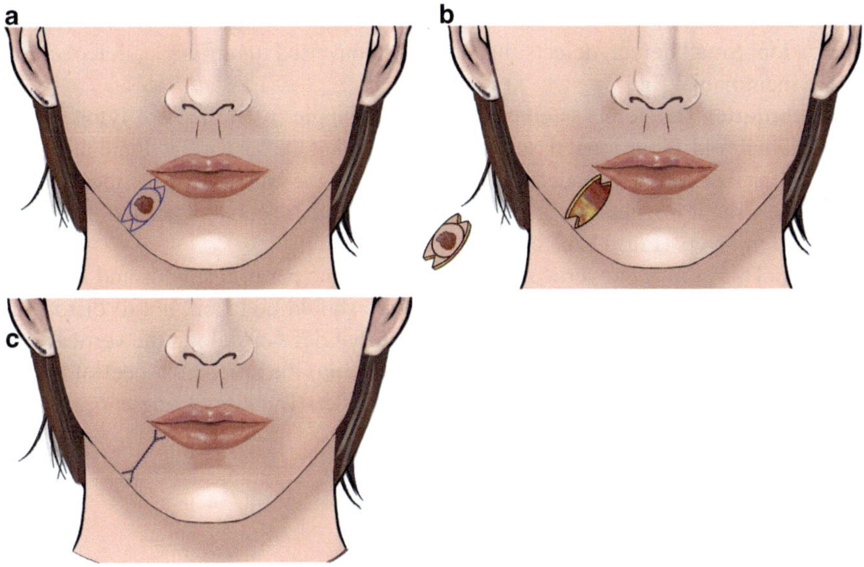

Fig. 11.3 M & W excision. (**a**) Markings for excision, (**b**) Excision defect, (**c**) Final closure

A-T Flap

Indication: Small defect, defects that could be converted to a triangle, defect closer to the mentolabial fold.

Technique: The defect is converted into a triangle, with the base lying on the mentolabial fold. Additional tissue can be removed at the base to facilitate this. Two curvilinear incisions are made from the margins of the base, along the mentolabial fold. The wound margins are undermined in the subcutaneous plane, and the defect is closed in layers (Fig. 11.4a–c, d–l).

Tips: This allows the vertical scar to lie along the perioral rhytids and the horizontal section along the mentolabial fold. Care should be taken, not to distort the vermillion border. Any lengthening or dog ear that develops along the vertical section of the scar can be corrected by extending it into the mucosal aspect of the lip and accurately approximating the vermillion border. The lateral dog ears are corrected along the mentolabial fold.

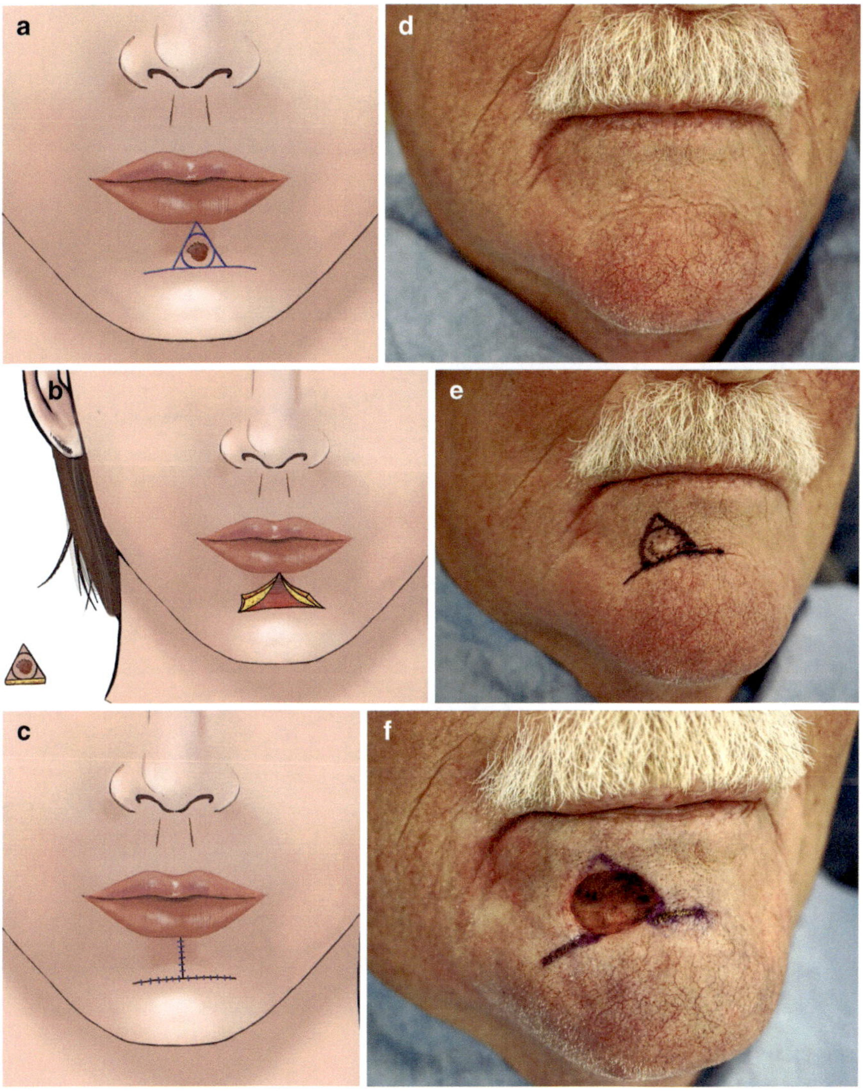

Fig. 11.4 A-T closure. (**a**) Markings for excision and flap, (**b**) Excision defect and flap raised, (**c**) Final closure, (**d**) Lesion lower lip, (**e**) Markings for excision and flap, (**f**) Excision defect, (**g**) Flap incisions, (**h**) Flaps raised, (**i**) Trail mobilisation of flaps, (**j**) Delineation of dog ears, (**k**) markings for dog ear excisions, (**l**) Final closure

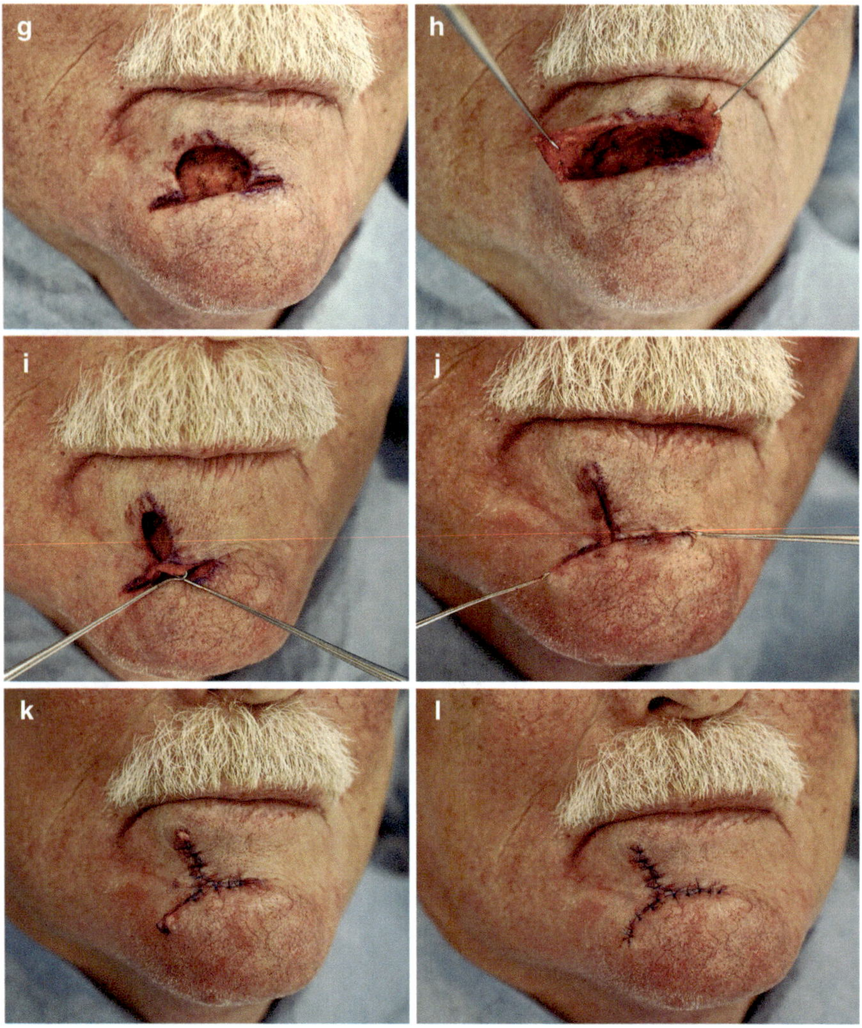

Fig. 11.4 (continued)

Superiorly-Based Nasolabial Flap

This is a random pattern flap, though it overlies the course of the facial vessels.

Indications: Medium-sized defect of a variety of shapes.

Technique: The flap is raised along the nasolabial fold, with one of its margins also forming the margin of the defect. A trial transfer and template can help determine the size of the flap. The overall length of the flap is planned to be longer to accommodate any loss of effective length, and the tip triangulated to help primary closure. The base of the flap is designed to be wider than the tip to maintain vascularity. The flap is raised in the subcutaneous plane. The wound margins are undermined in the subcutaneous plane, and the wound is closed in layers (Fig. 11.5a–d).

Tips: There is a tendency for "pin cushioning" with circular defects, and it also makes it difficult to place the scars along RSTL. Consideration should be given to modifying the defect to include parallel margins and extending it to make the final scar lie along aesthetic boundaries and RSTL (see inferiorly based nasolabial flap—Fig. 11.6a–d). The medial dog ear of the flap can also be excised along the vermillion border for better placement of the scar. The width of the flap should be adequate to prevent displacement of the vermillion. There are often more appropriate alternatives.

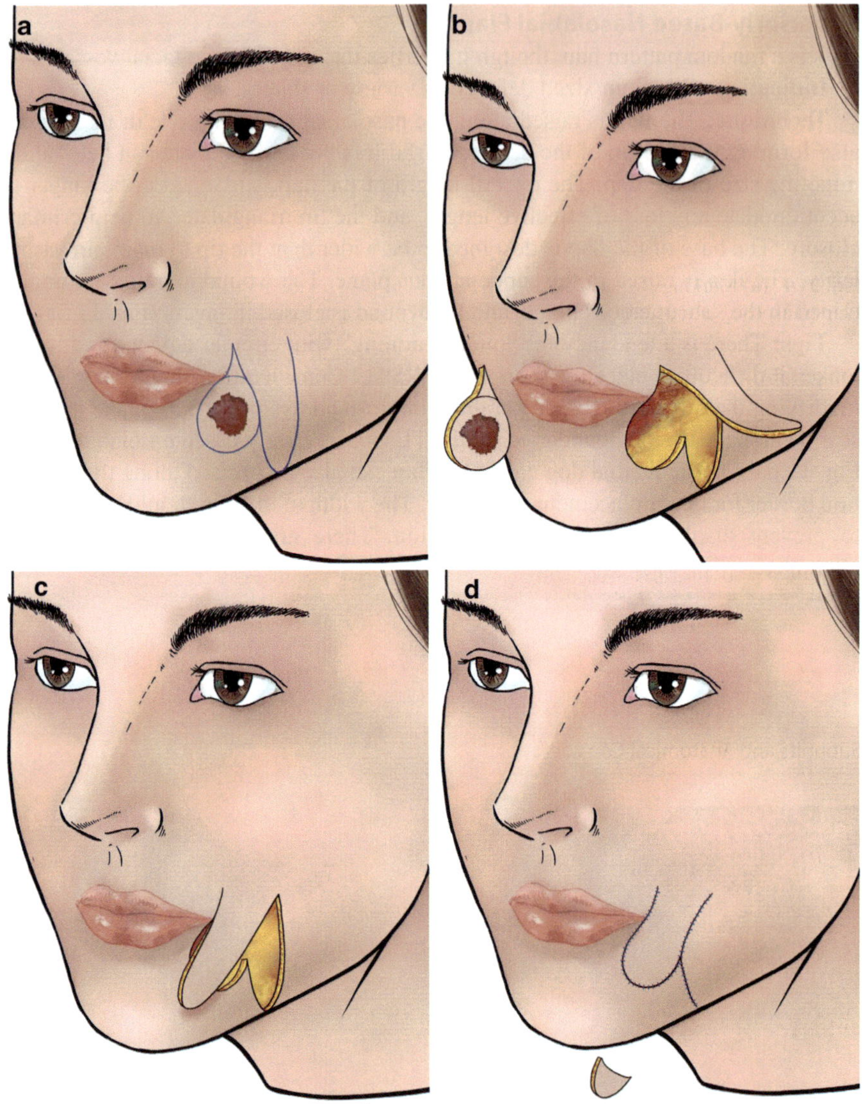

Fig. 11.5 Superiorly based nasolabial flap. (**a**) Markings for excision and flap, (**b**) Excision defect and flap raised, (**c**) Flap transposed into defect, (**d**) Final closure

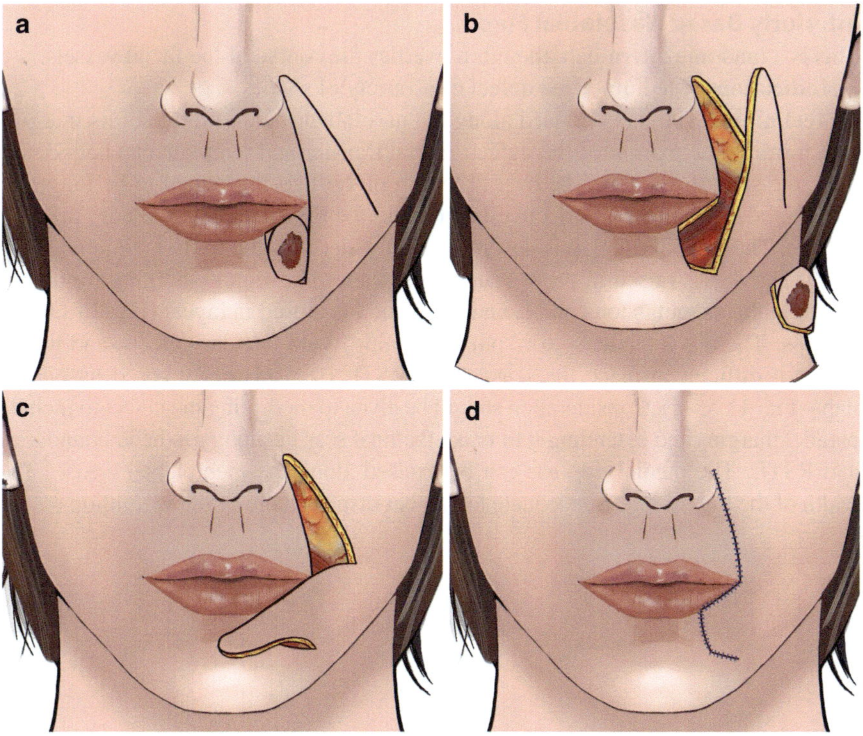

Fig. 11.6 Inferiorly based nasolabial flap. (**a**) Markings for excision and flap, (**b**) Excision dfect and flap raised, (**c**) Mobilisation of flap into defect, (**d**) Final closure

Inferiorly Based Nasolabial Flap

This is a random pattern flap, though it overlies the course of the facial vessels.

Indications: Medium-sized defect of a variety of shapes.

Technique: The flap is raised along the nasolabial fold, with one of its margins also forming the margin of the defect. A trial transfer and template can help determine the size of the flap. The overall length of the flap is planned to be longer to accommodate any loss of effective length, and the tip triangulated to help primary closure. The base of the flap is designed to be wider than the tip to maintain vascularity. The flap is raised in the subcutaneous plane. The wound margins are undermined in the subcutaneous plane, and the wound is closed in layers (Fig. 11.6a–d).

Tips: There is a tendency for "pin cushioning" with circular defects, and it also makes it difficult to place the scars along RSTL (see superiorly based nasolabial flap—Fig. 11.5a–d). Consideration should be given to modifying the defect to include parallel margins and extending it to make the final scar lie along aesthetic boundaries and RSTL. The medial dog ear can be excised along the mentolabial crease. The width of the flap should be adequate to prevent displacement of the vermillion.

Mucosa Only

Primary Closure

Indications: Small defects.

Technique: The defect is converted to a vertical ellipse, and the wound margins minimally undermined and the defect closed in layers.

Tips: Try and avoid "horizontal" incisions to minimise damage to the sensory nerve supply of the lips and distortion of the vermillion border.

Mucosal Advancement Flap

Indication: Large mucosal defects, whole lower lip mucosal defect (lip shave).

Technique: The margins of the mucosal defect are modified if necessary, to leave even/straight wound edges. The mucosa of the inner surface of the lip is raised as a flap with its base at the labial sulcus. The flap is raised on the surface of the muscle, deep to the plane of the minor salivary glands This is best done by alternate blunt and sharp dissection, in a vertical direction to create channels, prior to division. Care is taken not to "button hole" the flap. Frequent attempts are made to assess the mobility and adequacy of the flap and if possible, the "intervening" tissue is retained between the channels to preserve some sensation. Once adequate mobility is obtained, the flap is sutured accurately to create a new vermillion border (Fig. 11.7a–e, f–k).

Tips: There is a tendency for scar contracture to result in a decrease in vermillion exposure. This can be partly accommodated by placing the new vermillion border at a more anterior location. The lateral margins of the defect are frequently narrow, and it is therefore not necessary to dissect widely in this area, which can prevent additional damage to the mental nerves.

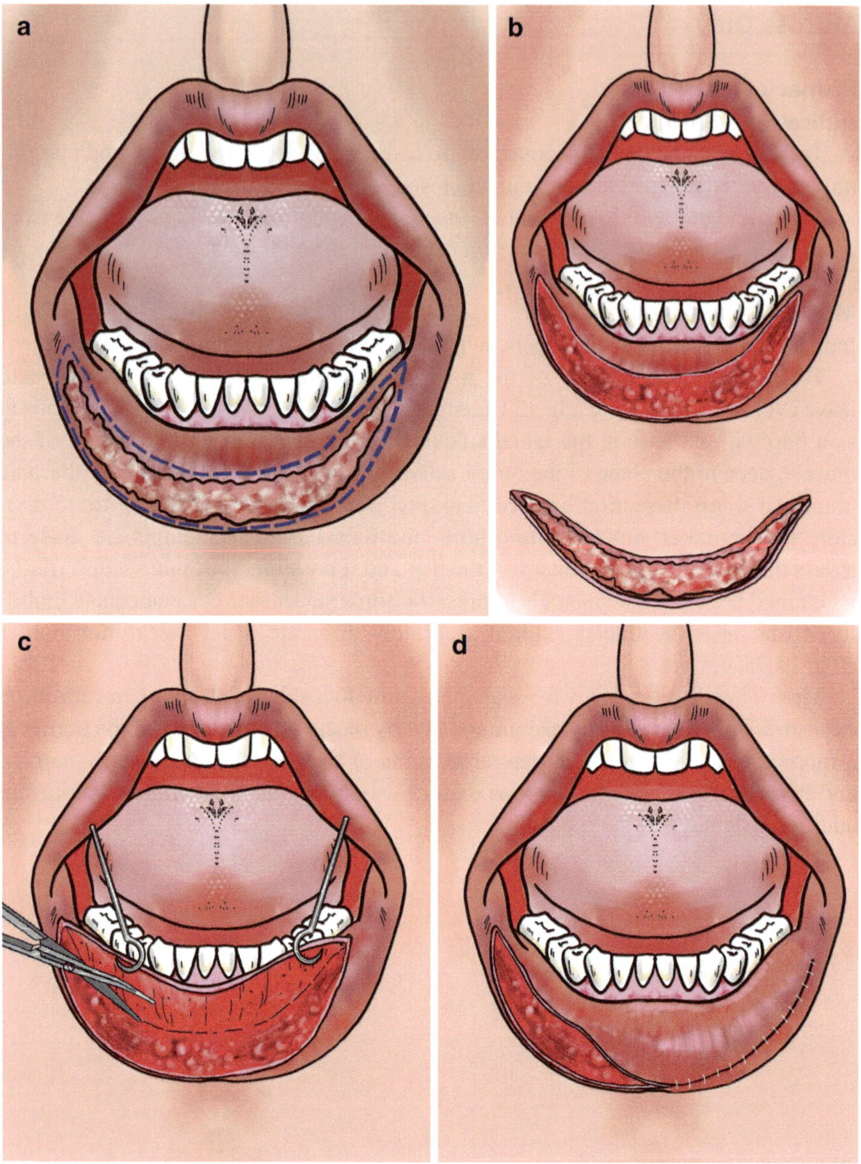

Fig. 11.7 Mucosal advancement flap. (**a**) Markings for excision, (**b**) Excision defect, (**c**) Mucosal flap raised, (**d**) Initial closure, (**e**) Final closure, (**f**) Lesion lower lip, (**g**) Markings for excision, (**h**) Mucosal excision, (**i**) Excision defect, (**j**) Mucosa raised, (**k**) Final closure

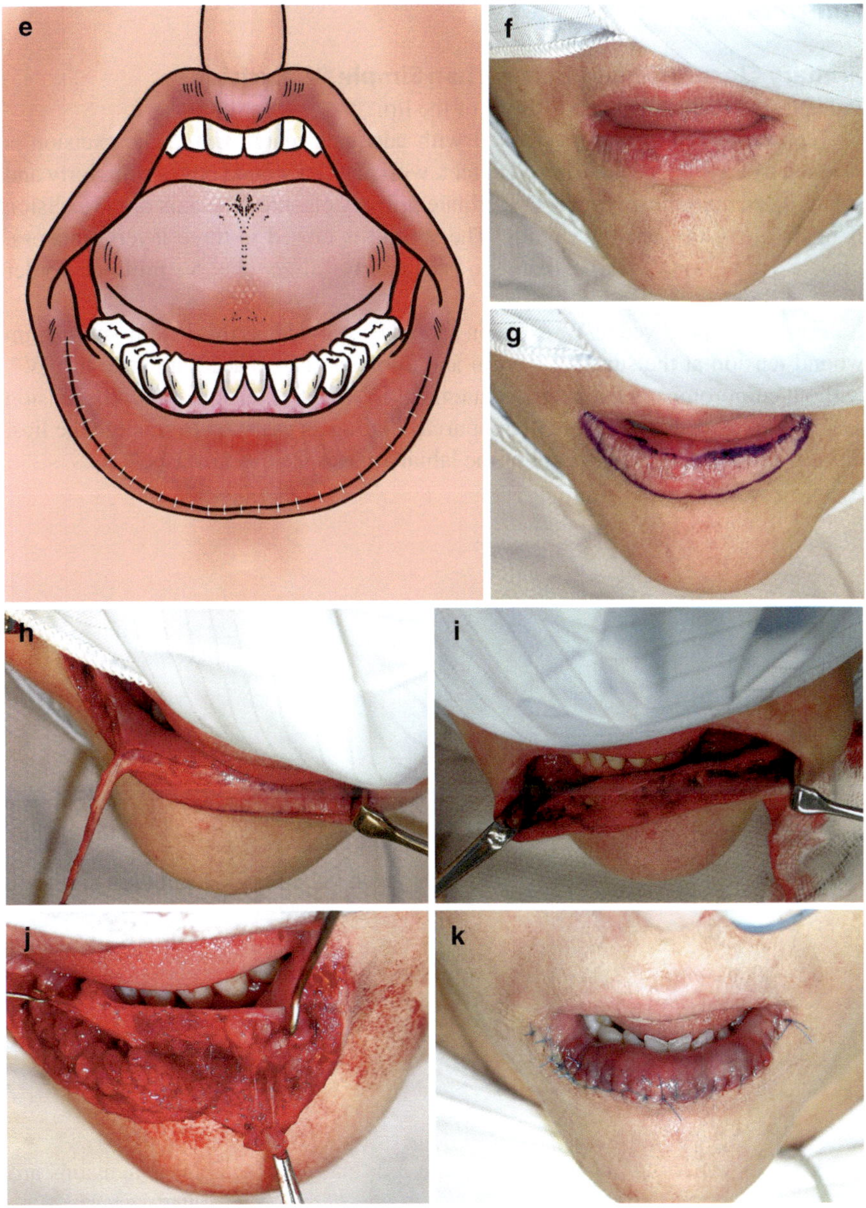

Fig. 11.7 (continued)

Full-thickness Defects

Primary Closure (Shield Rather Than Simple "V" Excision)

Indication: Small defects up to 1/3rd of the lip.

Technique: The lesion is marked with adequate margins, and the excision is planned to leave a "shield" shaped defect, with parallel wound edges superiorly and triangulated margins inferiorly to facilitate primary closure. The axis of the excision is made along the perioral rhytids. The wound is closed in three layers (mucosa, muscle and skin), taking care to accurately align the vermillion border (Fig. 11.8a–c, d–i).

Tips: A simple "wedge/V" excision should be avoided, as this leads to maximum wound tension at the superior margin and a longer scar to accommodate the "V", without compromising the excision margins. A "shield" excision allows the tension to be evenly distributed across a larger area. Getting an assistant to squeeze the lips, during the resection aids control of the labial arteries for haemostasis.

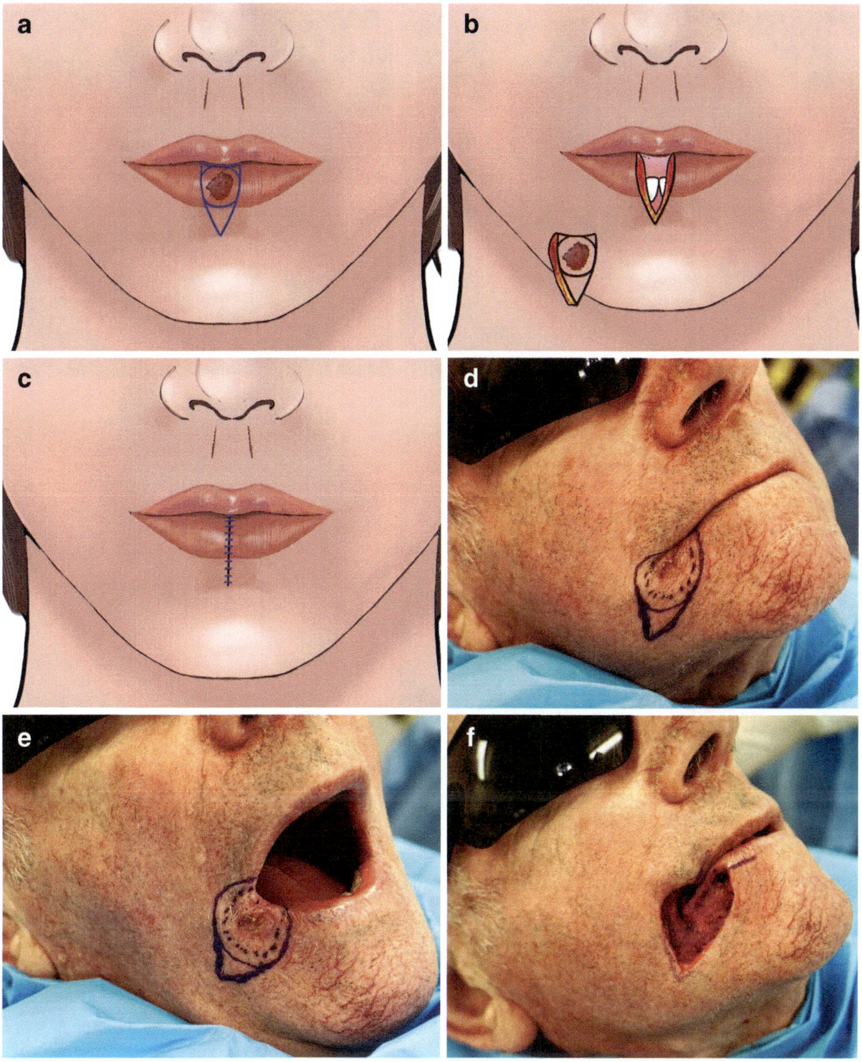

Fig. 11.8 Shield excision and primary closure. (**a**) Markings for excision, (**b**) Excision defect, (**c**) Final closure, (**d**) Markings for excision, (**e**) Markings for excision - open mouth, (**f**) Excision defect, (**g**) Excision defect - open mouth, (**h**) Final closure, (**i**) Final closure - open mouth

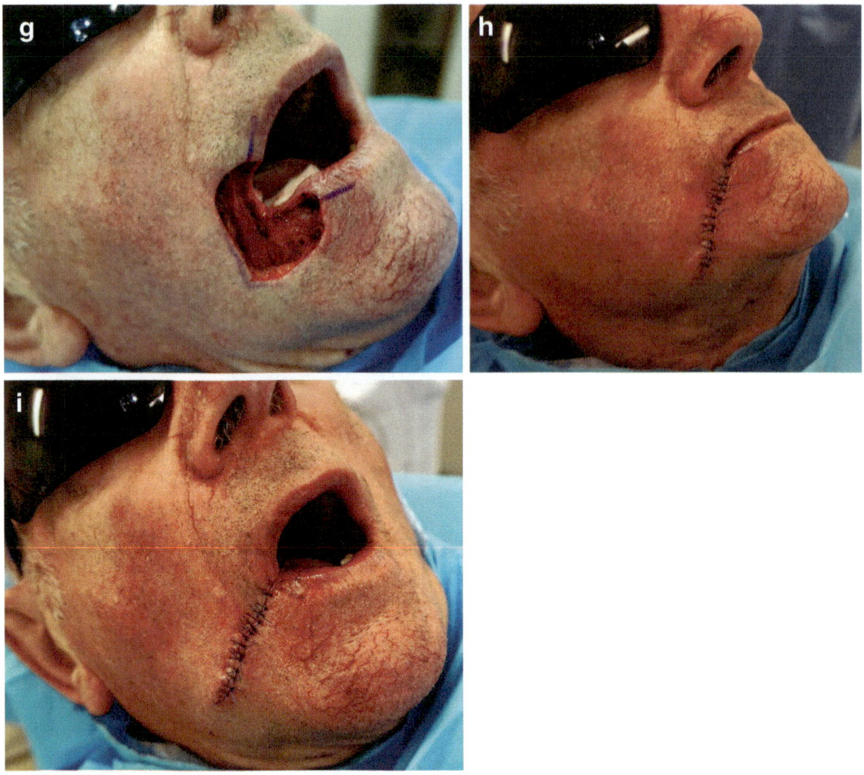

Fig. 11.8 (continued)

"W" Excision

Indication: Small lesions, up to 1/3rd of the lip.

Technique: The lesion is marked with adequate margins, and the excision is planned to leave a defect with parallel wound edges superiorly and "W" margins inferiorly to facilitate primary closure. The axis of the excision is made along the perioral rhytids. The wound is closed in three layers (mucosa, muscle and skin), taking care to accurately align the vermillion border (Fig. 11.9a–c, d–g).

Tips: A simple "wedge/V" excision should be avoided, as this leads to maximum wound tension at the superior margin and a longer scar to accommodate the "V", without compromising the excision margins. A "W" excision allows the tension to be evenly distributed across a larger area and importantly the overall length of the scar to be reduced, so that it does not transgress the adjacent aesthetic boundaries. Getting an assistant to squeeze the lips, during the resection aids control of the labial arteries for haemostasis.

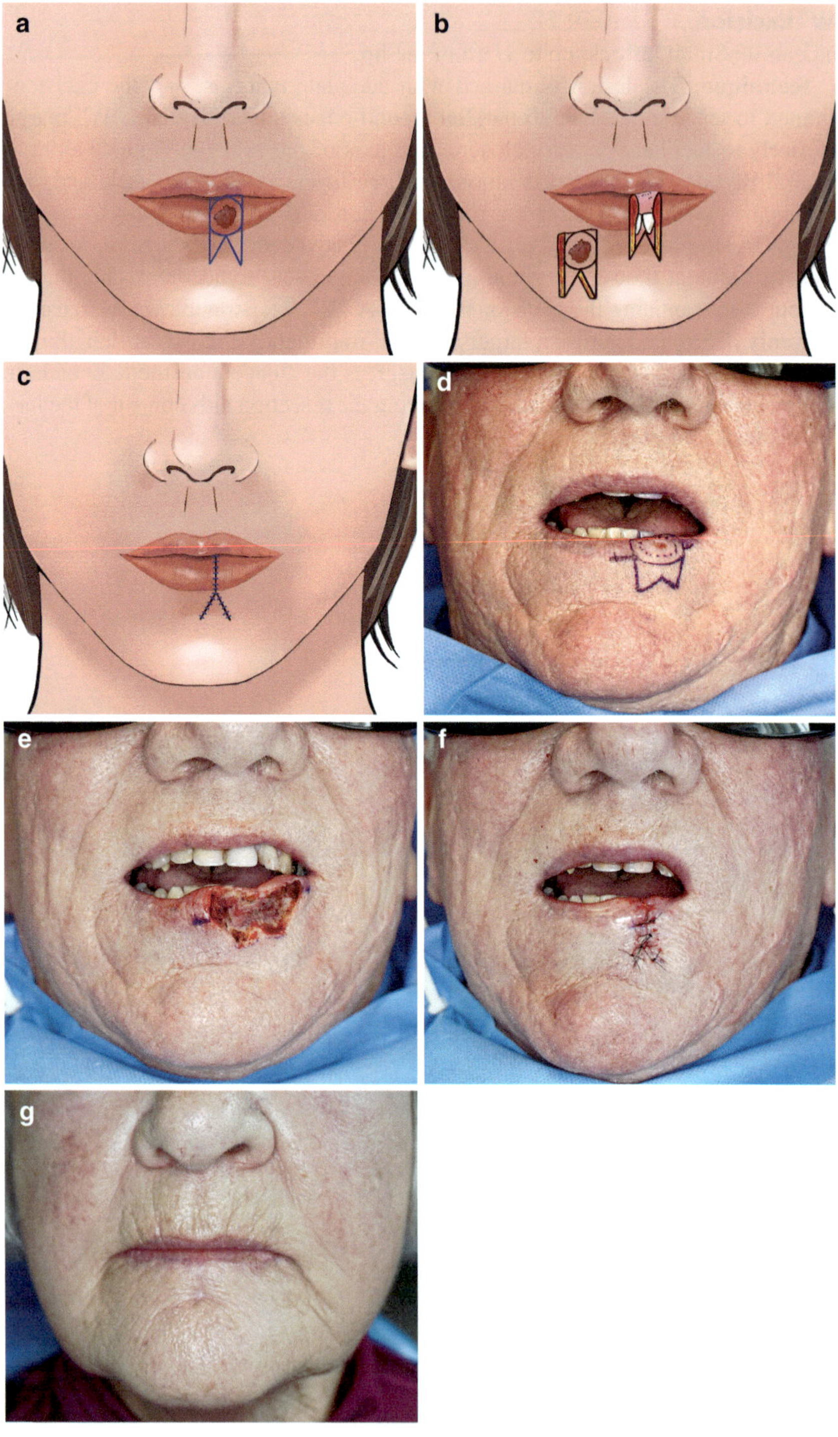

Fig. 11.9 "W" excision and primary closure. (**a**) Markings for excision, (**b**) Excision defect, (**c**) Final closure, (**d**) Markings for excision, (**e**) Excision defect, (**f**) Final closure, (**g**) Post operative appearance

Bilateral Advancement Flap

Indications: Medium defects.

Technique: The defect is modified to have parallel margins. The base is extended, if necessary, to lie on the mentolabial fold. A curvilinear incision is made from the base of the defect, along to mentolabial fold through skin only. The subcutaneous tissues dissected by alternate blunt and sharp dissection, until sufficient mobility is obtained to achieve primary closure of the defect, without excessive tension. It is often not necessary to make additional relieving incisions along the vestibular sulcus, to facilitate closure. If required, these can often be limited to a fraction of the corresponding skin incision. The wound is closed in three layers (mucosa, muscle, skin) (Fig. 11.10a–c).

Tips: The blunt dissection of the subcutaneous tissue helps to minimise neuro vascular damage to the flap and preserve sensory/motor innervation. The difference in length of the adjacent skin edges along the mentolabial fold can be accommodated by differential suturing or excision of dog ear along the chin rhytids, inferiorly.

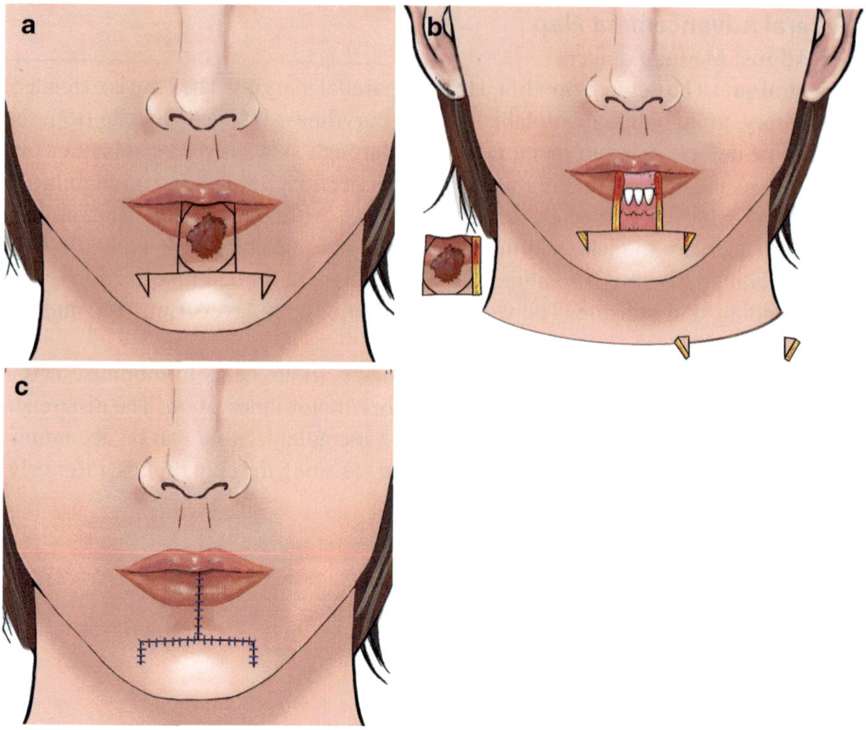

Fig. 11.10 Bilateral advancement flap. (**a**) Markings for excision, (**b**) Excision defect and flap incisions, (**c**) Final closure

Abbe Flap

Indications: Medium-sized defects, away from the commissure, two-stage flap.

Technique: The defect is modified to have parallel wound edges. The flap is marked to have a similar height of the donor defect, but the width can be reduced by up to 30%, to make use of the redundancy of the remaining lip. A full-thickness incision is made along one of the borders of the flap (skin, muscle, mucosa), but the incision along the other border is stopped short of the vermillion, to avoid damage to the vascular pedicle (labial artery). The flap is rotated into the defect, and the wounds are closed in layers, taking care to protect the labial artery (Fig. 11.11a–d). The donor site is closed primarily. The pedicle is divided in 3–4 weeks, and any revision to accurately approximate the vermillion border carried out at this stage (Figs. 11.11e).

Tips: Patient compliance is vital, and the patient should be counselled appropriately, prior to the procedure. The initial incision on the side of the flap with the vascular pedicle should stop short of the vermillion border. With extreme care, further dissection can be carried out through the skin and part of the muscle, to help accurately approximate the vermillion border during the primary reconstruction. As discussed at the beginning of the chapter, the labial artery runs along the free border of the lip, below the mucosa on the posterior aspect of the orbicularis oris and maintaining a portion of the muscle above the vessels offers some additional protection. An Abbe flap is better suited for reconstruction of upper lip defects, and other flaps should be considered before deciding on harvesting an Abbe flap from the upper lip to reconstruct a lower lip defect.

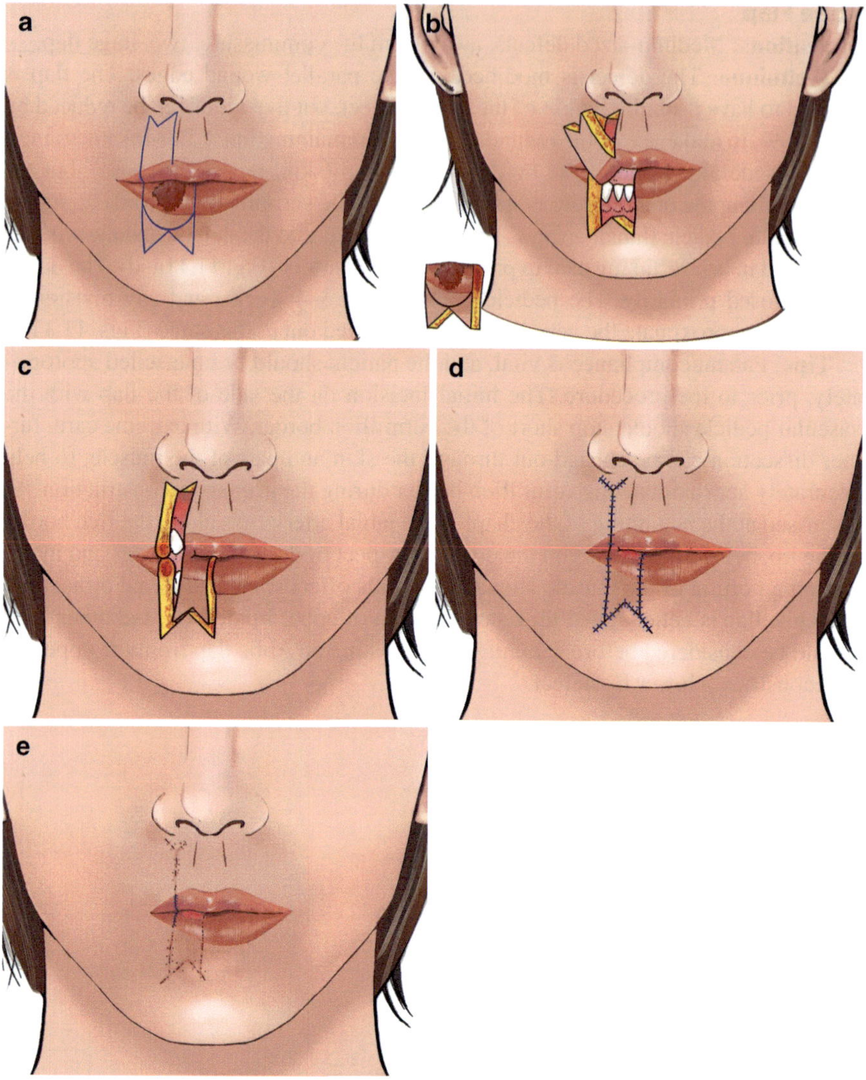

Fig. 11.11 Abbe flap. (**a**) Markings for excision and flap, (**b**) Excision defect and flap raised, (**c**) Flap mobilised into defect, (**d**) Final closure of first stage, (**e**) Final closure after second stage

Abbe–Estlander Flap

Indications: Medium-sized defects involving the commissure.

Technique: The flap is marked to have a similar height of the donor defect, but the width can be reduced by up to 30%, to make use of the redundancy of the remaining lip. A full-thickness incision is made along the lateral border of the flap (skin, muscle, mucosa), but the incision along the media border is stopped short of the vermillion, to avoid damage to the vascular pedicle (labial artery). The flap is rotated into the defect, and the wounds are closed in layers, taking care to protect the labial artery (Fig. 11.12a–d). The donor site defect is closed primarily. The intact medial border now forms the new commissure.

Tips: The initial incision on the side of the flap with the vascular pedicle should stop short of the vermillion border. With extreme care, further dissection can be carried out through the skin and part of the muscle, to help accurately approximate the vermillion border during the primary reconstruction. As discussed at the beginning of the chapter, the labial artery runs along the free border of the lip, below the mucosa on the posterior aspect of the orbicularis oris and maintaining a portion of the muscle above the vessels offers some additional protection. The residual asymmetry of the commissure improves with time and might need revision at a later date.

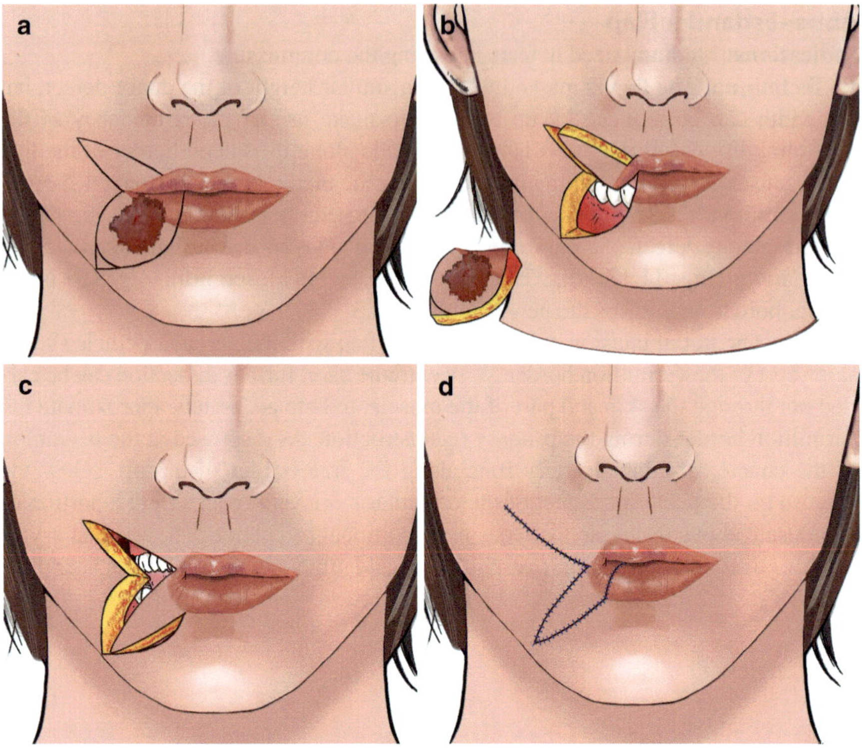

Fig. 11.12 Abbe-Eslander flap. (**a**) Markings for excision and flap, (**b**) Excision defect and flap raised, (**c**) Flap mobilised into defect, (**d**) Final closure

Karapandzic Flap

Indications: Medium and large defects (upper/lower lips).

Technique: The defect is modified to have parallel sides. The base of the defect can be extended if necessary to place it on the mentolabial fold. Curvilinear incisions are made from the base of the defect, extending laterally along the nasolabial/mentolabial fold, at an equivalent distance from the base of the defect to the free margin of the lip. The incision is made only through the skin, and the underlying tissue released by blunt and sharp dissection. The blunt dissection is carried out in a radial fashion around the stoma to preserve the incoming neurovascular bundles. The degree of mobilisation is assessed at regular intervals and if necessary, the skin incision can be extended, along the base of the nose, to completely circumscribe the stoma. Sufficient mobility is obtained to achieve primary closure of the defect, without excessive tension. It is often not necessary to make additional relieving incisions along the vestibular sulcus, to facilitate closure. If required, these can often be limited to a fraction of the corresponding skin incision. The wound is closed in layers (mucosa, muscle, skin) (Fig. 11.13a–d, e–k).

Tips: The unequal lengths of the wound edges can be accommodated by differential suturing. Any resultant dog ear can be excised along the perioral skin creases/nasolabial folds. The rounding of the commissures often improves with time and if necessarily can be corrected by commissuroplasty at a later date. The preservation of motor and sensory nerve supply and avoiding additional transection of the orbicularis oris improve function of the residual stoma.

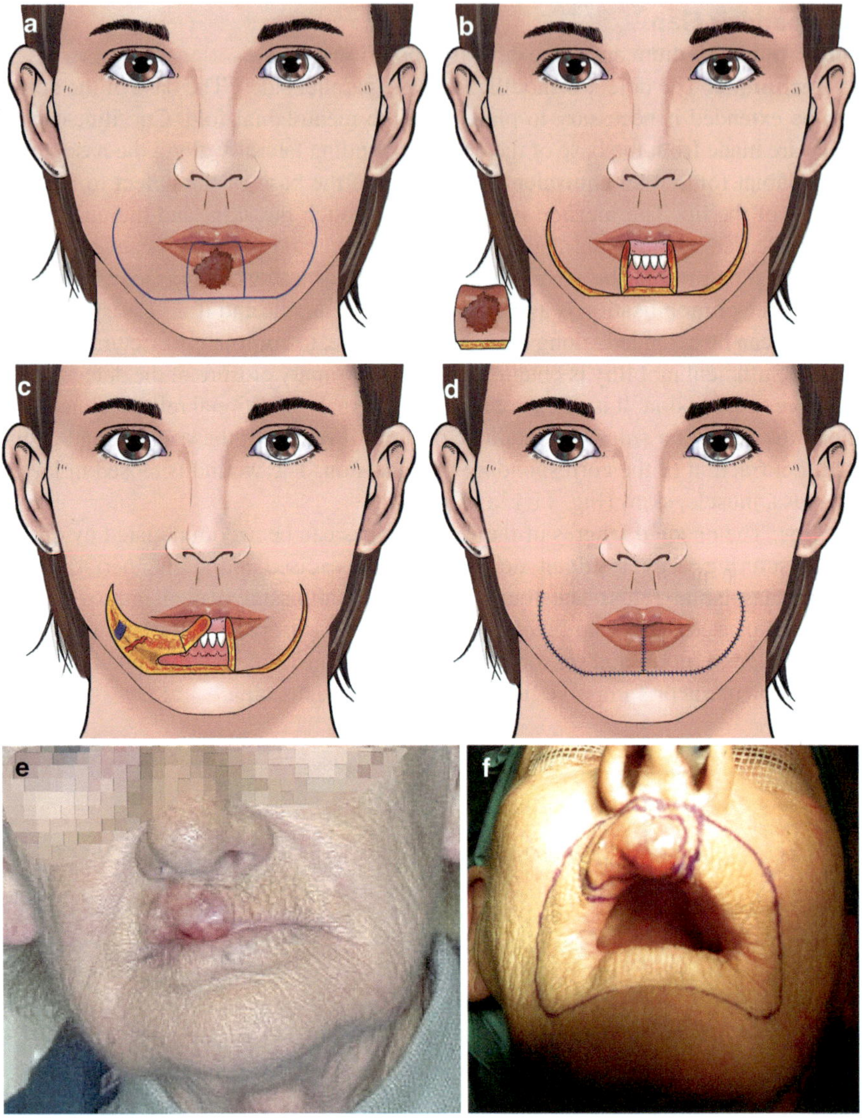

Fig. 11.13 Karapandzic flap. (**a**) Markings for excision and flap, (**b**) Excision defect and flap incisions, (**c**) Identification and preservation of vessels and nerves, (**d**) Final closure, (**e**) Lesion in the upper lip, (**f**) Markings for excision and flap, (**g**) Excision defect, (**h**) Flap incisions, (**i**) Flap mobilised into defect, (**j**) Final closure, (**k**) Post operative appearance

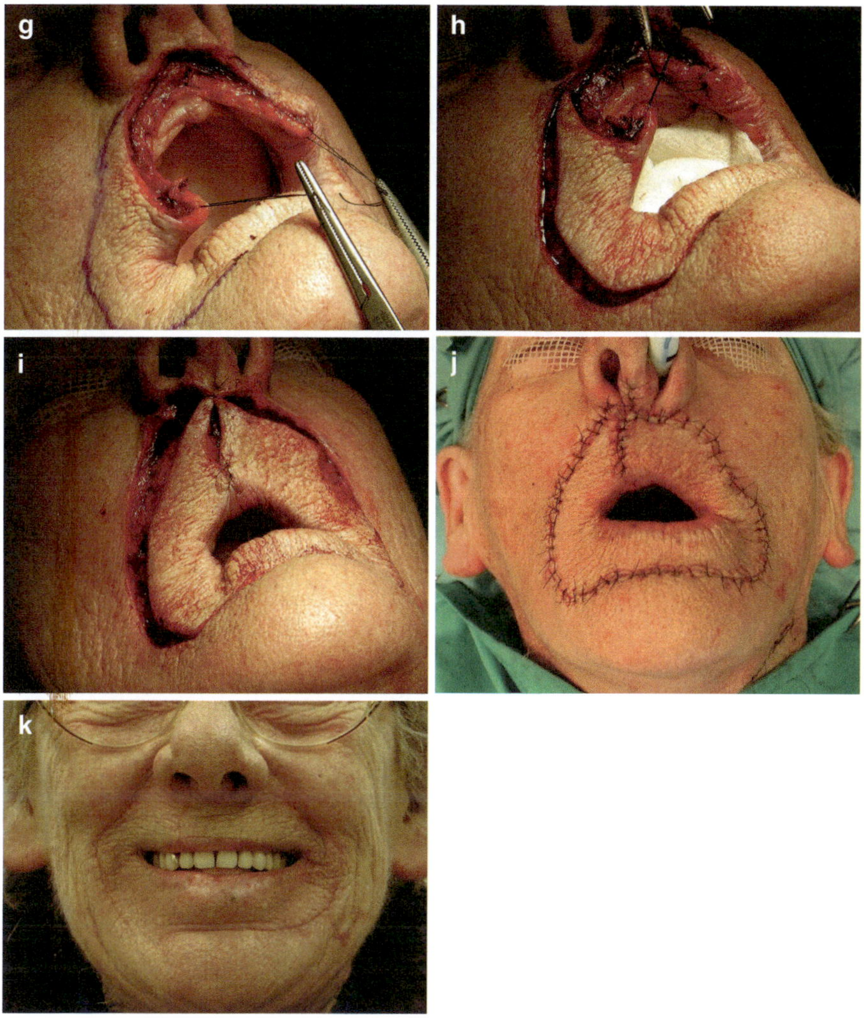

Fig. 11.13 (continued)

Bilateral Advancement Flap

Indications: Large defects.

Technique: The defect is modified to obtain parallel sides. An incision is made from the superior edge of the defect, curving upwards past the nasolabial fold and the inferior edge along the mentolabial fold. This incision is made only through skin and deeper tissues mobilised by blunt dissection. Corresponding incisions are made in the mucosa, to obtain the necessary mobilisation. The flaps edges are mobilised, and the wound is closed in layers (Fig. 11.14a–d).

Tips: The dog ears created are excised along the nasolabial and mentolabial folds. Care should be taken to prevent danaage to the mental nerves. Additional release of tissue from their mandibular attachements may be required. The advanced buccal mucosa can be used to resurface the lips, but a tongue flap may be necessary to obtain the necessary bulk.

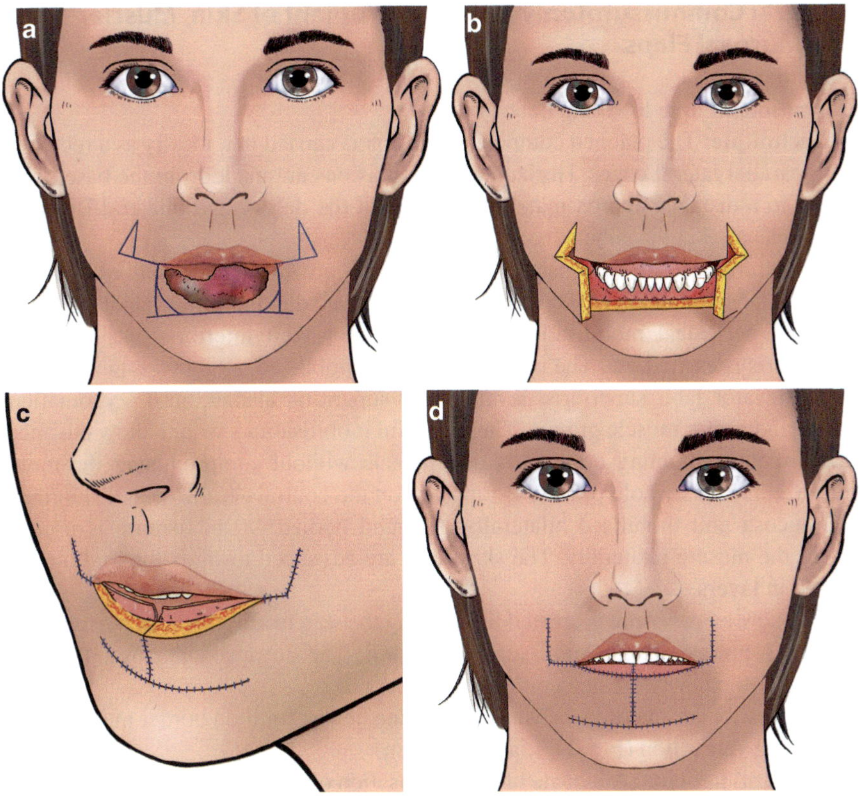

Fig. 11.14 Bilateral advamcement flaps. (**a**) Markings for excision and flap, (**b**) Excision defect and flaps raised, (**c**) Myocutaneous/mucosal flaps mobilsed into defect, (**d**) Final closure

Bilateral Commissurotomy and Advancement of Skin, Muscle, and Mucosal Flaps

Indications: Large lower lip defects.

Technique: The planned composite excision is carried out, ideally as a rectangle with parallel lateral edges. Horizontal skin incisions are made from the base of the defect to a distance approximately twice that of the defect, and bilateral Burrow's flap is elevated in the subcutaneous plane.

Bilateral mucosal commissurotomy incisions are then made and extended to same distance bilaterally. The mucosal flap is elevated to the lower labial sulcus.

Supra-periosteal mobilisation of the depressor labii inferioris and depressor anguli oris is carried out. The risorius is bluntly mobilised, along with mobilisation of the levator labii superioris, levator labii superioris alaeque nasi, zygomaticus major and minor muscle groups. These careful mobilisations would allow advancement of the remaining orbicularis oris muscle without compromising the motor innervation. This whole process is repeated on the contralateral side and skin/muscle/mucosa unit mobilised bilaterally. A round bodied 4/0 pds suture is used to repair the muscle bilaterally. The skin flaps are advanced towards the midline and closed in layers.

The new commissure is created by suturing the skin to the advanced muscle, with the same preoperative commissure dimension. The advanced mucosal flaps are sutured to the newly created commissure bilaterally.

The vestibular mucosa is advanced to create new vermillion border matching the remaining vermillion (Fig. 11.15a–d, e–i, j–m).

Tips and benefits: Adequate blunt mobilisation of the muscle group will provide the necessary lip volume. The commissurotomy only involves the orbicularis oris musculature. The mobilised muscle group based on the risorius will be sutured to the cut ends of orbicularis oris musculature, thus re-creating the new orbicularis oris aperture with intact motor innervation. Blunt dissection aids preservation of the motor and sensory innervations in addition to the vascularity of the mobilised tissue. As "additional" tissue is brought into the defect, it reduces the risk of microstomia associated with "redistribution" flaps. Round bodied needles are preferably used for suturing the muscle layer.

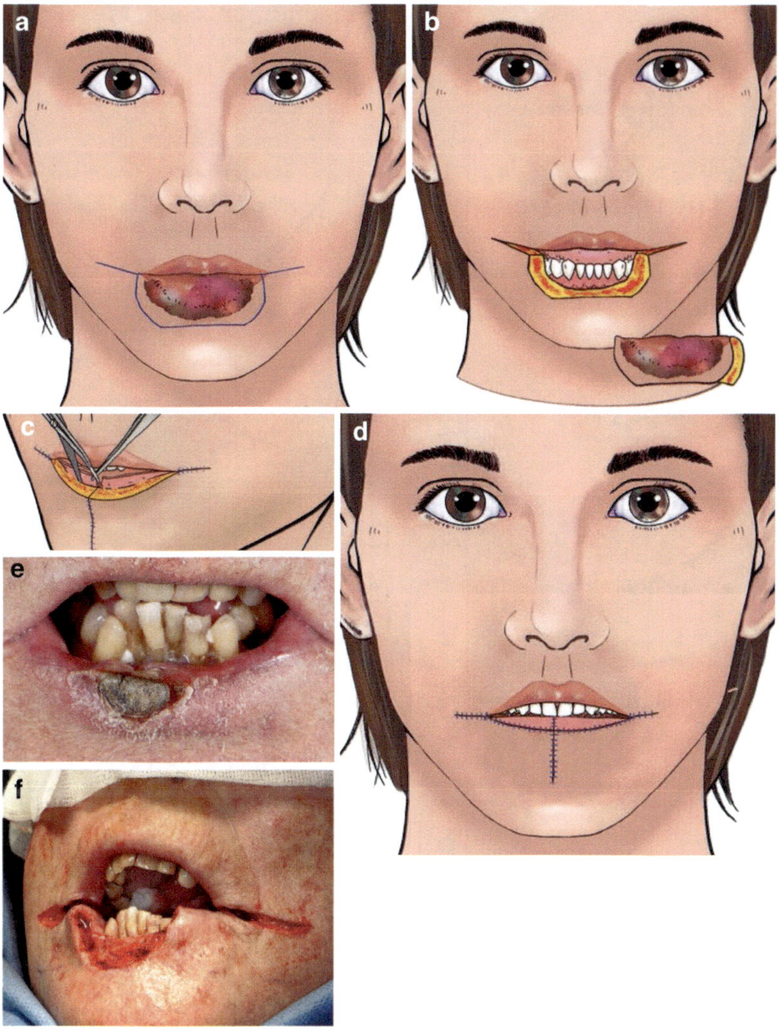

Fig. 11.15 Bilateral commisurotomyand advancement of skin, muscle and mucosal flaps. (**a**) Markings for excision and flaps, (**b**) Excision defect and flap incisions, (**c**) Mobilisation of myocutaneous and mucosal flaps into defect, (**d**) Final closure, (**e**) Large lesion lower lip, (**f**) Excision defect and flap incisions, (**g**) Final closure, (**h**) Post operative appearance - rest, (**i**) Post operative apperance - smiling, (**j**) Markings for excision and flap, (**k**) Excision defect and flap markings, (**l**) Fianl closure, (**m**) Early post operative appearance

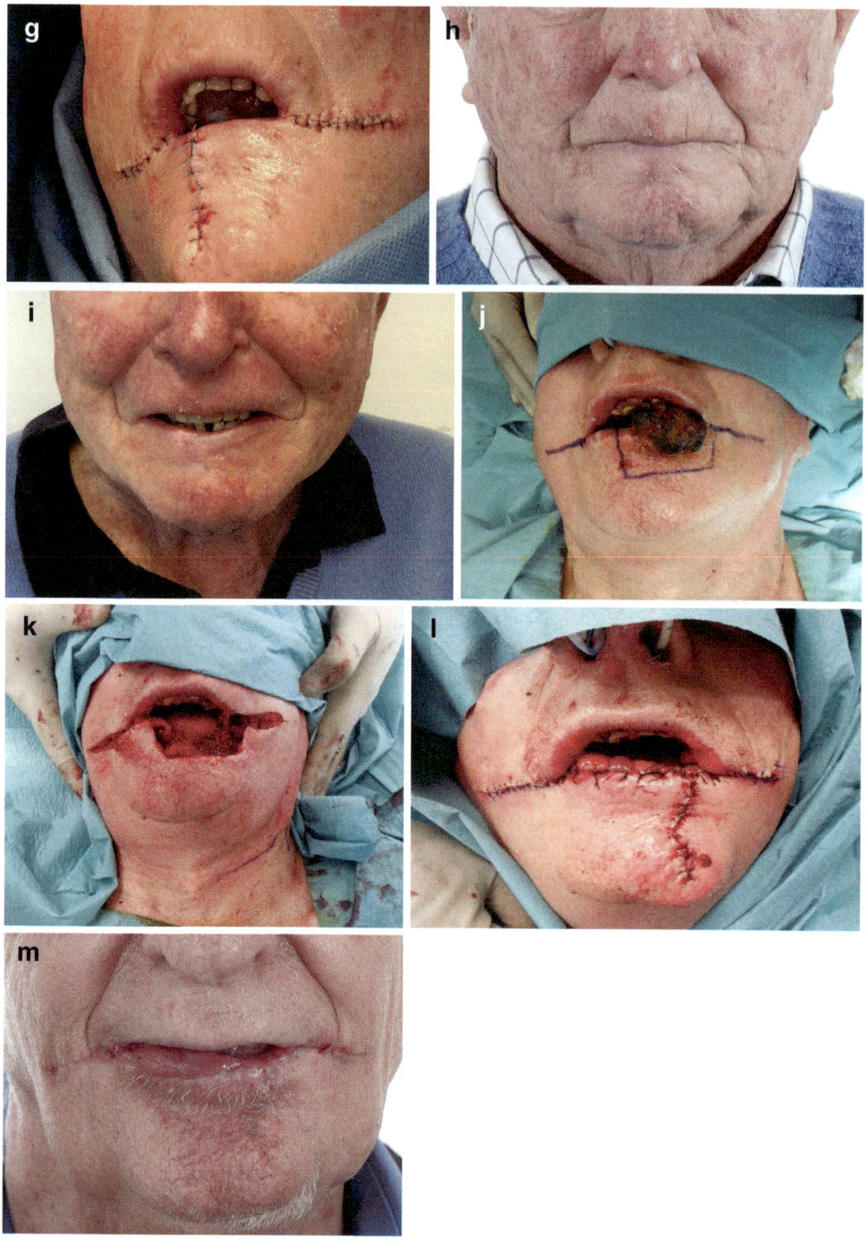

Fig. 11.15 (continued)

Karapandzic + Abbe Flap

Indications: Large defects.

Technique: (See Abbe (Fig. 11.1a–d) and karapandzic flaps (Fig. 11.13a–d) for additional details). The defect is modified to obtain parallel margins. An abbe flap based laterally and a karapandzic flap predominantly based on the contral lateral side are raised, taking particular care not to compromise the vascularity of the Abbe flap. The wounds are closed in layers (Fig. 11.16a–d). The Abbe flap is divided in 3–4 weeks time, and any revision of the vermillion border carried out at this stage (Fig. 11.16e).

Tips: (See Figs. 11.11a–d, 11.13a–d) This combination allows the donor sites to be more equally distributed between the upper and lower lip. A decrease in the size of the oral aperture is inevitable, as it is still a "lip redistribution" flap, which does not bring additional tissue to reconstruct the defect.

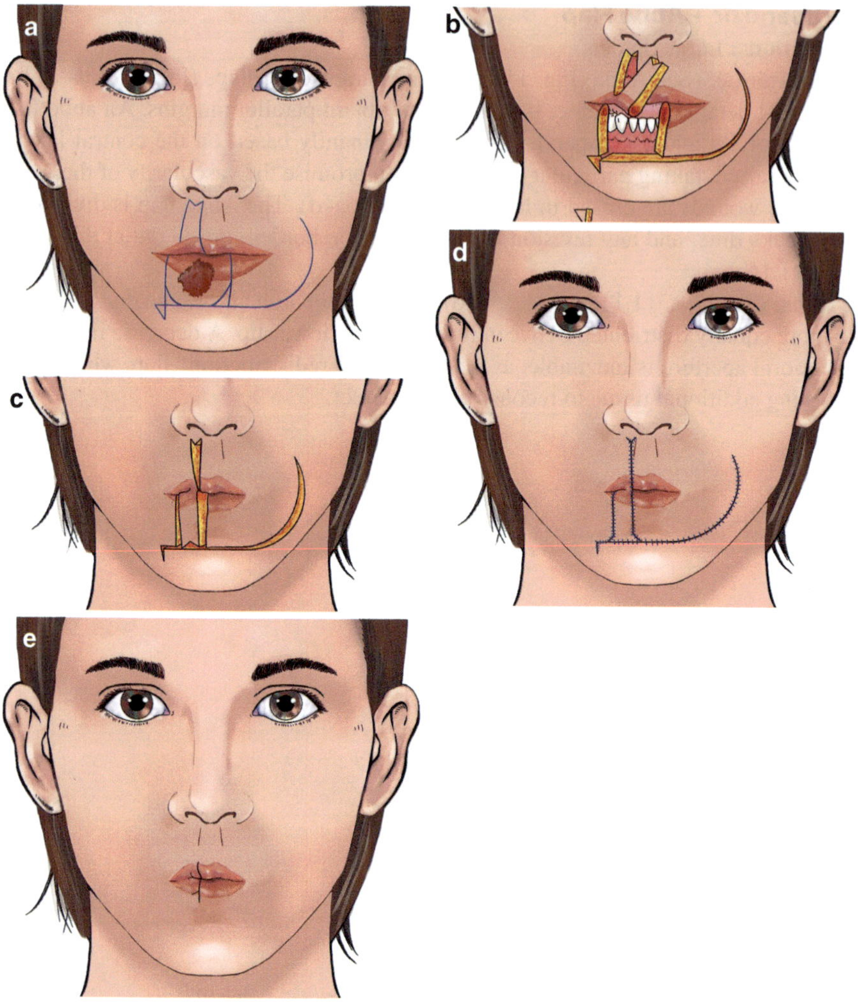

Fig. 11.16 Karapandzic and Abbe flap. (**a**) Markings for excision and flap, (**b**) Excision defect and flap raised, (**c**) Flaps mobilised into defect, (**d**) Final closure at first stage, (**e**) Final closure after second stage

Bilateral Fan Flap

Indications: Total lower lip defect.

Technique: The margins of the defect are modified to obtain parallel edges. The rectangular fan flap is marked out immediately lateral to the defect, with the width of the rectangle equal to the size of the hemi lip defect. The length (height) of the rectangle is twice the width and based along the nasolabial fold. The medial back cut is marked to stop short of the upper lip vermillion, to preserve the superior labial vessels and acts as a pivot point for the flap rotation. A full-thickness incision is made along the inferior, lateral and upper medial margins, and the flap mobilised into the defect. The wound is closed in layers. The vermillion is reconstructed with a tongue flap (Fig. 11.17a–d).

Tips: The fan flap imports "new" cheek tissue into the defect, and the reduction in size of the oral aperture is minimised. The motor and sensory nerve supply is divided (unlike a karapandzic flap) though partial ingrowth occurs over a period of time. The corners of the rectangle can be rounded to facilitate rotation and wound closure. The position of the commissure is often preserved. The defect margins are of different length and should be accommodated by differential suturing. It is often possible to place the final suture line along the nasolabial and mentolabial folds.

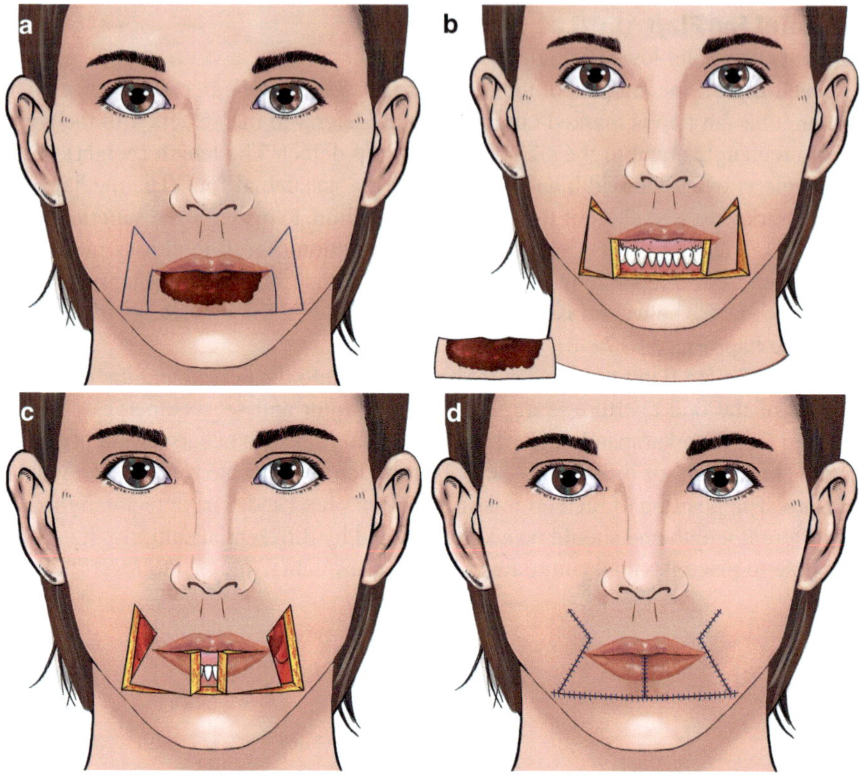

Fig. 11.17 Bilateral fan flaps. (**a**) Markings for excision and flaps, (**b**) Excision defect and flaps raised, (**c**) Flaps mobilised into defect, (**d**) Final closure

Upper Lip (Philtrum/Lateral)

Skin Only (Consider Converting to Full Thickness)

Primary Closure

Indications: Small defects.

Technique: The defect is converted into an ellipse to orient the scar along the perioral rhytids. The wound margins are undermined in the sub-cuatneous plane and closed in layers (Fig. 11.18a, b).

Tips: Closure of elliptical defects leads to increase in length of the scar and can cause distortion of the vermillion border. This can be overcome by utilising an alternate method of reconstruction or extending the wound into the mucosa and accurately approximating the vermillion border. Consideration should be given to converting the defect into a full-thickness defect to aid closure.

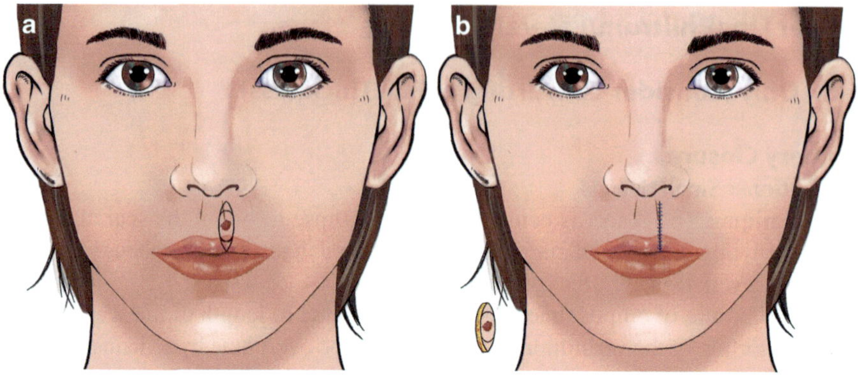

Fig. 11.18 Excison and primary closure. (**a**) Markings for excision, (**b**) Final closure

Bilateral/Unilateral Advancement Flap

Indications: Small- and medium-sized defects.

Technique: The defect is modified to obtain parallel lateral edges and extended superiorly and inferiorly to place the final suture line along the vermillion and base of nose, alar facial sulcus. The lateral flaps are raised in the subcutaneous plane, and any dog ears excised along the alar facial sulcus. The wounds are closed in layers (Fig. 11.19a–d).

Tips: The difference is length of the wound margins can be accommodated by differential suturing. Any dog ears that develop are excised along the alar facial sulcus and commissural rhytids. Accurate approximation of the vermillion is mandatory. In unilateral flaps, the medial suture line can be placed along the philtral ridge or perioral rhytids. Excision of muscle and mucosa is often needed to accommodate the excess tissue but is less than the skin excision.

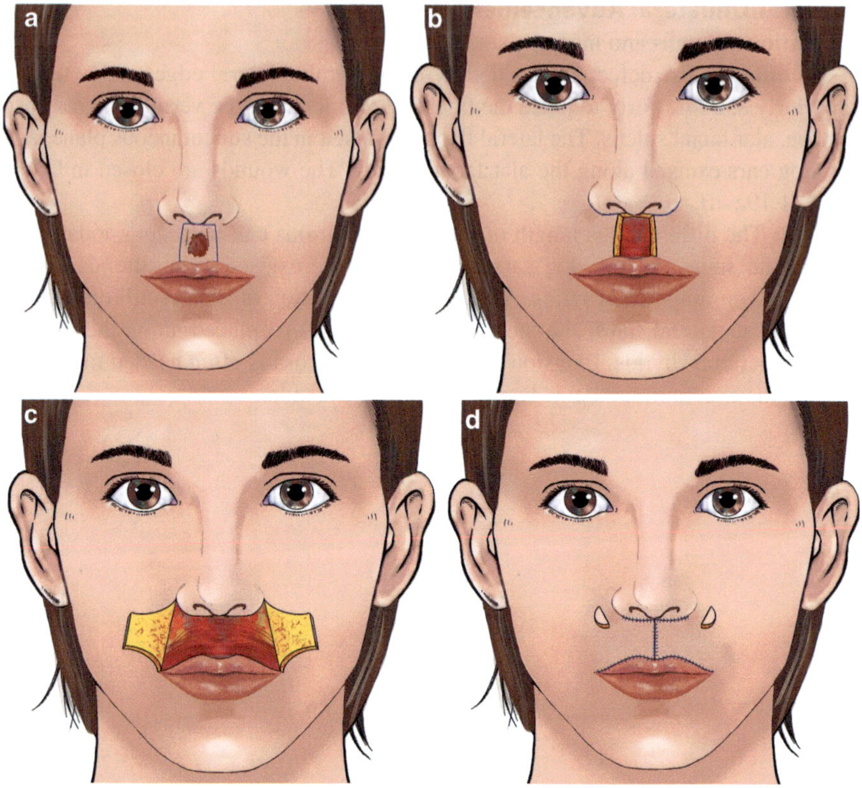

Fig. 11.19 Bilateral advancement flaps. (**a**) Markings for excision, (**b**) Excision defect, (**c**) Flaps raised, (**d**) Final closure

A-T Flap

Indications: Small defects, close to vermillion.

Technique: The defect is converted to a triangle, with the base along the vermillion border. Skin incisions are made laterally from the base of the triangle, along the vermillion border. The flaps are raised in a subcutaneous plane and mobilised into the defect. The wound is closed in layers (Fig. 11.20a–c).

Tips: The difference is length of the wound margins can be accommodated by differential suturing. Any dog ears that develop are excised along the perioral and commissural rhytids and by extending the vertical limb into the mucosal aspect. Accurate approximation of the vermillion is mandatory. Consideration can be given for converting to full-thickness defects.

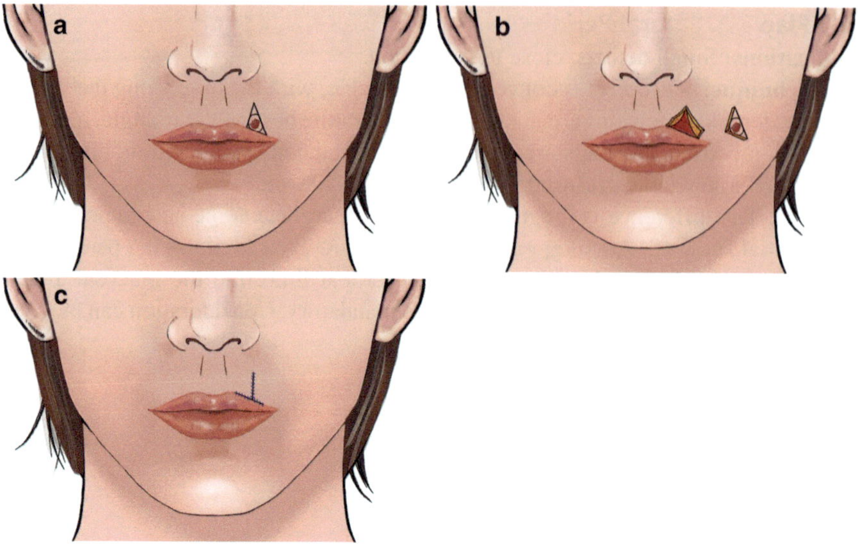

Fig. 11.20 A-T flap. (**a**) Markings for excision, (**b**) Excision defect and flaps raised, (**c**) Final closure

Unilateral/Bilateral Perialar Crescentic Advancement Flap

Indications: Medium-sized defects.

Technique: The defect is modified to obtain parallel lateral edges and extended superiorly and inferiorly to place the final suture line along the vermillion and base of nose, alar facial sulcus. The lateral flaps are raised in the subcutaneous plane, and any dog ears planned for excision along the alar facial sulcus. The wounds are closed in layers (Fig. 11.21a–d, e–g).

Tips: The difference is length of the wound margins can be accommodated by differential suturing. Any dog ears that develop are excised along the alar facial sulcus and commissural rhytids. Accurate approximation of the vermillion is mandatory. In unilateral flaps, the medial suture line can be placed along the philtral ridge or perioral rhytids. Excision of muscle and mucosa is often needed to accommodate the excess tissue but is less than the skin excision.

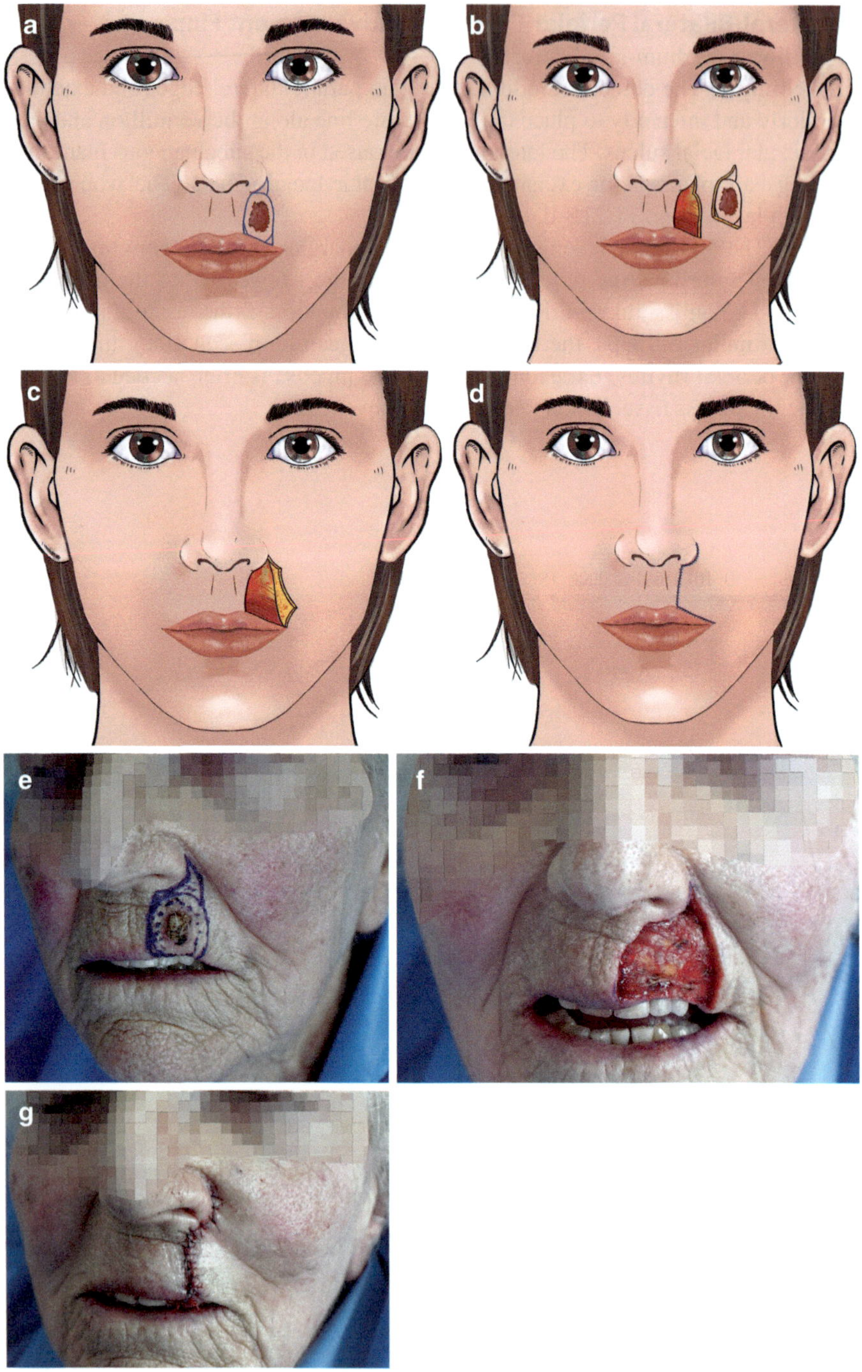

Fig. 11.21 Perialar cresentric advanceement flap. (**a**) Markings for excison and flap, (**b**) Excision defect, (**c**) Flap raised, (**d**) Final closure, (**e**) Markings for excision, (**f**) Excision defect, (**g**) Final closure

Laterally Based Rotation Flap

Indications: Small defects, away from vermillion.

Technique: The defect is modified into a triangle to place base along the nasal base/nasolabial fold. A curvilinear incision is made from the base of the defect, along the nasolabial fold. The flap is raised in a subcutaneous plane, and the dissection extended inferiorly to the vermillion junction. The wound is closed in layers (Fig. 11.22a–c, d–k).

Tips: The difference is length of the wound margins can be accommodated by differential suturing. Any dog ears that develop are excised along the alar facial sulcus. Accurate approximation of the vermillion is mandatory, and the wound can be extended inferiorly into the mucosa, to accommodate for any increase in length of the vertical component.

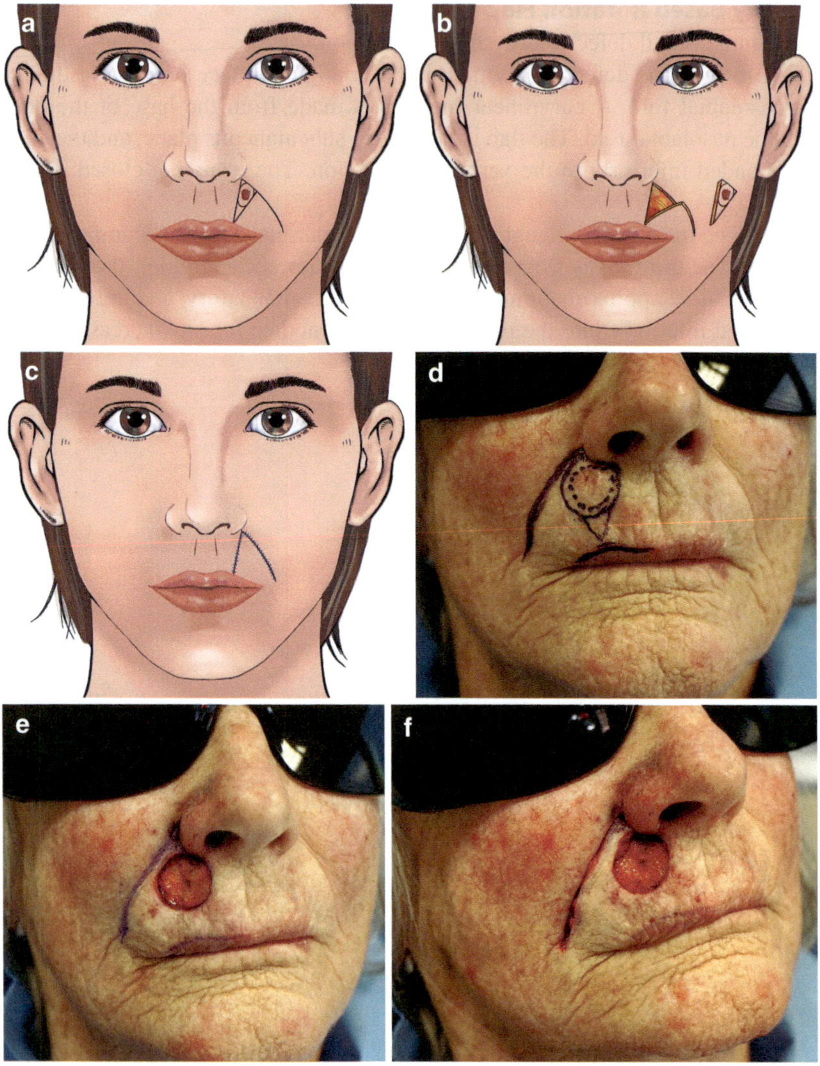

Fig. 11.22 Laterally based rotation flap. (**a**) Markings for excision and flap, (**b**) Excision defect and flap raised, (**c**) Final closure, (**d**) Markings for excision and flap, (**e**) Excision defect, (**f**) Flap incisions, (**g**) Flap raised, (**h**) Trial mobilisation, (**i**) Initial closure with delineation of dog ears, (**j**) Final closure, (**k**) Post operative appearance

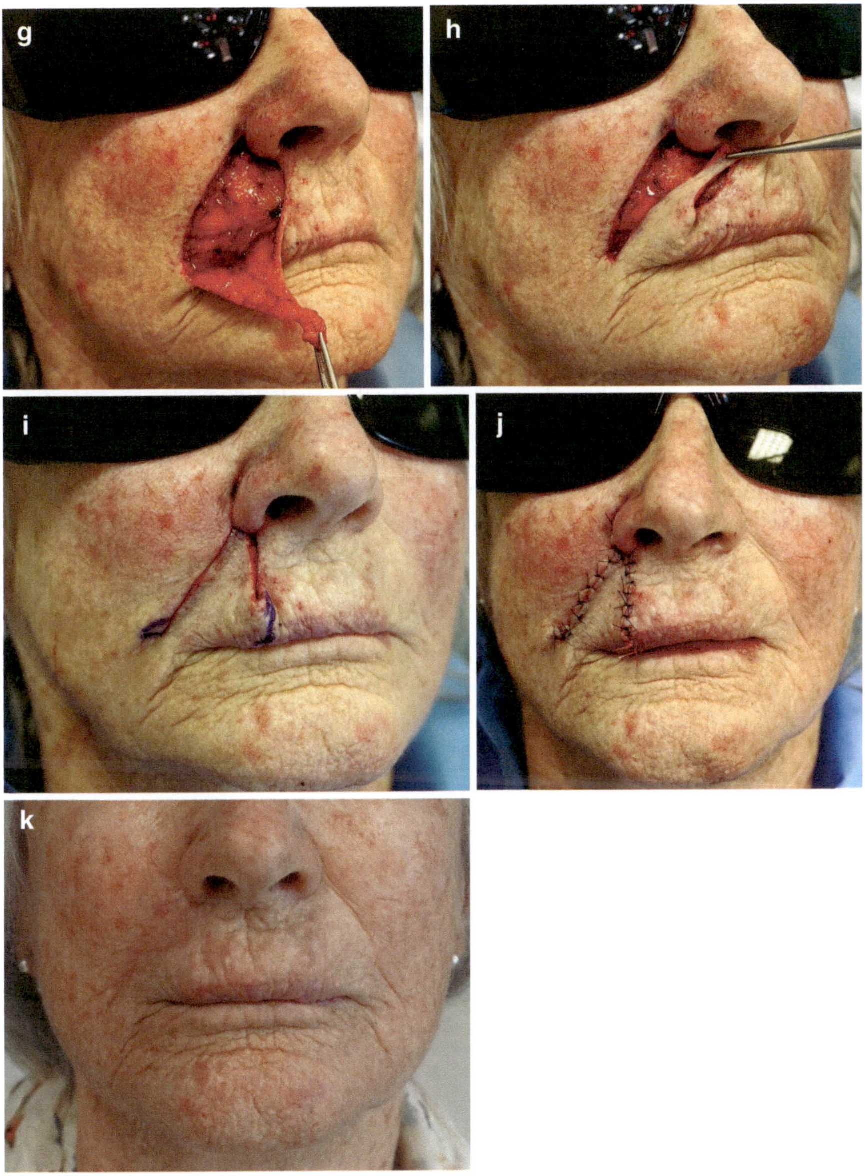

Fig. 11.22 (continued)

Island Advancement Flap

Indications: Medium-/large-sized defects.

Technique: The defect is modified to obtain parallel lateral margins and extended superiorly and inferiorly to the base of nose and vermillion border, if necessary, to best camouflage the scars. Curvilinear incisions are made from the superior and inferior margins of the defect, to delineate a triangular skin island, at least two to three times the length of the defect. The flap is oriented along the melolabial fold. The incision is deepened only through the skin along the entire outline of the flap. The central subcutaneous tissue, beneath the flap is preserved to provide the vascularity. The flap subcutaneous tissue closest and furthest from the defect is released incrementally to obtain the necessary mobility. The flap is mobilised into the defect, and wound is closed in layers (Fig. 11.23a–c, d–h, i–o).

Tips: The defect can be enlarged to occupy the whole subunit for best positioning of the scars. Maintain adequate width of the flap to avoid distortion of the vermillion border and nasal base. The size of the skin pedicle will also determine the extent of safe subcutaneous dissection. It is mandatory to retain an adequate subcutaneous island pedicle, the size of which needs to take into account additional tissue release that might be required to obtain the necessary mobility.

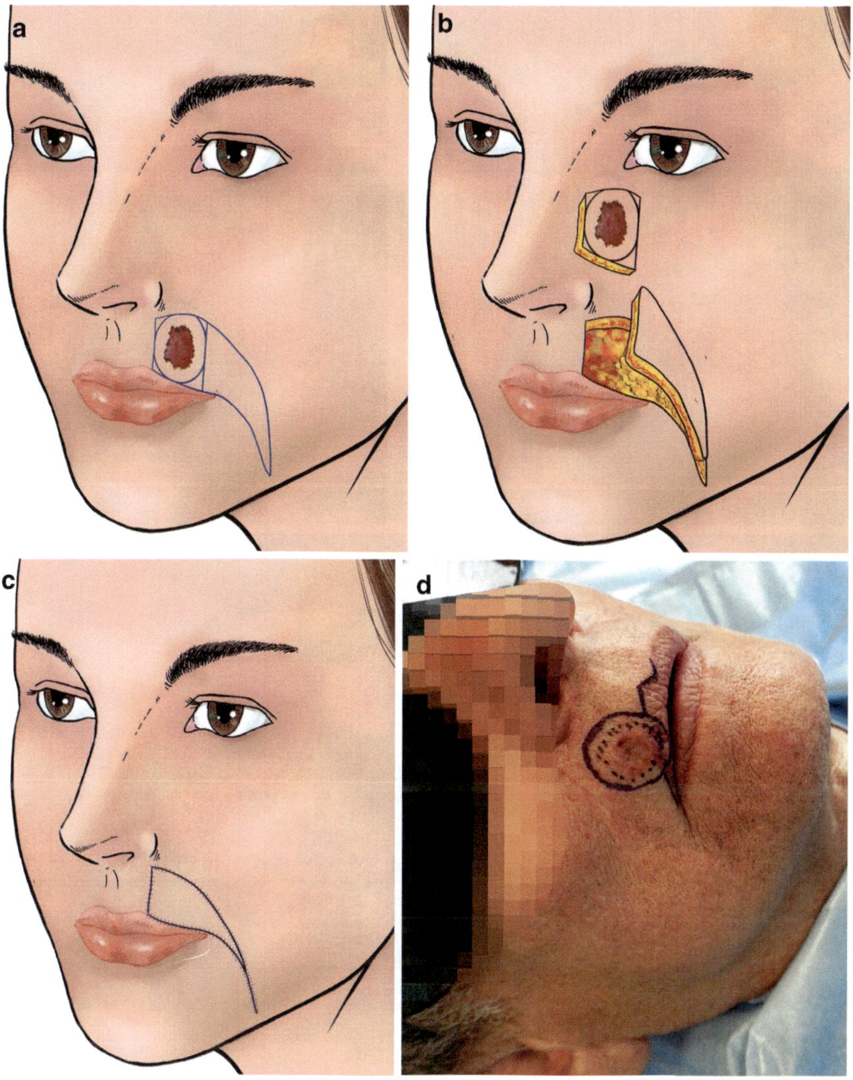

Fig. 11.23 Island advancement flap. (**a**) Markings for excision and flap, (**b**) Excision defect and flap raised, (**c**) Final closure, (**d**) Markings for excision, (**e**) Markings for excision and flap, (**f**) Excision defect, (**g**) Flap mobilised into defect, (**h**) Final closure, (**i**) Markings for excision, (**j**) Markings for excision and flap, (**k**) Excision defect, (**l**) Flap incisions, (**m**) Subcutaneous pedicle, (**n**) Flap mobilised into defect, (**o**) Final closure

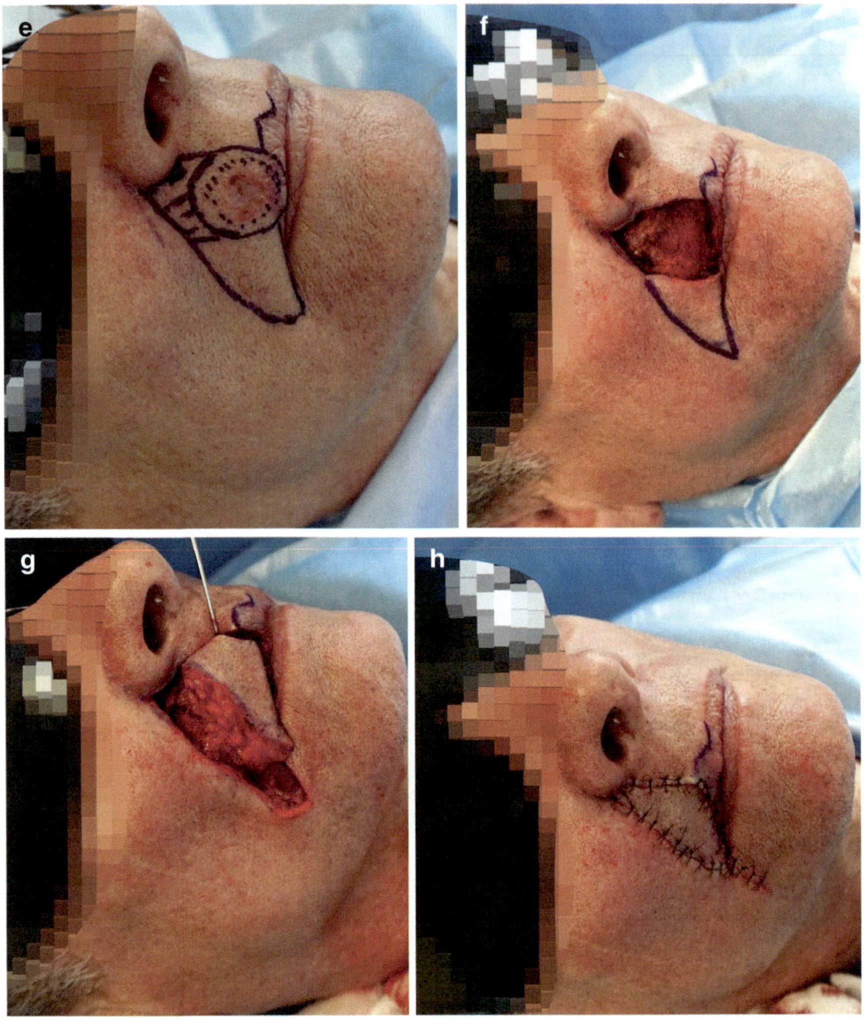

Fig. 11.23 (continued)

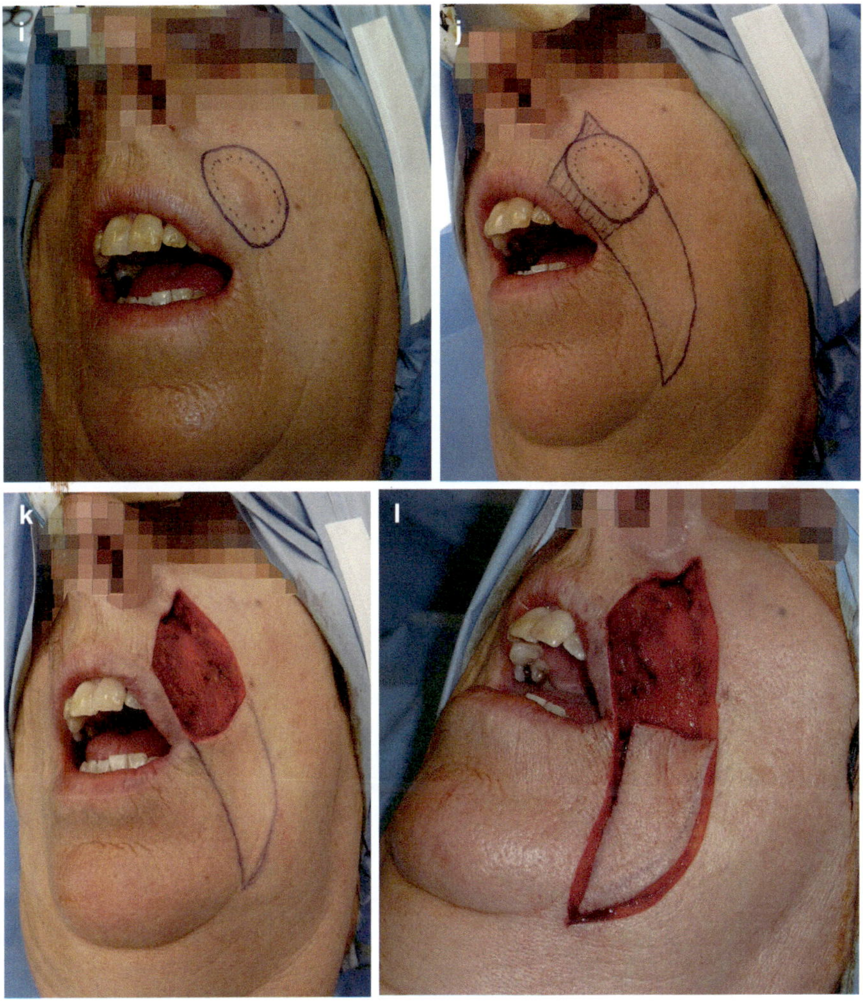

Fig. 11.23 (continued)

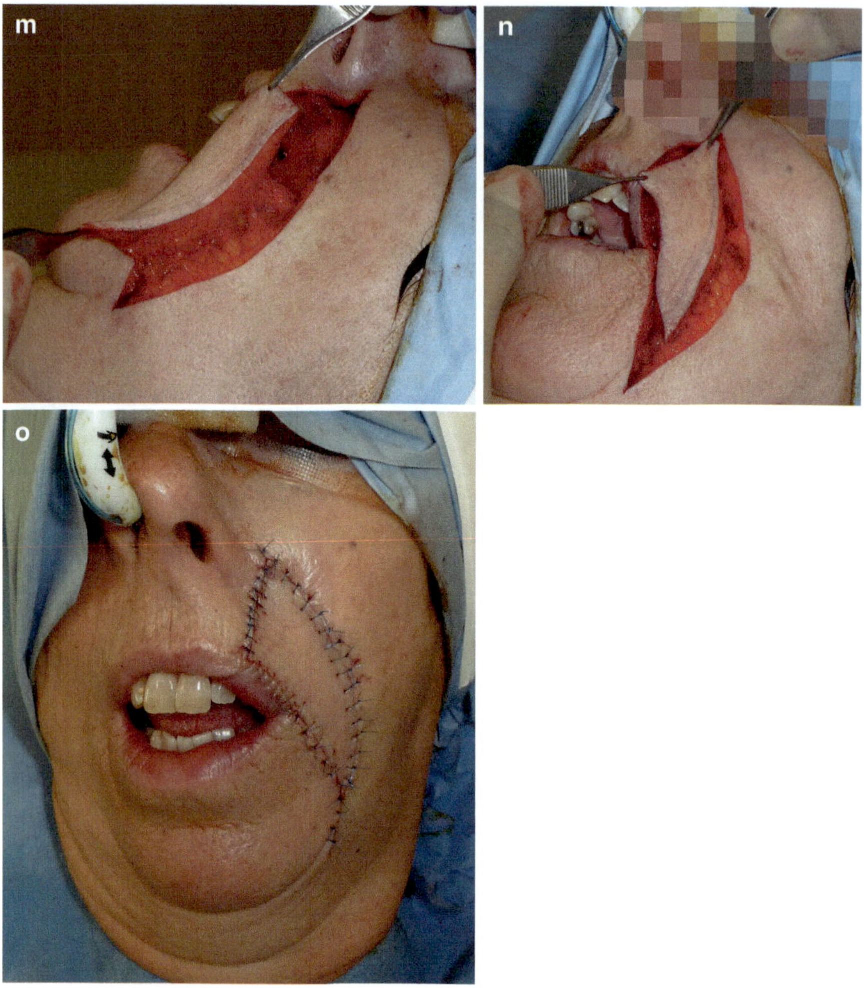

Fig. 11.23 (continued)

Inferiorly Based Nasolabial Flap

This is a random pattern flap, though it overlies the course of the facial vessels.

Indications: Medium-sized defect of a variety of shapes.

Technique: The defect is modified to obtain parallel lateral wound edges and extended inferiorly and superiorly to the vermillion border and nasal base. The flap is raised along the nasolabial fold, with one of its margins also forming the margin of the defect. A trial transfer and template can help determine the size of the flap. The overall length of the flap is planned to be longer to accommodate any loss of effective length and the tip triangulated to help primary closure. The base of the flap is designed to be wider than the tip to maintain vascularity. The flap is raised in the subcutaneous plane. The wound margins are undermined, the flap is mobilised into the defect, and the wound is closed in layers (Fig. 11.24a–d, e–i).

Tips: There is a tendency for "pin cushioning" with circular defects, and it also makes it difficult to place the scars along RSTL (see superiorly based nasolabial flap—Fig. 11.5a–d). The width of the flap should be adequate to prevent displacement of the vermillion and nasal base.

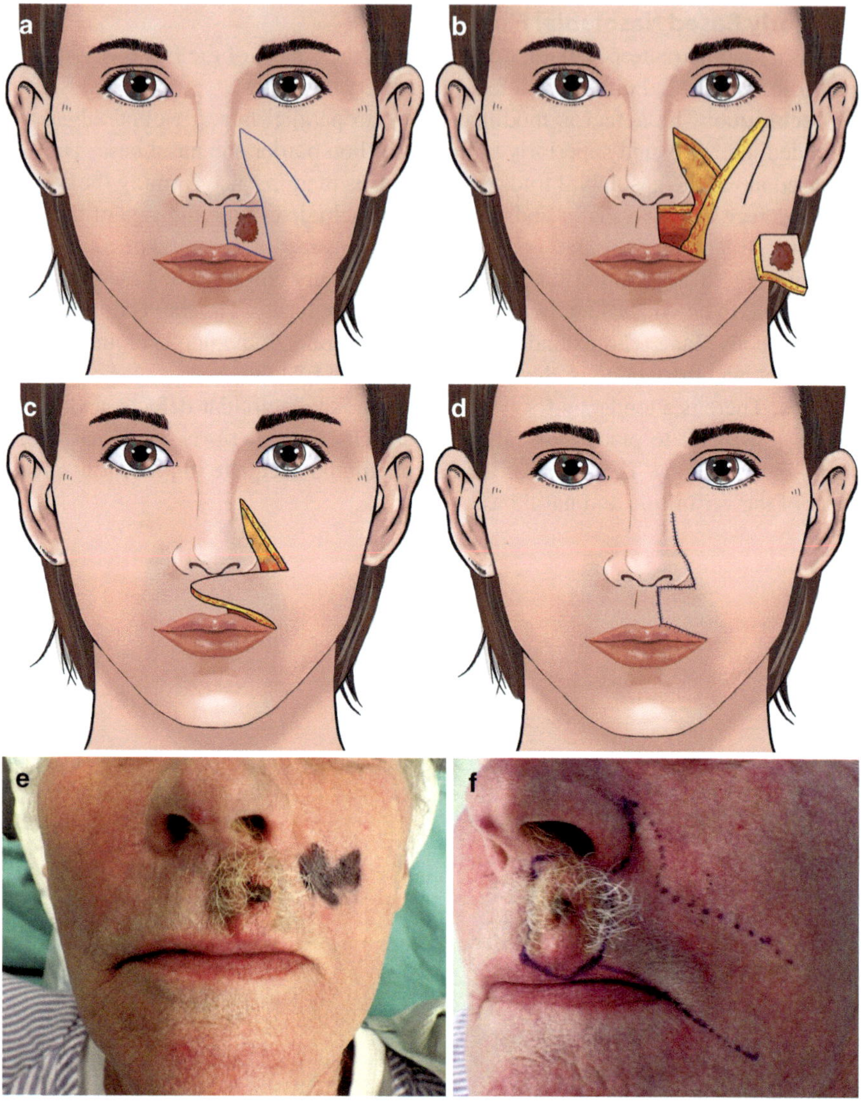

Fig. 11.24 Inferiorly based nasolabial flap. (**a**) Markings for excision and flap, (**b**) Excision defect and flap raised, (**c**) Flap mobilised into defect, (**d**) Final closure, (**e**) Lesion upper lip, (**f**) Markings for excision and flap, (**g**) Excision dfect and flap raised, (**h**) Fianl closure, (**i**) Early post operative appearance

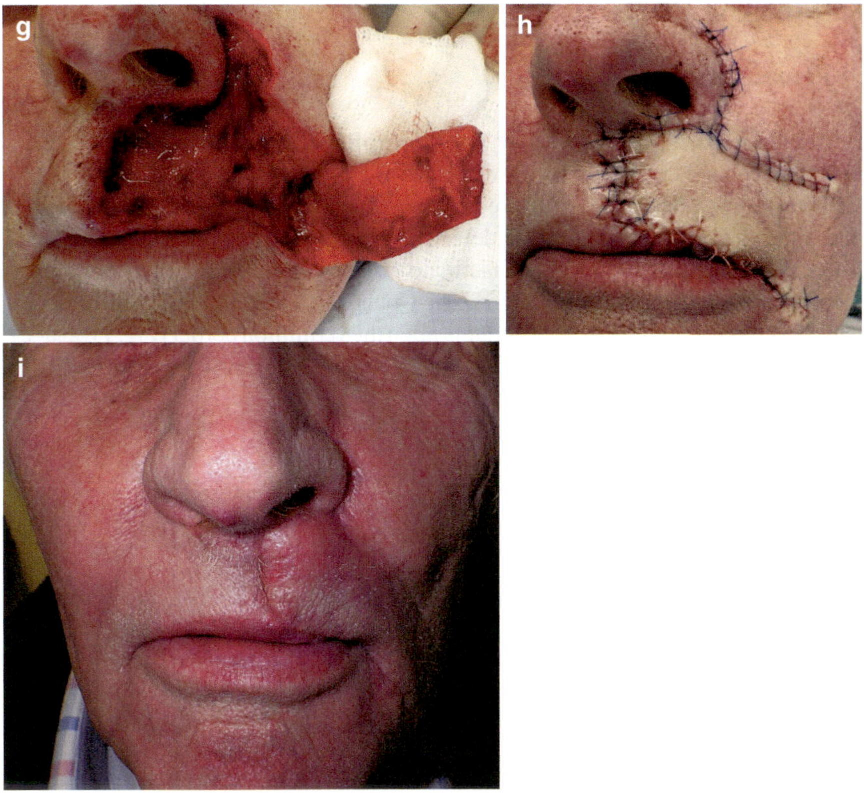

Fig. 11.24 (continued)

Full-Thickness Defects

Philtrum/Lateral Defects

Primary Closure (Shield Rather Than Simple "V" Excision)

Indication: Small defects up to 1/3rd of the lip.

Technique: The lesion is marked with adequate margins, and the excision is planned to leave a "shield" shaped defect, with parallel wound edge inferiorly and triangulated margins superiorly to facilitate primary closure. The axis of the excision is made along the perioral rhytids. The wound is closed in three layers (mucosa, muscle and skin), taking care to accurately align the vermillion border (Fig. 11.25a–c).

Tips: A "shield" excision rather than a "V" allows the tension to be evenly distributed across a larger area. Getting an assistant to squeeze the lips, during the resection aids control of the labial arteries for haemostasis.

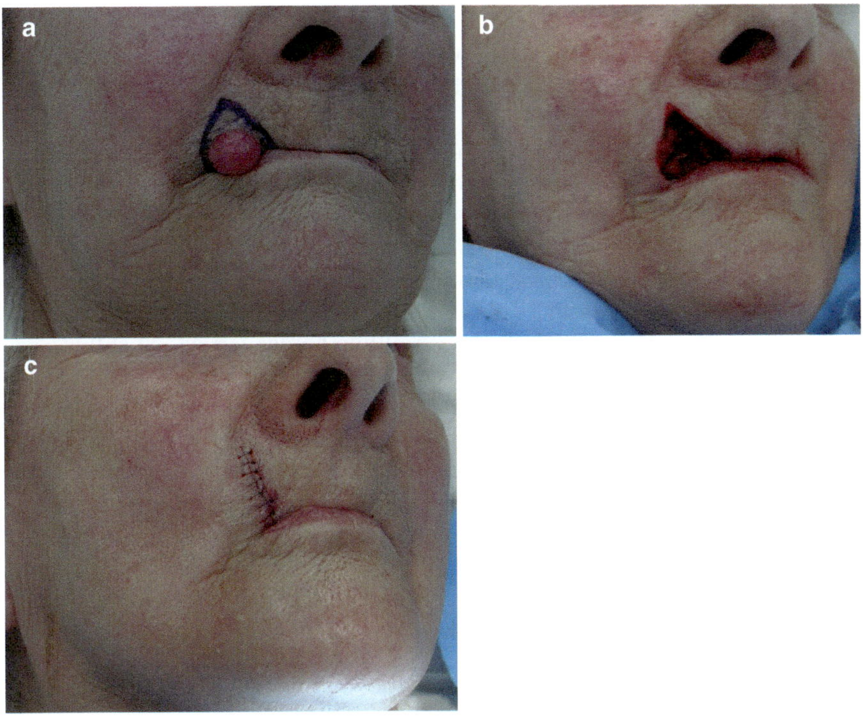

Fig. 11.25 Excision and primary closure. (**a**) Markings for excision, (**b**) Excision defect, (**c**) Final closure

Abbe Flap

Indications: Medium-sized defects, away from the commissure, two-stage flap.

Technique: The defect is modified to have parallel wound edges. The flap is marked to have a similar height of the donor defect, but the width can be reduced by up to 30%, to make use of the redundancy of the remaining lip. A full-thickness incision is made along one of the borders of the flap (skin, muscle, mucosa), but the incision along the other border is stopped short of the vermillion, to avoid damage to the vascular pedicle (labial artery). The flap is rotated into the defect, and the wounds are closed in three layers, taking care to protect the labial artery. The donor site is closed primarily. The pedicle is divided in 3–4 weeks, and any revision to accurately approximate the vermillion border carried out at this stage (Figs. 11.26a–d, e–l).

Tips: Patient compliance is vital, and the patient should be counselled appropriately, prior to the procedure. The initial incision on the side of the flap with the vascular pedicle should stop short of the vermillion border. With extreme care, further dissection can be carried out through the skin and part of the muscle, to help accurately approximate the vermillion border during the primary reconstruction. As discussed at the beginning of the chapter, the labial artery runs along the free border of the lip, below the mucosa on the posterior aspect of the orbicularis oris and maintaining a portion of the muscle above the vessels offers some additional protection.

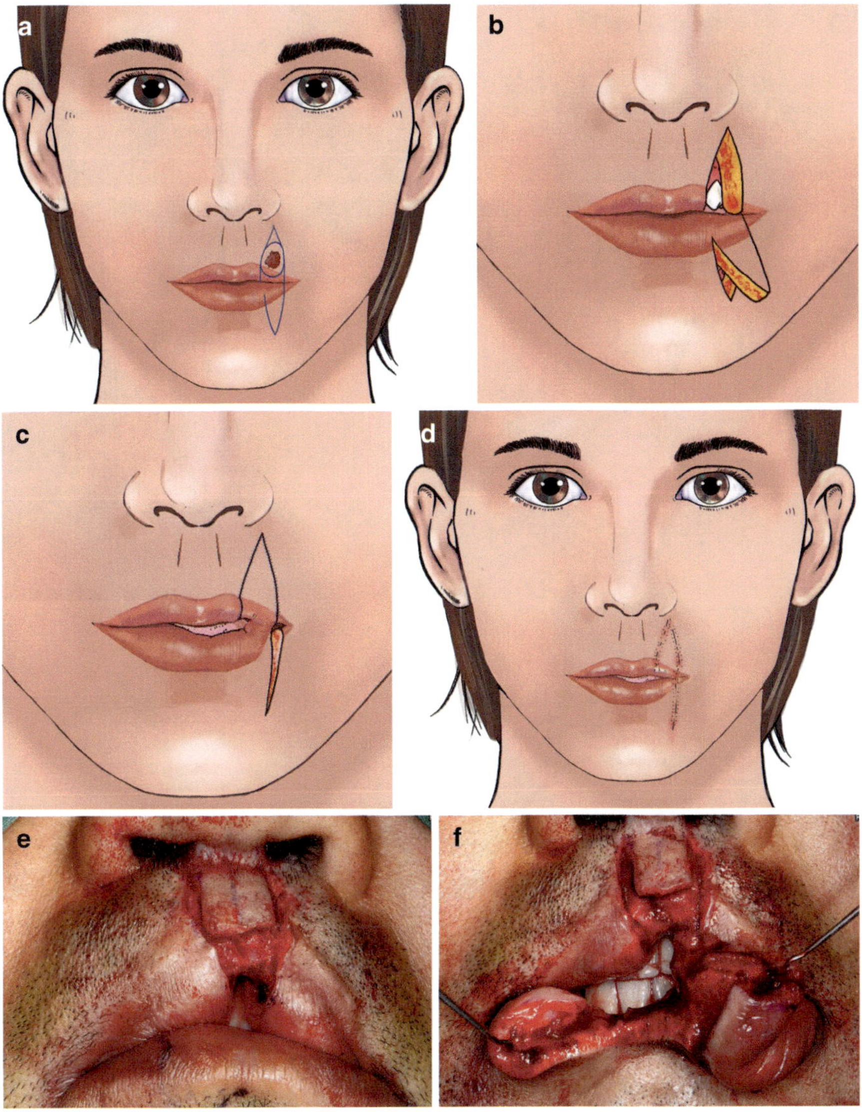

Fig. 11.26 Abbe flap. (**a**) Markings for excision and flap, (**b**) Excision defect and flap raised, (**c**) First stage flap inset and suturing, (**d**) Second stage after flap division, (**e**) Defect upper lip, (**f**) Flap raised lower lip, (**g**) Initial closure distal flap edge, (**h**) subsequent closure proximal flap edge, (**i**) Closure donar site - final appearance first stage, (**j**) Final appearance - first stage lateral view, (**k**) Apperanace after second stage flap division, (**l**) Post operative appearance

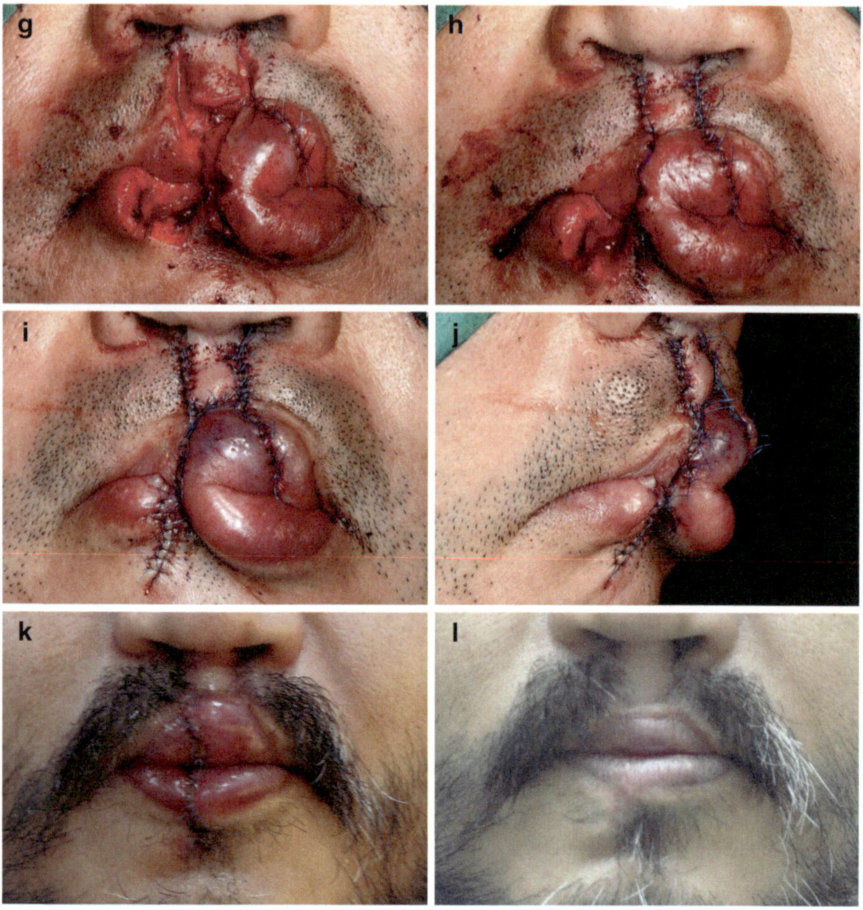

Fig. 11.26 (continued)

Abbe–Estlander Flap

Indications: Medium-sized defects involving the commissure.

Technique: The flap is marked to have a similar height of the donor defect, but the width can be reduced by up to 30%, to make use of the redundancy of the remaining lip. A full-thickness incision is made along the lateral border of the flap (skin, muscle, mucosa), but the incision along the media border is stopped short of the vermillion, to avoid damage to the vascular pedicle (labial artery). The flap is rotated into the defect, and the wounds are closed in three layers, taking care to protect the labial artery (Fig. 11.27a–d). The donor site defect is closed primarily. The intact medial border now forms the new commissure.

Tips: The initial incision on the side of the flap with the vascular pedicle should stop short of the vermillion border. With extreme care, further dissection can be carried out through the skin and part of the muscle, to help accurately approximate the vermillion border during the primary reconstruction. As discussed at the beginning of the chapter, the labial artery runs along the free border of the lip, below the mucosa on the posterior aspect of the orbicularis oris and maintaining a portion of the muscle above the vessels offers some additional protection. The residual asymmetry of the commissure improves with time and might need revision at a later date.

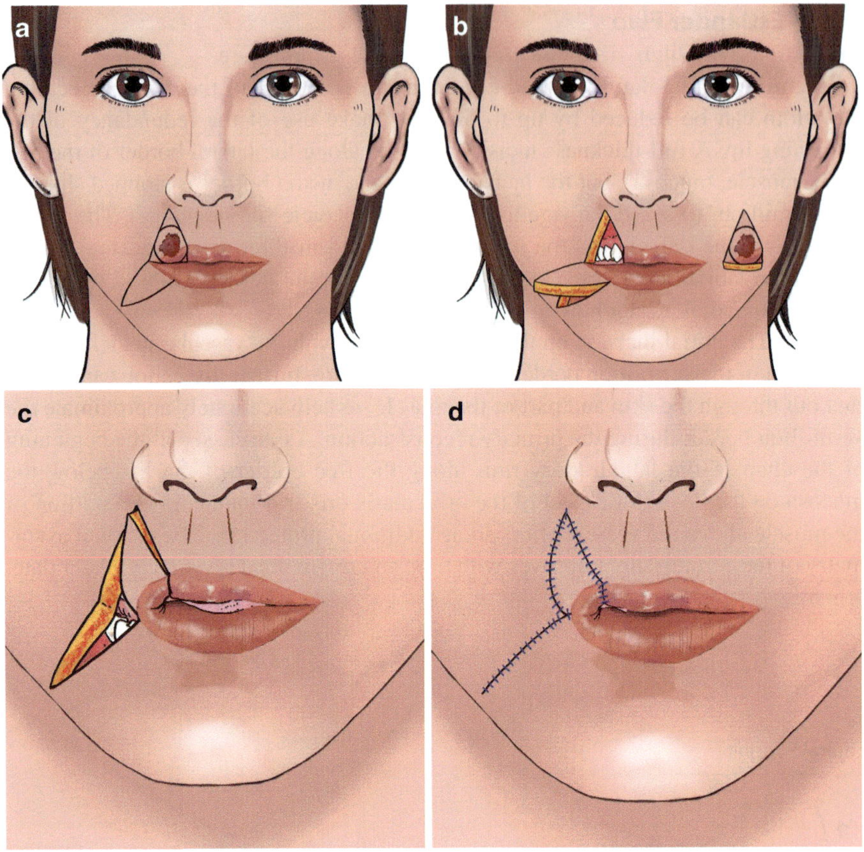

Fig. 11.27 Abbe-Estlander flap. (**a**) Markings for excision and flap, (**b**) Excision defect and flap raised, (**c**) Flap mobilised into defect, (**d**) Final closure

Unilateral/Bilateral Perialar Crescentic Advancement Flap

Indications: Medium-sized defects.

Technique: The defect is modified to obtain parallel lateral edges and extended superiorly, to place the suture line along the base of nose, alar facial sulcus. An incision is made from the base of the defect, along the base of the nose and extended laterally around the alar facial sulcus. The dissection is through skin, subcutaneous tissue and muscle, but the mucosa along the depth of the labial sulcus is initially preserved. The flaps are mobilised medially and the mucosa at the base released at this stage as required. Burrows triangles are excised along the alar facial sulcus. The wound is closed in three layers, taking care to accurately approximate the vermillion border (Fig. 11.28a–d).

Tips: The difference is length of the wound margins can be accommodated by differential suturing. Any dog ears that develop are excised along the alar facial sulcus. Accurate approximation of the vermillion is mandatory. In unilateral flaps, the medial suture line can be placed along the philtral ridge or perioral rhytids. Mucosal incisions can often be smaller than the corresponding skin component.

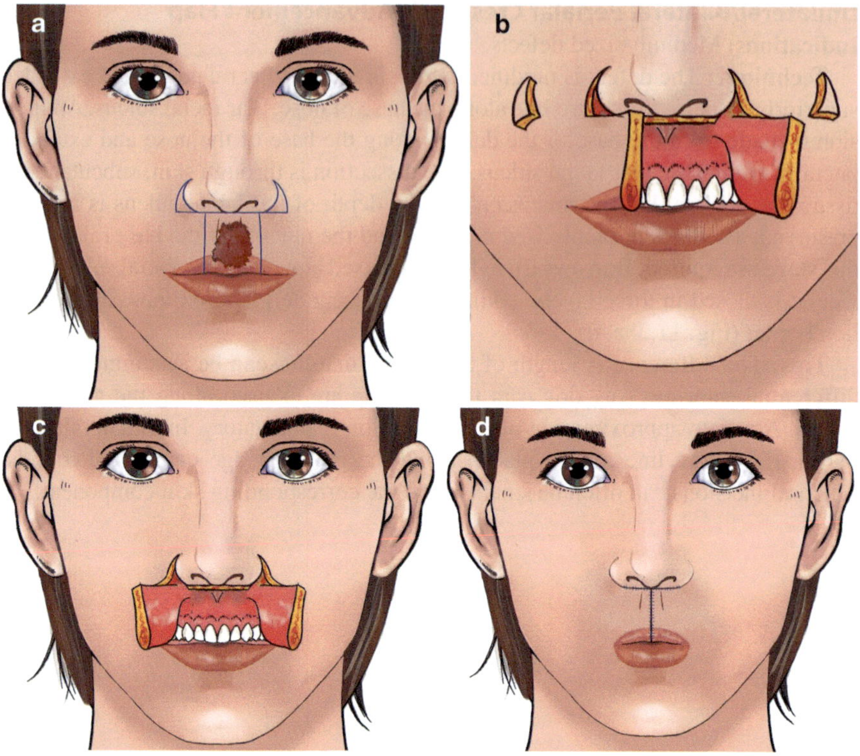

Fig. 11.28 Perialar cresentric advancement flap. (**a**) Markings for excision and flap, (**b**) Excision defect and flap incisions, (**c**) Flaps raised, (**d**) Final closure

Nasolabial Flap + Abbe Flap

Indications: Total upper lip defect.

Technique: An Abbe flap is raised to reconstruct the philtrum (see Fig. 11.26). Two inferiorly based nasolabial flap are raised, with the inferior extent of the medial incision stopping at the level of the planned commissure. A trail transfer will help determine the size of the flap, and the tip is triangulated to facilitate primary closure of the secondary defect. The dissection is deepened up to the periosteum superiorly and mucosa inferiorly. The flaps are mobilised, and the mucosa at the depth of the vestibule is released laterally to reconstruct the inner layer. The nasolabial flaps are sutured to the Abbe flap in layers (Fig. 11.29a–e). The Abbe flap is divided in 3–4 weeks, and any additional revision of the vermillion undertaken at this stage (Fig. 11.29f).

Tips: The nasolabial flaps imports "new" cheek tissue into the defect, and the reduction in size of the oral aperture is minimised. The motor and sensory nerve supply is divided (unlike a karapandzic flap) though partial ingrowth occurs over a period of time. The reconstruction of the lateral vermillion is however often less than ideal.

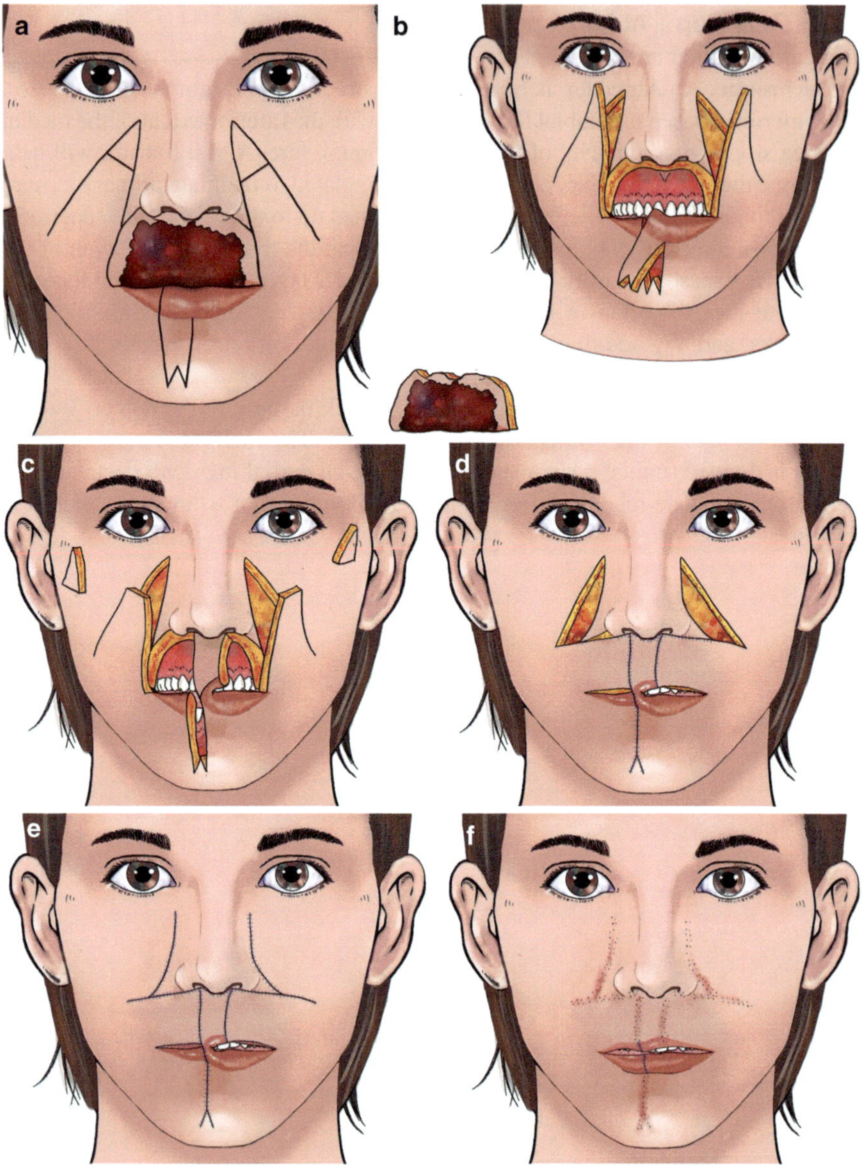

Fig. 11.29 Nasolabial flap + Abbe flap. (**a**) Markings for excision and flaps, (**b**) Excision defect and flaps raised, (**c**) Initial inset of Abbe flap, (**d**) Subsequent closure of lower lip donar site, (**e**) Final closure - first stage, (**f**) Second stage division of pedicle and closure

Chin Defects

The chin unit is defined by the mentolabial fold superiorly and laterally and the lower border of the mandible inferiorly. The RSTLs are arranged in a curvilinear pattern, and scars are ideally designed to lie parallel to these (See Figs. 11.1, 11.2).

Primary Closure

Indications: Small defects.

Technique: The defect is modified to an ellipse, to orient the eventual scar along the RSTLs. The wound margins are undermined, and the defect is closed in layers (Fig. 11.30a–c).

Tips: Care should be taken to avoid distortion of the mentolabial fold/lower lip, associated with the lengthening of the scar following elliptical excision.

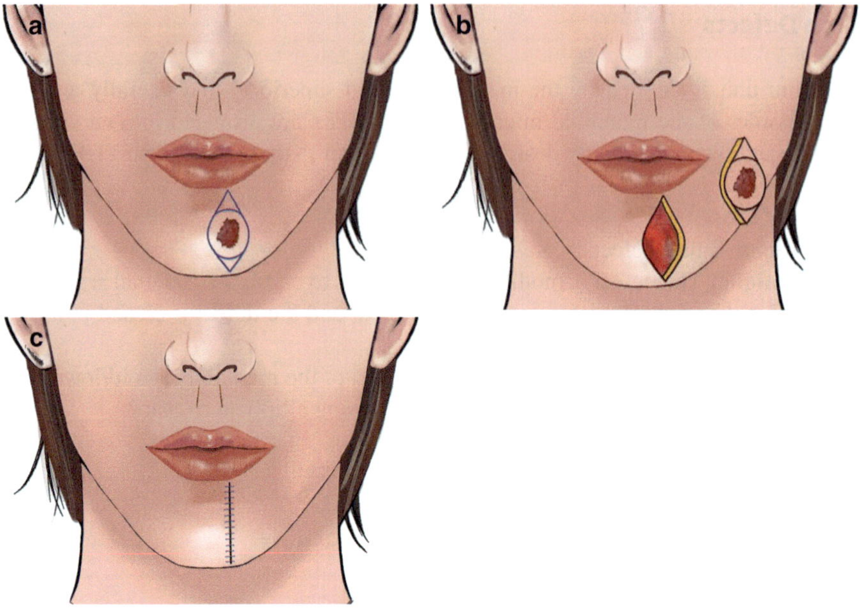

Fig. 11.30 Excision and primary closure. (**a**) Markings for excision, (**b**) Excision defect, (**c**) Final closure

V-T Transposition Flap

Indications: Small and medium defects, triangular defects, defects that can be modified into a triangle.

Technique: The defect is modified into a triangle, with the base along the mentolabial fold and its long axis along the chin RSTLs. Two curvilinear incisions are made from the base of the triangle, along the mentolabial folds. The flaps are raised in the subcutaneous flap and mobilised into the defect. The wound is closed in layers (Fig. 11.31a–c).

Tips: The difference is length and thickness of the wound margins can be accommodated by differential suturing. Any dog ears that develop are excised along the RSTLs.

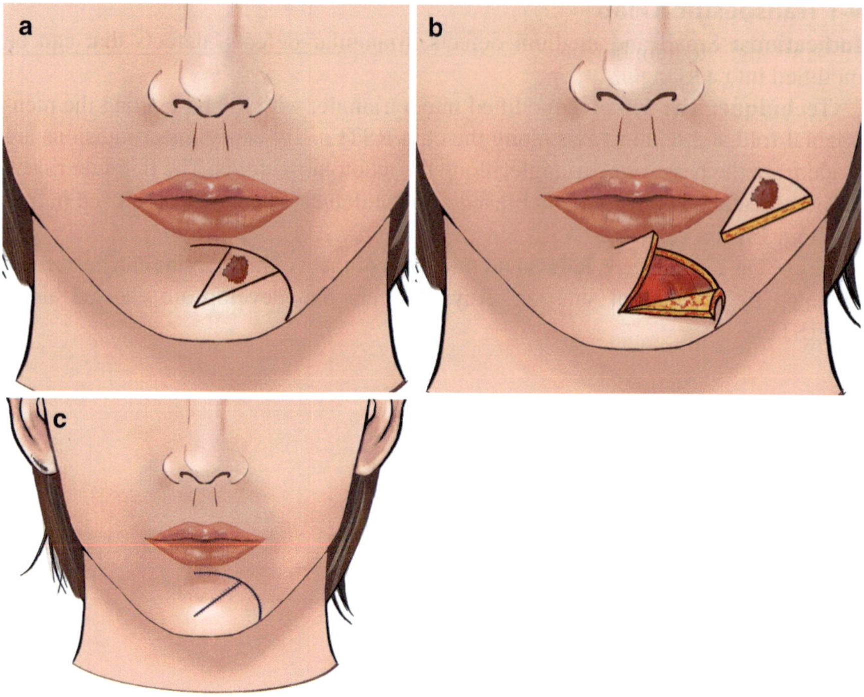

Fig. 11.31 V-T flap. (**a**) Markings for excision and flap, (**b**) Excision dfect and flaps raised, (**c**) Final closure

Rotation Flap

Indications: Medium defects.

Technique: The defect is modified into a triangle, with the base along the mentolabial fold and its long axis along the chin RSTLs. A curvilinear incision is made from the base of the defect, along the mentolabial fold. The flap is raised in the subcutaneous plane and mobilised into the defect. The wound is closed in layers (Fig. 11.32a–d).

Tips: The difference is length and thickness of the wound margins can be accommodated by differential suturing. Any dog ears that develop are excised along the RSTLs, preferably in the submental region. A back cut, if necessary, is best made outside the circumference of the flap rather than inside to avoid vascular compromise.

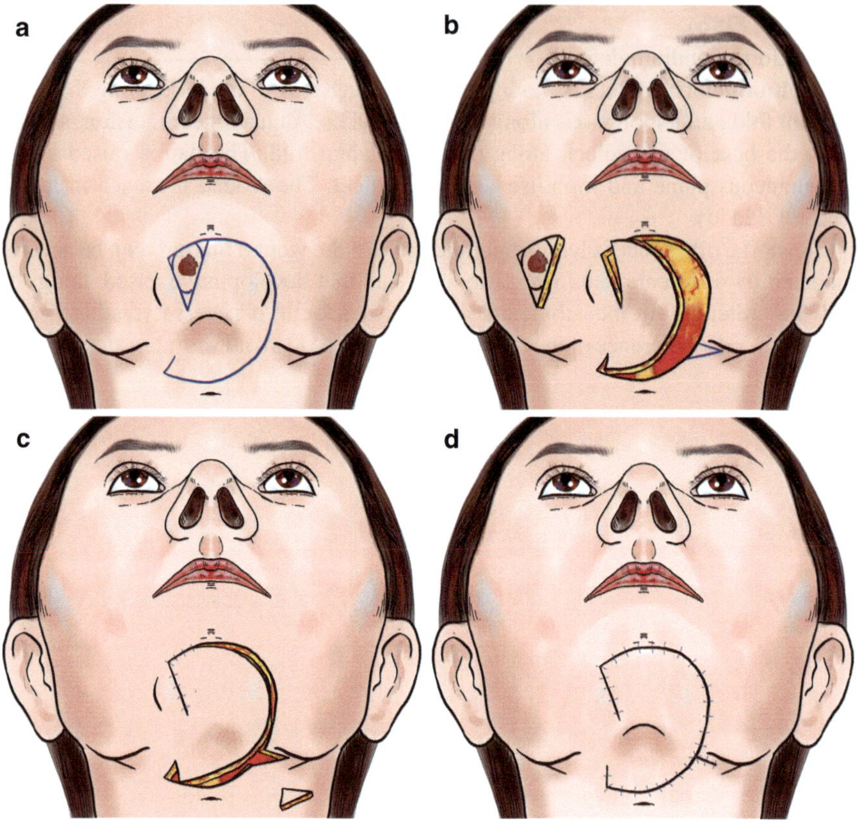

Fig. 11.32 Rotation flap. (**a**) Markings for excision and flap, (**b**) Excision defect and flap raised, (**c**) Flap mobilised into defect, (**d**) Final closure

Bilobed Flap

Indications: Medium-sized defects, circular defects.

Technique: The first lobe is designed to be of similar dimensions to the defect, and the second lobe can be made slightly narrower, but longer to accommodate triangulated ends on the summit, to facilitate primary closure. The flap is raised in the subcutaneous plane. The wound margins are widely undermined, and the defect is closed in layers. Closure of the primary defect often results in a dog ear at its base that will have to be corrected. The additional length of the second limb is excised, and the tertiary defect is closed primarily (Fig. 11.33a–d).

Tips: The flap is best designed lateral to the defect to utilise the tissue laxity and accommodate the scars in the submental area. Due to curvilinear incisions, it is not possible to place all the scars along RSTLs, and there is a tendency for "pin cushioning" of the flap. This can be partly mitigated by modifying the defect and flap margin to include right-angled corners and parallel wound margins.

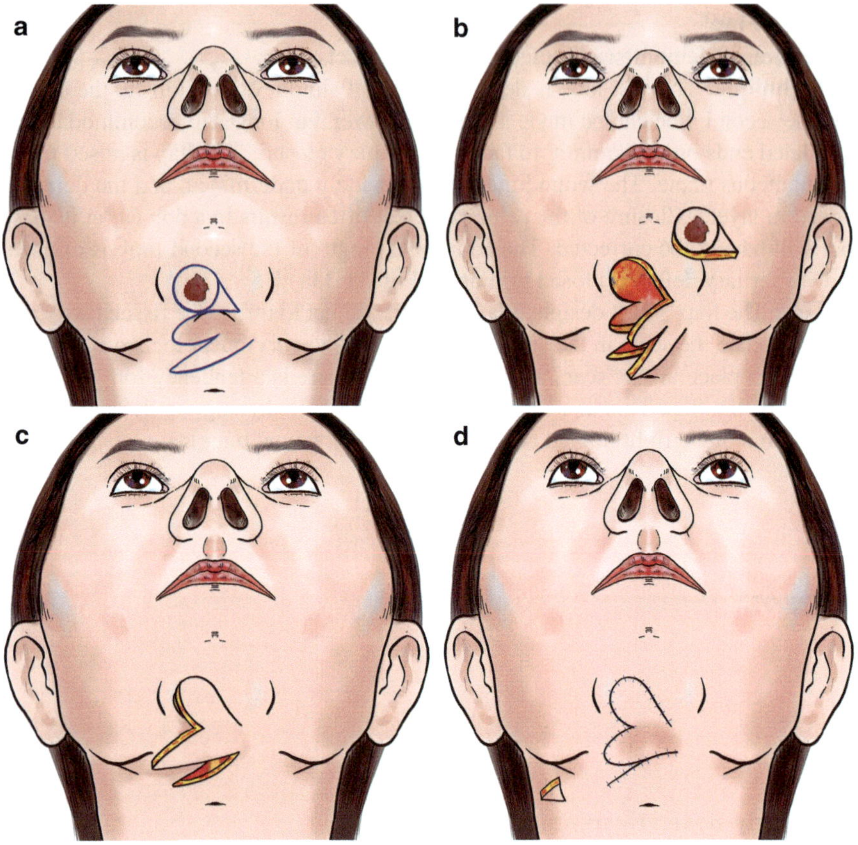

Fig. 11.33 Bilobed flap. (**a**) Markings for excision and flap, (**b**) Excision defect and flaps raised, (**c**) Flap mobilised into defect, (**d**) Final closure

Rhombic Flap

Indications: Medium-sized defects.

Technique: The defect is modified into a rhombus with 60° and 120° internal angles. The lateral/superior limbs are placed along the mentolabial fold, if possible. An inferiorly based rhomboid flap is designed by extending the short diagonal to a distance equal to one of the sides, and a further line is drawn from its extremity, parallel to the adjacent side of the defect. The flap is raised in the subcutaneous plane and mobilised into the defect. The wound is closed in layers (Fig. 11.34a–d).

Tips: Though four flaps could be raised for any given defect, inferiorly based flaps are able to best utilise the tissue laxity in the submental region. The flaps are ideally designed to place the superior/lateral margins along the mentolabial fold and along with inferiorly based flap, allow the scars to be placed in the most advantageous position.

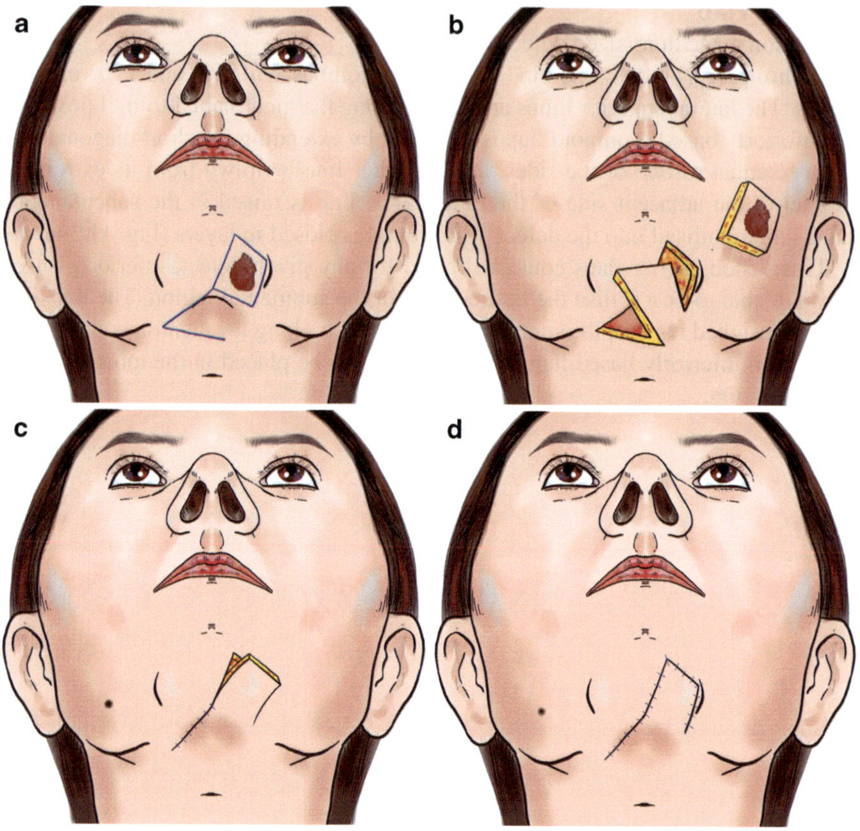

Fig. 11.34 Rhombic flap. (**a**) Markings for excision and flap, (**b**) Excision defect and flap raised, (**c**) Flap mobilsed into defect and closure of secondary defect, (**d**) Final closure

Nano Fat Grafting

Indications: Chronic non-healing vermillion ulcers, actinic cheilitis, chronic radiation induced ulcers, lip atrophy.

Technique: Nanofat has become an extremely useful material in perioral regeneration. It has more stem cells and the capacity to differentiate into an adipogenic lineage. This is an in vivo cellular therapy. A 27-gauge needle is used to inject very superficially, into reticular and papillary dermis in the cutaneous aspect. The goal on the mucosal aspect is to inject into the submucosal plane. The needle is inserted with the bevel facing upwards, and the nanofat is injected upon withdrawal of the needle. The nanofat injections are done in a layered fashion (two to three layers) along the vermillion border, areas of actinic keratosis and angular cheilitis (Fig. 11.35a–d). It can be repeated as necessary.

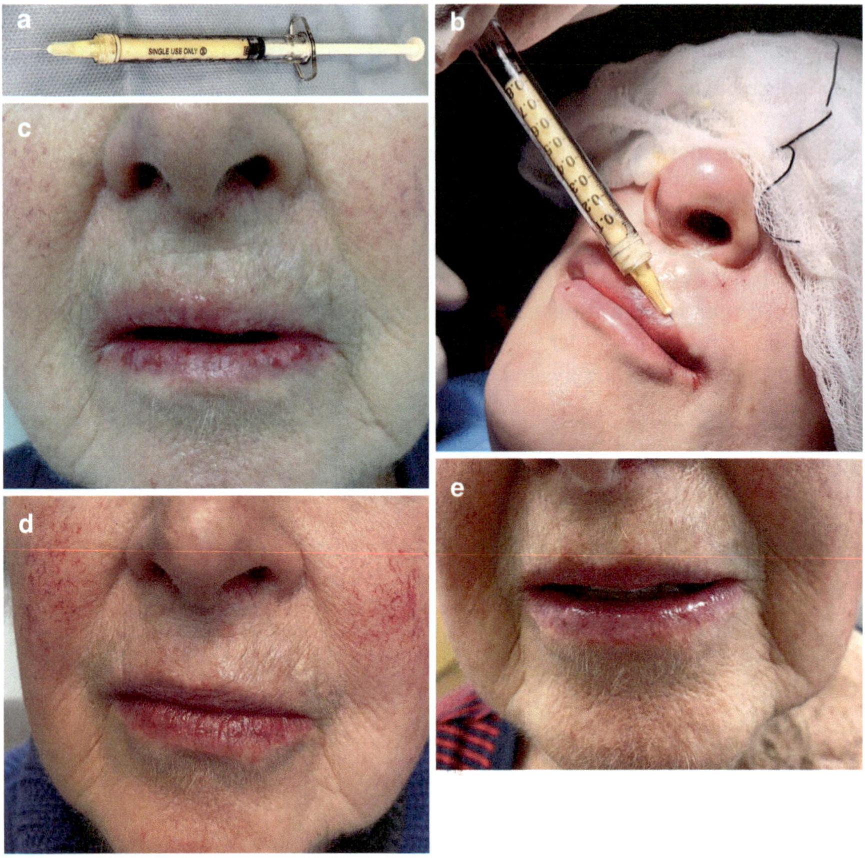

Fig. 11.35 Nanofat injection. (**a**) Harvested nanofat, (**b**) Nanofat injection, (**c**) Pre injection appearance, (**d** & **e**) Post injection appearance

Suggested Algorithm

Lips

Lower Lip

Skin Only

Small
1. Primary closure (along rhytids)
2. M/W closure

Medium
1. A-T, V-T flap
2. Inferiorly based nasolabial flap
3. Superiorly based nasolabial flap

Mucosa Only

Small
1. Primary closure

Medium/Large
1. Mucosal advancement flap

Full-thickness Defect

Small
1. Primary closure
2. W excision

Medium
1. Bilateral advancement flap
2. Karapandzic flap
3. Abbe flap
4. Abbe–Estlander flap

Large Defects
1. Karapandzic flap
2. Bilateral advancement flap
3. Karapandzic flap + Abbe flap
4. Fan flap

Upper Lip

Skin Only

Small
1. Primary closure
2. A-T flap

Medium
1. Laterally based rotation/transposition flap
2. Unilateral/bilateral perialar crescentic advancement flap
3. Island advancement flap
4. Inferiorly based nasolabial flap

Full Thickness

Small
1. Primary closure

Medium
1. Perialar crescentic advancement flap
2. Karapandzic flap
3. Abbe flap
4. Abbe–Estlander flap

Large
1. Bilateral nasolabial flap + Abbe flap

Upper/Lower Lip (Chronic Ulcers/Atrophy)

Nanofat injection

Chin Defects

Small
1. Primary closure

Medium
1. V-T flap
2. Rotation flap
3. Bilobed flap
4. Rhombic flap

Neck Defects

12

Subunits and Anatomical Considerations

The circumferential neck unit can be defined superiorly by the lower border of the mandible anteriorly and the hair line posteriorly. The inferior limits are the clavicle anteriorly and the upper border of the scapula posteriorly. The neck can be divided into anterior and posterior subunits, with the anterior subunit, being further divided into a midline and two lateral units (Fig. 12.1).

The thickness and mobility of the neck skin vary with the location and are often defined by the age of the person and general body habitus. The platysma muscle overlies the investing layer of the cervical facia and is often dehiscent in the midline. The anterior and external jugular veins lie immediately beneath the muscle. The nerves of the cervical plexus emerge from the posterior border of the sternomastoid muscle and along with the mandibular and cervical branches of the facial nerve also lie beneath the platysma. The RSTLs are obliquely and transversely oriented in the neck.

V. Ilankovan et al., *Local Flaps in Facial Reconstruction*,
https://doi.org/10.1007/978-3-031-49464-2_12

The skin of the posterior neck is thicker than that in the anterior/lateral neck and less mobile. The trapezius muscle enclosed by the investing layer lies beneath the skin.

The skin redundancy and the RSTLs allow flaps to be raised in the neck to reconstruct a variety of neck and adjacent defects, with good aesthetic outcomes. It also enables relatively large defects to be closed primarily.

Fig. 12.1 Neck subunits

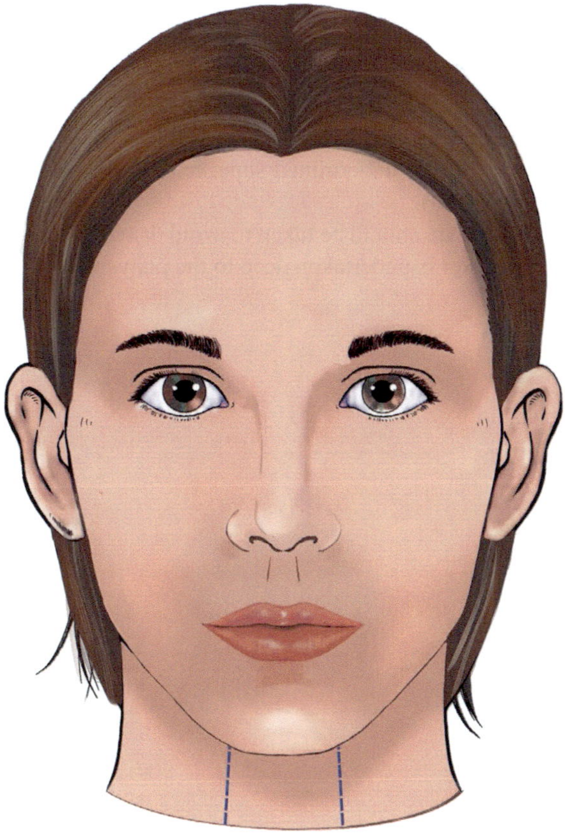

Central Neck

Primary Closure

Indications: Small and medium defects.

Technique: The defect is converted into an ellipse, along the RSTLs. The wound margins can be undermined superficial or deep the platysma and closed in layers (Fig. 12.2a–c).

Tips: Care should be taken to avoid damage to the underlying nerves and vessels if dissection is undertaken deep to the platysma.

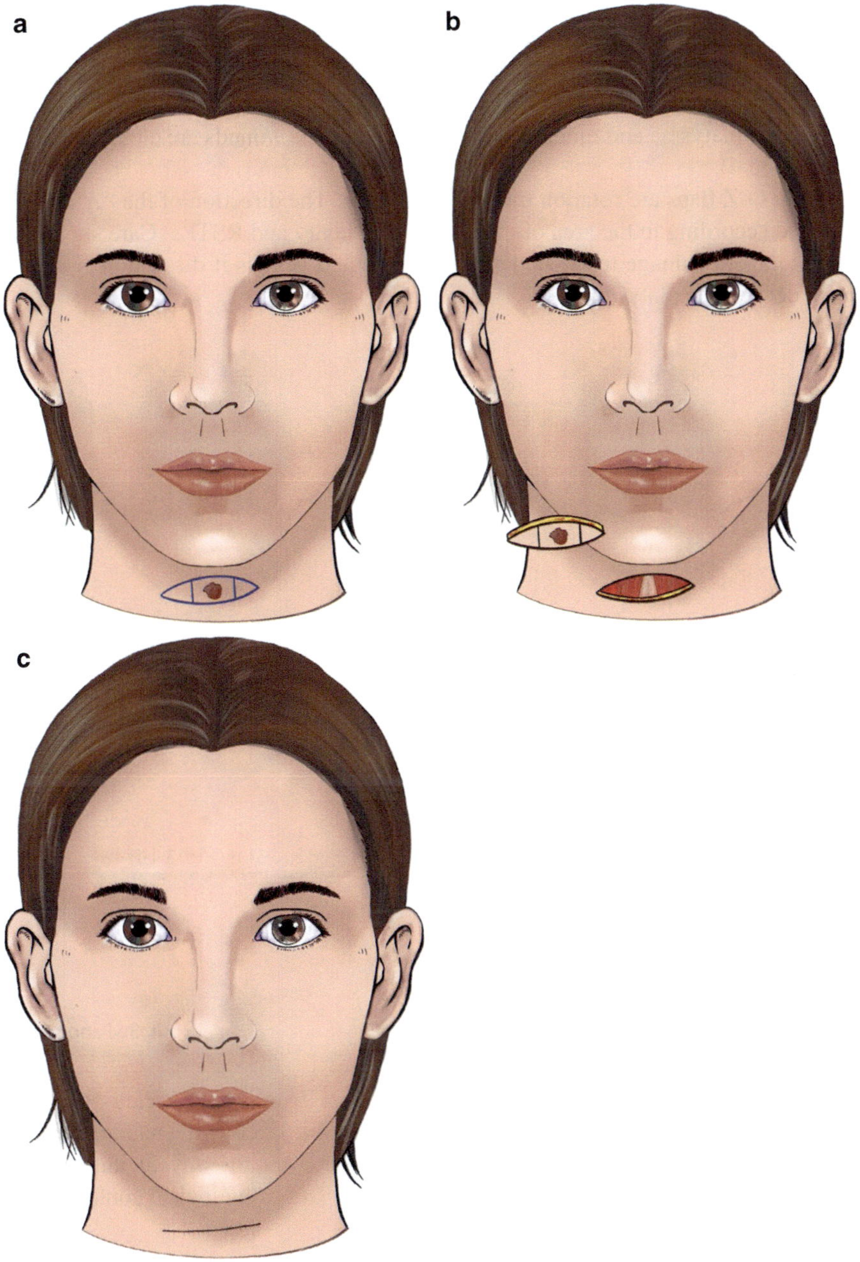

Fig. 12.2 Excision and primary closure. (**a**) Markings for excision, (**b**) Excision defect, (**c**) Final closure

O-Z Flap

Indications: Small- and medium-sized defects, circular defects.

Technique: The defect is modified into a circle. Two curvilinear incisions are made from the opposite poles of the defect. The flaps are elevated superficial or deep to the platysma and mobilised into the defect. The wounds are closed in layers (Fig. 12.3a–i).

Tips: O-Z flaps are rotation transposition flaps. The direction of the "Z" can be adjusted according to the area of maximum skin laxity and RSTLs. Care should be taken to avoid damage to the underlying nerves and vessels if dissection is undertaken deep to the platysma.

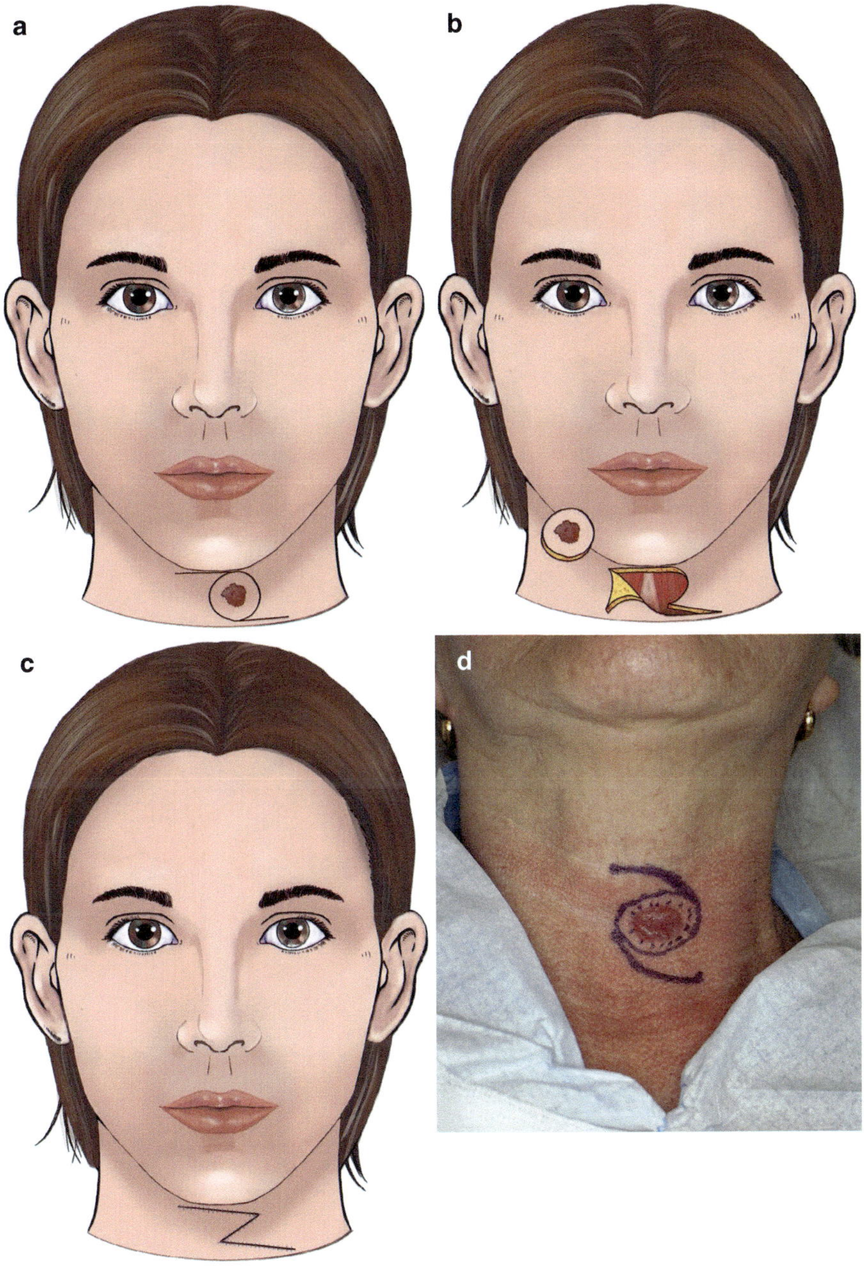

Fig. 12.3 O-Z flap. (**a**) Markings for excision and flap, (**b**) Excision defect and flaps raised, (**c**) Final closure, (**d**) Markings for excision and flap, (**e**) Excision defect, (**f**) Incisions for flap, (**g**) Undermining of edges, (**h**) Trial transposition, (**i**) Final closure

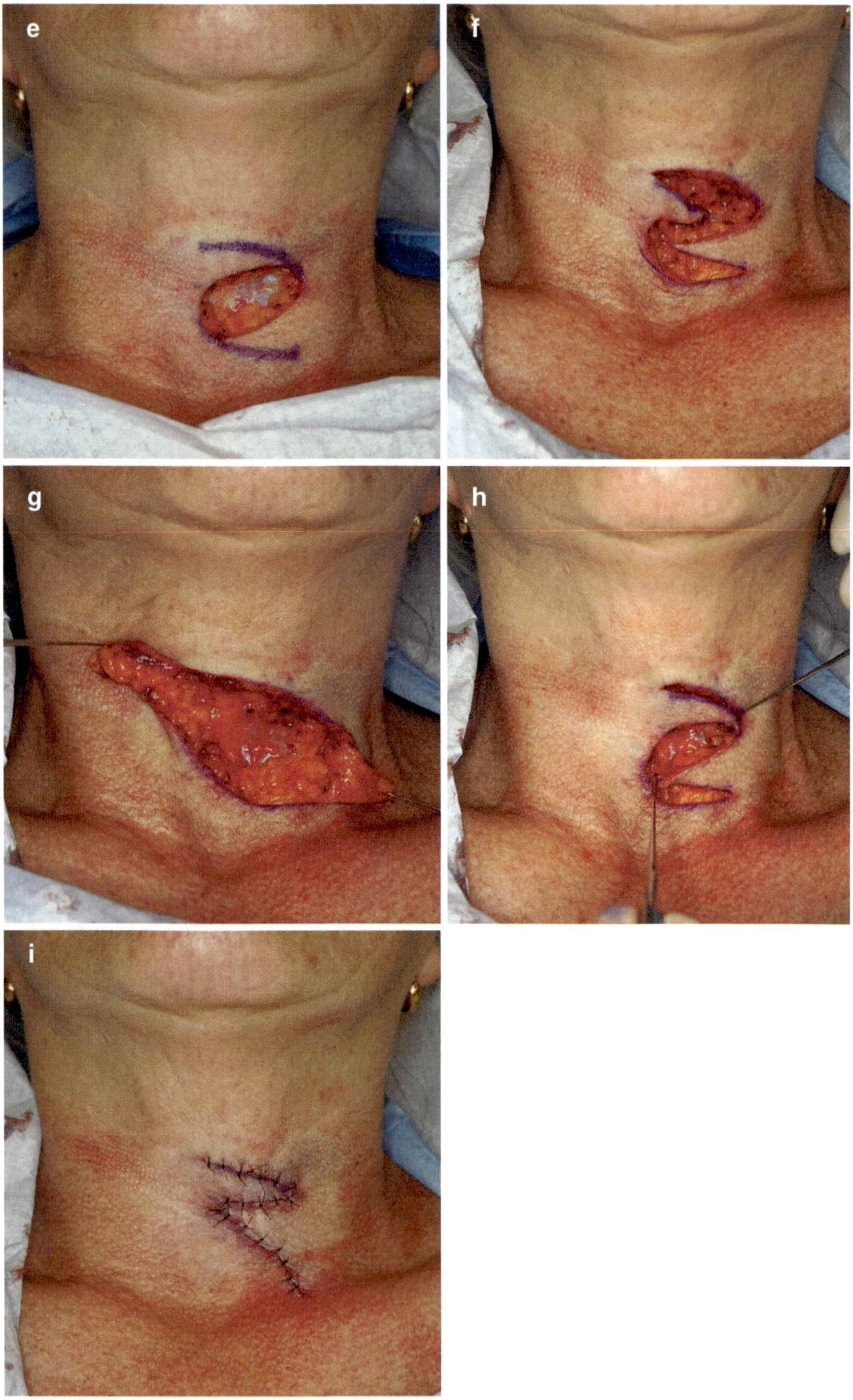

Fig. 12.3 (continued)

Rhombic Flap

Indications: Medium-sized defects.

Technique: The defect is modified into a rhombus with 60° and 120° internal angles. A rhomboid flap is designed by extending the short diagonal to a distance equal to one of the sides, and a further line is drawn from its extremity, parallel to the adjacent side of the defect. The flap is raised superficial or deep to the platysma and mobilised into the defect. The wound is closed in layers (Fig. 12.4a–d).

Tips: Though four flaps could be raised for any given defect, inferiorly based flaps are able to best utilise the tissue laxity and avoid damage to the mandibular branches of the facial nerve in the upper neck.

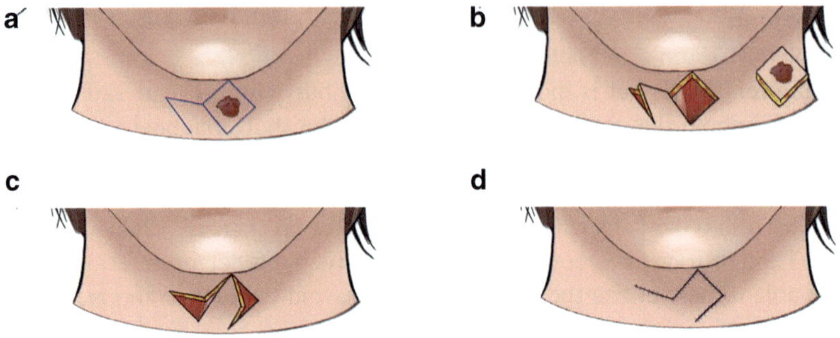

Fig. 12.4 Rhombic flap. (**a**) Markings for excision and flap, (**b**) Excision defect and flap raised, (**c**) Flap transposed into defect, (**d**) Final closure

Lateral Neck

Primary Closure

Indications: Small and medium defects.

Technique: The defect is converted into an ellipse, along the RSTLs. The wound margins can be undermined superficial or deep the platysma and closed in layers (Fig. 12.5a–e).

Tips: Care should be taken to avoid damage to the underlying nerves and vessels if dissection is undertaken deep to the platysma.

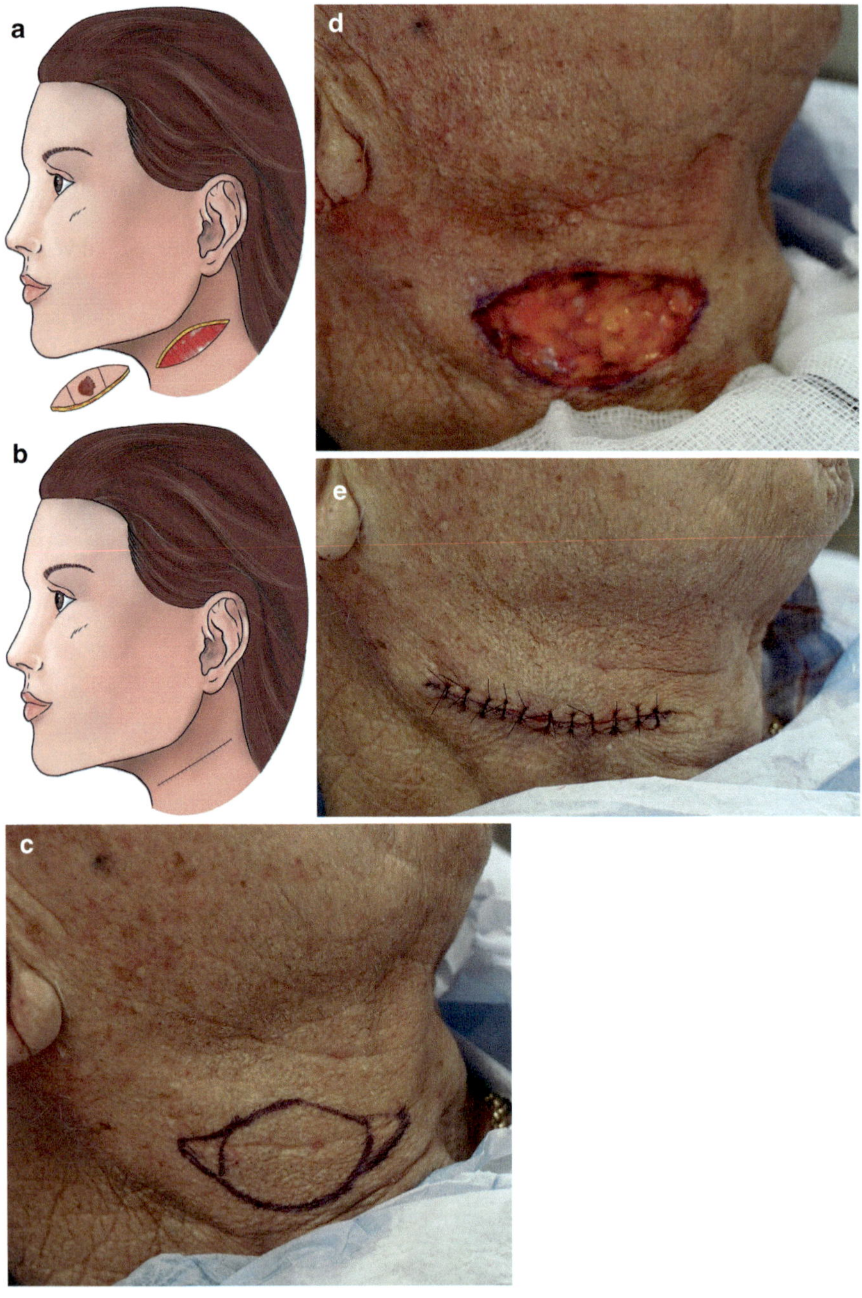

Fig. 12.5 Excision and primary closure. (**a**) Excision defect, (**b**) Final closure, (**c**) Markings for excision, (**d**) Excision defect, (**e**) Final closure

O-Z Flaps

Indications: Small- and medium-sized defects, circular defects.

Technique: The defect is modified into a circle. Two curvilinear incisions are made from the opposite poles of the defect. The flaps are elevated superficial or deep to the platysma and mobilised into the defect. The wounds are closed in layers (Fig. 12.6a–c).

Tips: O-Z flaps are rotation transposition flaps. The direction of the "Z" can be adjusted according to the area of maximum skin laxity and RSTLs. Care should be taken to avoid damage to the underlying nerves and vessels if dissection is undertaken deep to the platysma.

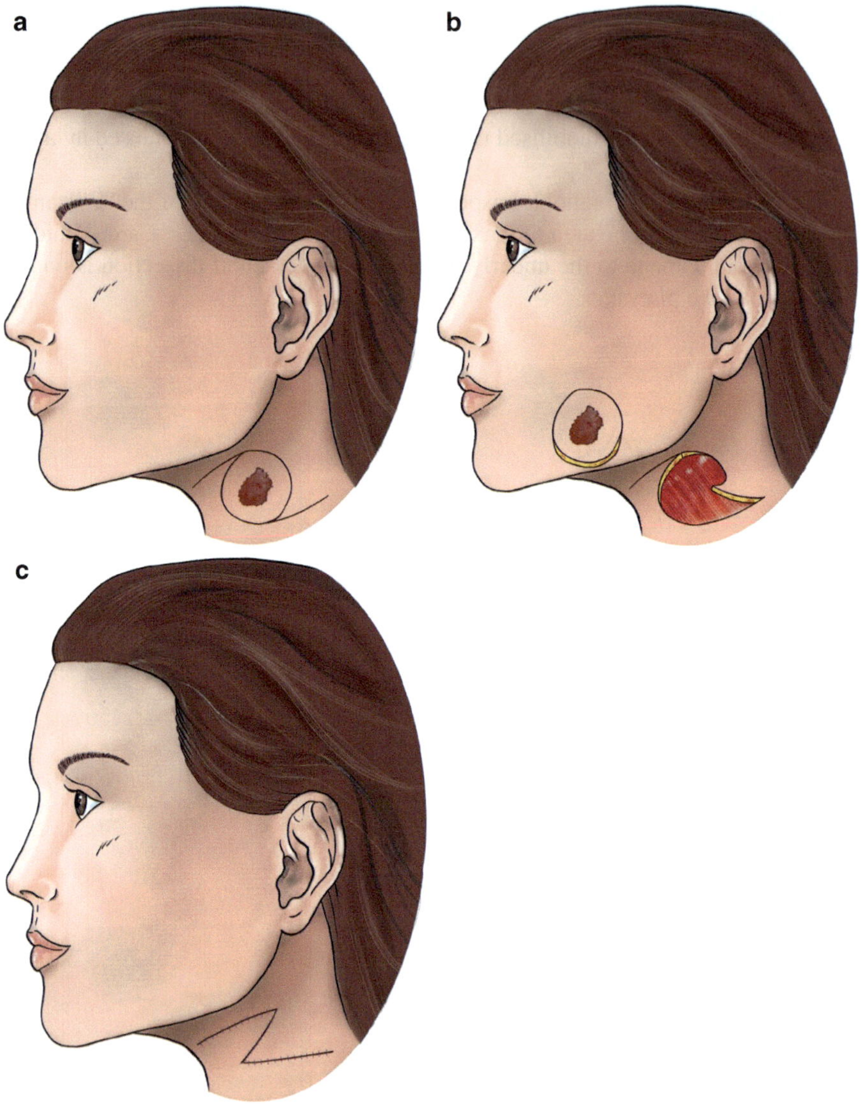

Fig. 12.6 O-Z flap. (**a**) Markings for excision and flaps, (**b**) Excision dfect and flaps raised, (**c**) Final closure

Rotation Transposition Flap

Indications: Medium defects.

Technique: The defect is modified into a triangle, and a curvilinear incision is made from the base of the defect. The flap is raised superficial or deep to the platysma and mobilised into the defect. The wounds are undermined widely and closed in layers (Fig. 12.7a–c, d–h).

Tips: The orientation of the curvilinear incision can be varied according to the adjacent tissue laxity and RSTLs. The flaps can be raised anterior or posterior to the defect. Care should be taken to avoid damage to the underlying nerves and vessels if dissection is undertaken deep to the platysma. The difference is length and thickness of the wound margins can be accommodated by differential suturing. Any dog ears that develop are excised along the RSTLs.

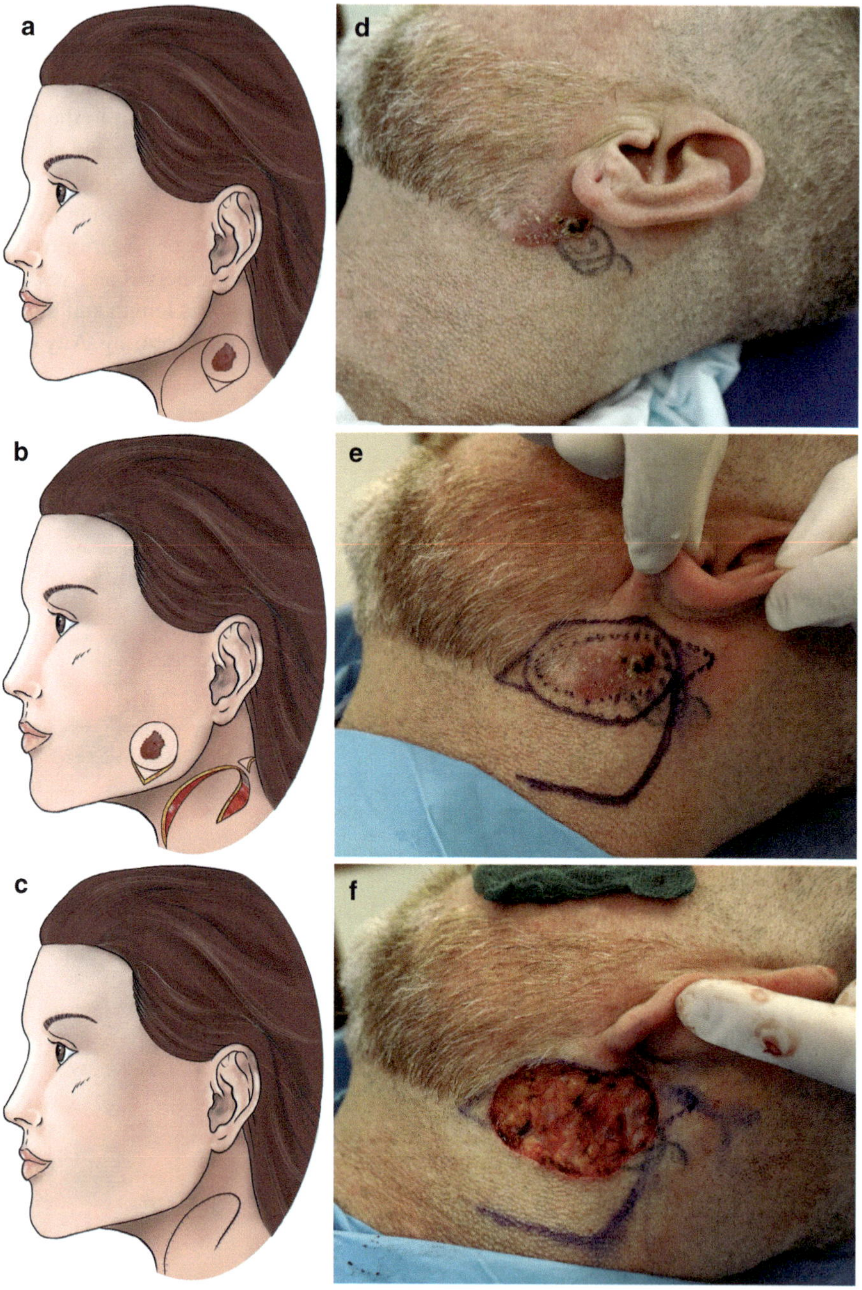

Fig. 12.7 Rotation/transposition flap. (**a**) Markings for excision and flap, (**b**) Excision defect and flap mobilised, (**c**) Final closure, (**d**) Lesion left neck, (**e**) Markings for excision and flap, (**f**) Excision defect, (**g**) Flap raised, (**h**) Final closure

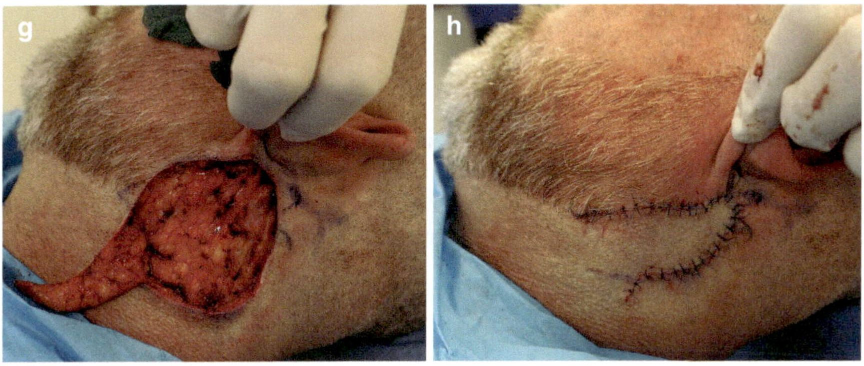

Fig. 12.7 (continued)

Posterior Neck

Primary Closure

Indications: Small and medium defects.

Technique: The defect is converted into an ellipse, and the wound margins undermined in the subcutaneous plane and closed in layers (Fig. 12.8a–c, d–g).

Tips: The ellipse can be oriented along a horizontal or vertical axis. A horizontal ellipse will have to take into account wound tension during neck flexion.

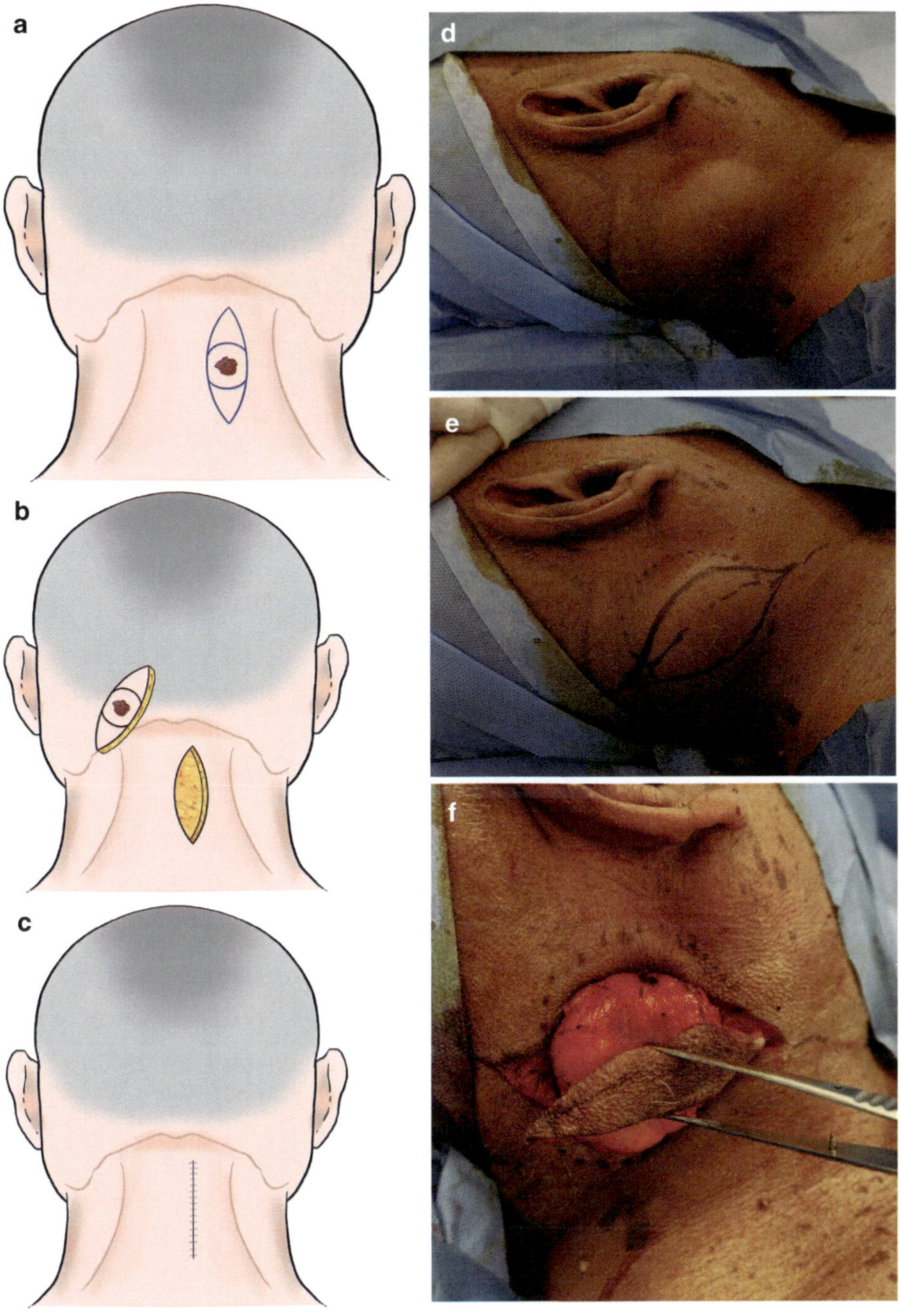

Fig. 12.8 Excision and primary closure. (**a**) Markings for excision, (**b**) Excision defect, (**c**) Final closure, (**d**) Lesion posterior neck, (**e**) Markings for excision, (**f**) Excision and defect, (**g**) Final closure

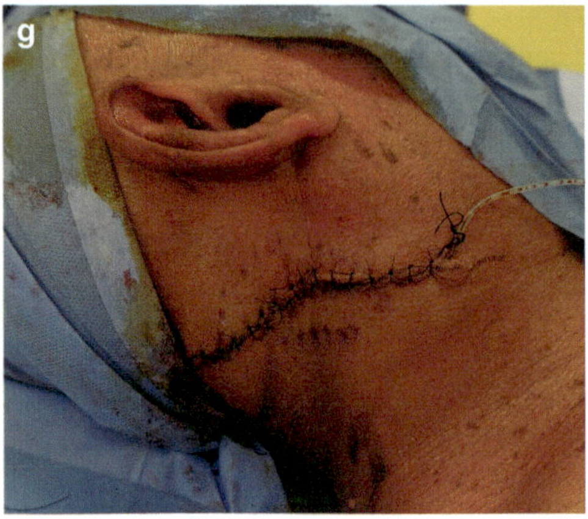

Fig. 12.8 (continued)

O-Z Flap

Indications: Small- and medium-sized defects, circular defects.

Technique: The defect is modified into a circle. Two curvilinear incisions are made from the opposite poles of the defect. The flaps are elevated in the subcutaneous plane and mobilised into the defect. The wounds are closed in layers (Fig. 12.9a–d).

Tips: O-Z flaps are rotation transposition flaps. The direction of the "Z" can be adjusted according to the area of maximum skin laxity and in the case of a horizontal orientation will have to take into account wound tension during neck flexion.

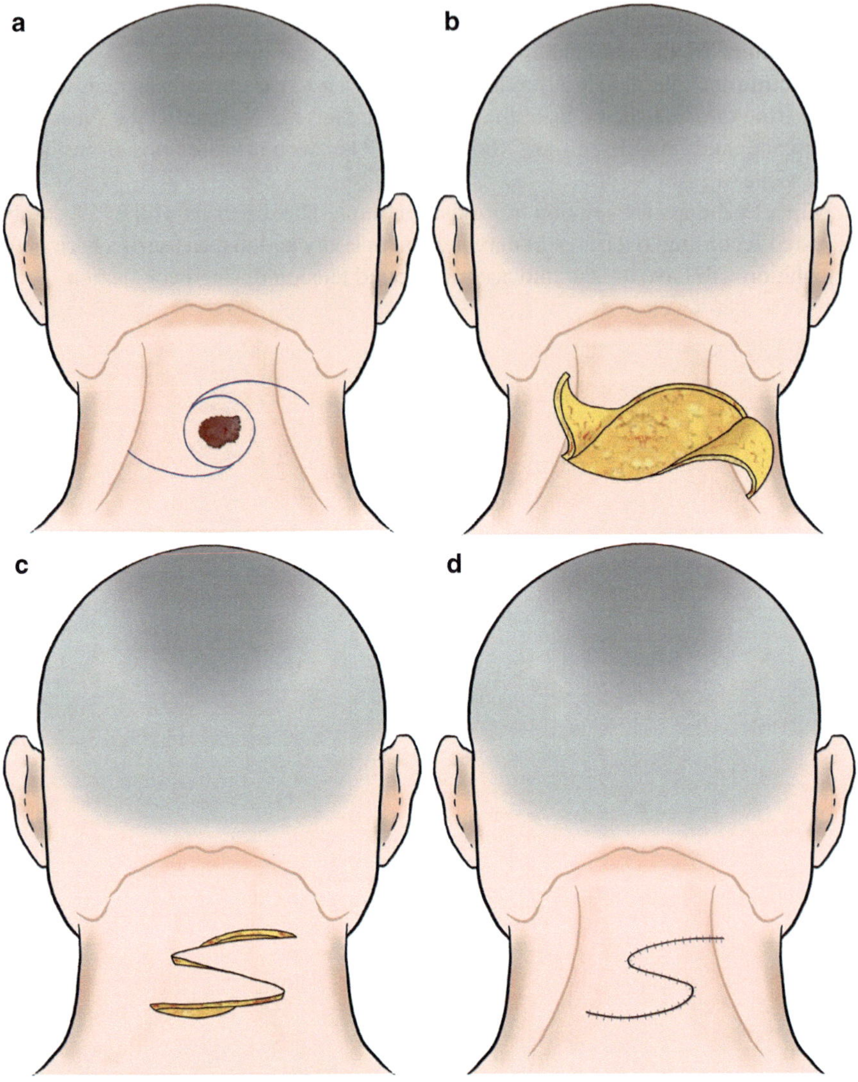

Fig. 12.9 O-Z flap. (**a**) Markings for excision and flap, (**b**) Excision defect and flaps raised, (**c**) Flaps mobilsed into defect, (**d**) Final closure

Rotation Transposition Flap

Indications: Medium defects.

Technique: The defect is modified into a triangle, and a curvilinear incision is made from the base of the defect. The flap is raised in the subcutaneous plane and mobilised into the defect. The wound is closed in layers (Fig. 12.10a–c).

Tips: The orientation of the curvilinear incision can be varied according to the adjacent tissue laxity, but is best placed vertically. A horizontal orientation will have to take into account wound tension during neck flexion. The difference is length and thickness of the wound margins can be accommodated by differential suturing. Any dog ears that develop are excised outside the margins of the flap to avoid vascular compromise.

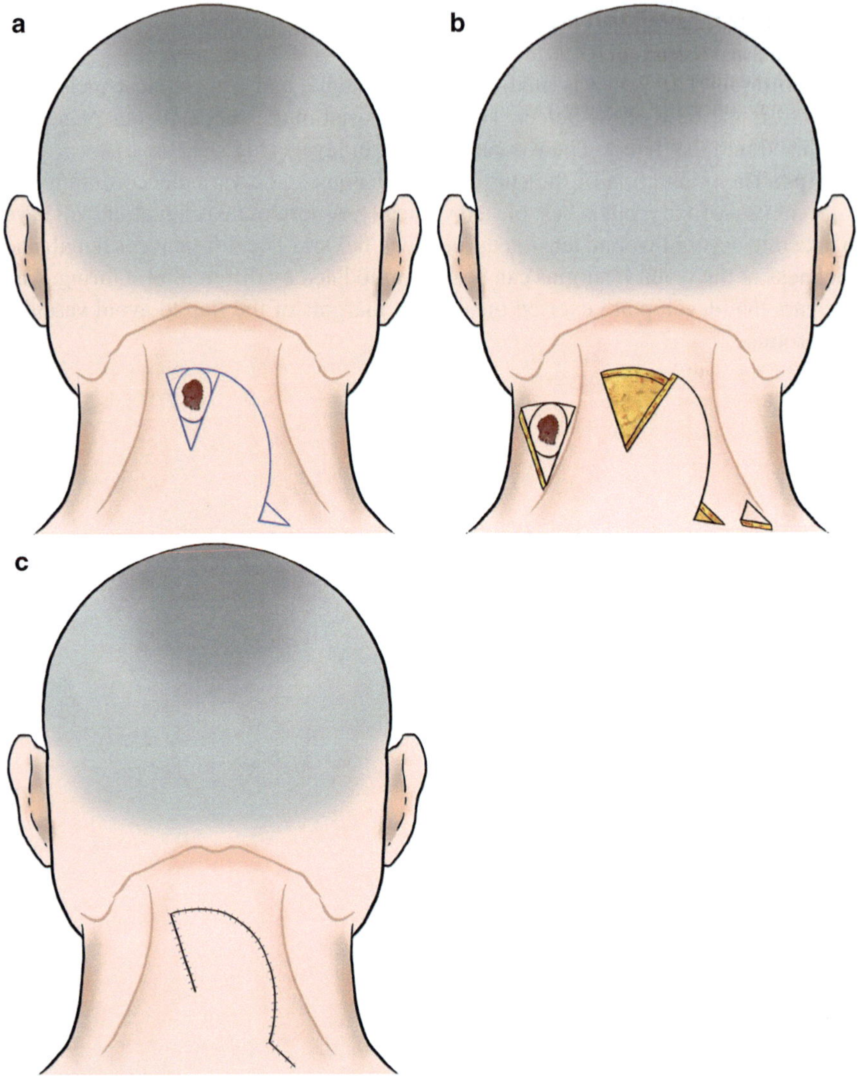

Fig. 12.10 Rotation transposition flap. (**a**) Markings for excision and flap, (**b**) Excision dfect and flap raised, (**c**) Final closure

Suggested Algorithm

Central Neck

1. Primary closure
2. O-Z flap
3. Rhombic flap

Lateral Neck

1. Primary closure
2. O-Z flap
3. Rotation/transposition flap

Posterior Neck

1. Primary closure
2. O-Z flap
3. Rotation/transposition flap

Algorithms for Specific Sites

Scalp

Central (Vertex) Defects

Small

1. Primary closure
2. Healing by secondary intention

Medium

1. Rotation/transposition flap
2. O-Z closure
3. Unilateral/bilateral advancement flap
4. Multiple rotation (pin wheel) flap
5. Multiple Limberg flap
6. Skin graft
7. RECELL®

Large

1. Skin graft
2. Skin graft with Integra®
3. Skin graft with pericranial flap
4. Multiple rotation flap
5. Rotation/transposition flap with skin graft to secondary defect

Lateral Defects

Small

1. Primary closure

V. Ilankovan et al., *Local Flaps in Facial Reconstruction*,
https://doi.org/10.1007/978-3-031-49464-2

Medium
1. Unilateral/bilateral advancement flap
2. Rotation/transposition flap
3. O-Z closure
4. Skin graft

Large
1. Rotation/transposition flap with skin graft to secondary defect
2. Skin graft
3. Skin graft with Integra®

Forehead

Central Defects

Small
1. Primary closure (vertical)
2. "M" excision (superior)
3. "W" excision (Inferior)

Medium

Upper
1. V-T flap
2. Unilateral/bilateral advancement flap

Lower
1. A-T flap
2. Unilateral/bilateral advancement flap

Paramedian

Small
1. Primary closure (vertical/horizontal)

Medium

Upper
1. V-T flap
2. Unilateral/bilateral advancement flap
3. Rotation/transposition flap

Lower

1. A-T, V-T flap
2. Unilateral/bilateral advancement flap

Temple/Lateral Forehead

Small

1. Primary closure (along crow's feet)

Medium

1. V-T flap
2. Rotation/transposition flap
3. Unilateral/bilateral advancement flap
4. Rhombic flap
5. Skin graft

Large

1. Multiple transposition flaps
2. Rotation/transposition flap with skin grafting of secondary defect
3. Skin graft
4. Skin graft with Integra®
5. Tissue expansion

Nose

Dorsum

Small

1. Primary closure (vertical/horizontal)

Medium

1. Glabella advancement flap
2. Glabella transposition flap
3. Skin graft

Nasal Tip

Small

1. Primary closure (vertical/horizontal)

Medium
1. Glabella advancement flap
2. Bilobed flap
3. Skin graft

Columella

1. Primary closure
2. Skin graft
3. Two-stage melolabial flap

Side Wall

Small
1. Primary closure (vertical)
2. Healing by secondary intention

Medium
1. Skin graft

Upper Side Wall
1. Glabella transposition flap

Lower Side Wall
1. Bilobed flap
2. Apron flap

Ala

Small
1. Island advancement flap

Medium
1. Bilobed flap (laterally based)
2. Bilobed flap (medially based)
3. Two-stage melolabial flap
4. Apron flap

Paramedian Forehead Flap
1. Large nasal defects involving multiple nasal subunits
2. Large nasal tip defects

3. Large ala defects
4. Large dorsal defects
5. Large side wall defects

Eyelids

Upper Eyelid

Anterior Lamellar Defects

1. Primary closure (horizontal/vertical)
2. Advancement flap
3. Fricke flap
4. Skin graft

Full-Thickness Defects

Small

1. Primary closure (vertical)

Medium

1. Primary closure with lateral canthotomy and superior cantholysis
2. Tenzel flap

Large

1. Cutler beard flap

Medial Canthus

1. Healing be secondary intention
2. Glabella transposition flap
3. Glabella island flap
4. Skin graft

Lower Eyelid

Anterior Lamella Defects

Small

1. Primary closure (vertical)
2. Tear drop

Medium
1. Advancement flap
2. Tripier flap
3. Rotation/transposition flap

Large
1. McGregor flap
2. Mustarde' flap

Full-Thickness Defects

Small
1. Primary closure

Medium
1. Primary closure with lateral canthotomy and inferior cantholysis
2. Tenzel flap

Large Defects
1. Hughes flap
2. Macgregor flap
3. Mustarde' flap

Ear

Concha

Partial Thickness
1. Healing by secondary intention
2. Skin graft

Partial Thickness/Full Thickness
1. Revolving door flap
2. Post-auricular artery island flap
3. Post-auricular transposition flap
4. Pre-auricular transposition flap

Antihelix/Helix

Partial Thickness

1. Healing by secondary intention (antihelix)
2. Skin graft (antihelix)

Full Thickness
1. Wedge excision
2. Helical rim advancement
3. Two-stage post-auricular flap

Triangular Fossa

1. Healing by secondary intention
2. Skin graft
3. Superiorly based pre-auricular flap

Tragus
1. Superiorly based pre-auricular flap
2. Advancement flap

Posterior Surface of Pinna

1. Healing by secondary intention
2. Primary closure
3. Skin graft
4. Post auricular advancement/transposition flap
5. Rhombic flap

Lobule

1. Primary closure

Cheek

Medial

Small
1. Primary closure

Medium
1. Island advancement flap
2. Rotation/transposition flap (lateral)
3. Rotation/transposition flap (Inferior)

Buccal

Small
1. Primary closure

Medium
1. Primary closure
2. Rhombic flap
3. Rotation/transposition flap (lateral)
4. Rotation/transposition flap (inferior)
5. Island advancement flap
6. Bilobed flap

Zygomatic Unit

Small
1. Primary closure

Medium
1. Rhombic flap
2. Rotation/transposition flap
3. Mustarde' flap

Mandibular

Small
1. Primary closure

Medium
1. Rhombic flap
2. Rotation/transposition flap
3. Bilobed flap

Lateral Unit

Small

1. Primary closure

Medium

1. Asymmetric primary closure
2. Rhombic flap
3. Rotation/transposition flap
4. Bilobed flap

Lips

Lower Lip

Skin Only

Small

1. Primary closure (along rhytids)
2. M/W closure

Medium

1. A-T flap
2. Inferiorly based nasolabial flap
3. Superiorly based nasolabial flap

Mucosa Only

Small

1. Primary closure

Medium/Large

1. Mucosal advancement flap

Full-Thickness Defect

Small

1. Primary closure
2. W excision

Medium

1. Bilateral advancement flap (Commissurotomy)
2. Karapandzic flap
3. Abbe flap
4. Abbe– Estlander flap

Large Defects

1. Bilateral advancement flap (Commissurotomy)
2. Karapandzic flap
3. Karapandzic flap + Abbe flap
4. Fan flap

Upper Lip

Skin Only

Small

1. Primary closure
2. A-T flap

Medium

1. Laterally based rotation/transposition flap
2. Unilateral/bilateral perialar crescentic advancement flap
3. Island advancement flap
4. Inferiorly based nasolabial flap

Full Thickness

Small

1. Primary closure

Medium

1. Perialar crescentic advancement flap
2. Karapandzic flap
3. Abbe flap
4. Abbe–Estlander flap

Large

1. Bilateral nasolabial flap + Abbe flap

Upper/Lower Lip (Chronic Ulcers/Atrophy)

Nanofat injection

Chin Defects

Small

1. Primary closure

Medium

1. V-T flap
2. Rotation flap
3. Bilobed flap
4. Rhombic flap

Neck

Central Neck

1. Primary closure
2. O-Z flap
3. Rhombic flap

Lateral Neck

1. Primary closure
2. O-Z flap
3. Rotation/transposition flap

Posterior Neck

1. Primary closure
2. O-Z flap
3. Rotation/transposition flap

Index

A
Abbe-Estlander flap, 399, 437
Abbe flap, 397, 409, 434, 441, 491
Accessory nerve, 20
Advancement flaps
  bilateral, 45, 46, 112, 132, 150, 395, 404, 415, 419
  island, 45, 59, 195, 424
  rotation, 343, 347
  unilateral, 45, 110, 130, 150, 415, 419, 439
Aesthetic borders, 23, 29, 33, 51, 328, 376
Aesthetic subunits, 25
Aesthetic units, 23, 25, 375
Algorithms
  auricle/pinna, 488–489
  cheek, 373–374
  chin, 493
  eyelid, 487–488
  forehead, 484–485
  lips, 491–493
  neck, 493
  nose, 485–487
  scalp, 483–484
Anterior lamella, 215, 218, 235, 254
Antihelix/helix, 282, 286–302
  helical rim advancement, 264, 286–302, 304
  lobule, primary closure, 322
  partial thickness defect
    healing by secondary intention, 312
    skin graft, 264, 304
    superiorly based pre auricular transposition flap, 280, 304
  posterior surface pinna
    advancement flap, 290, 299
    healing by secondary intention, 312
    post auricular advancement/transposition flap, 315, 318
    primary closure, 312
    rhombic flap, 320
    skin graft, 312
  tragus
    advancement flap, 308
    transposition flap, 318
  triangular fossa
    healing by secondary intention, 304
    skin graft, 304
    superiorly based pre-auricular flap, 304
  two stage post auricular flap, 302
  wedge excision, 286, 390, 393
Anti tragus, 280, 299
Apron flap, 190
A-T flap, 128, 138
Auricle/pinna
  anatomy, 16
  local anaesthesia, 17
  nerve supply, 17
Auriculotemporal nerve, 9, 10, 16, 18, 76

B
Bilateral advancement flap, 45, 46, 132
Bilateral fan flap, 411, 412
Bilateral perialar crescentic advancement flap, 439
Bilobed flap, 51, 104, 176, 184, 187, 198, 200, 370
Buccal subunit, 29, 328, 339–347
Burrow's triangles, 45, 110, 112, 126, 132, 136, 142, 145, 150, 152, 154, 169

C
Cantholysis (inferior), 243, 247
Cantholysis (superior), 231
Canthotomy (lateral), 231, 243, 247, 251
Cavum concha, 264–280

V. Ilankovan et al., *Local Flaps in Facial Reconstruction*,
https://doi.org/10.1007/978-3-031-49464-2

Cheek
  aesthetic subunits, 29, 30
  aesthetic unit, 29
  buccal subunit
    bilobed flap, 184, 198
    island advancement flap, 45, 334, 358
    primary closure, 176, 184, 198, 339
    rhombic flap, 341
    rotation/transposition flap (inferiorly based), 347–349
    rotation/transposition flap (laterally based), 364
  infra-orbital subunit
    primary closure, 360
    rotation/transposition flap (inferiorly based), 364
    rotation/transposition flap (laterally based), 364
  lateral subunit
    asymmetric primary closure, 367
    bilobed flap, 370
    primary closure, 367
    rhombic flap, 370
    rotation/transposition flap, 114
  local anaesthesia, 11
  mandibular subunit
    bilobed flap, 370
    primary closure, 360
    rhombic flap, 360
    rotation/transposition flap, 364
  medial subunit
    Island advancement flap, 334
    primary closure, 330
    rotation/transposition flap (inferiorly based), 347
    rotation/transposition flap (laterally based), 343
  nerve supply, 411, 441
  zygomatic subunit
    primary closure, 350
    rhombic flap, 352
    rotation/transposition flap, 355
Cheek advancement flap
  inferiorly based, 347
  laterally based, 343
Chin
  aesthetic unit, 25
  bilobed flap, 449
  local anaesthesia, 14
  nerve supply, 441
  primary closure, 443
  rhombic flap, 451
  rotation flap, 447
  V-T transposition flap, 445
Columella
  primary closure, 211
  skin graft, 211
  two stage melolabial flap, 213–214
Concha (cymba/cavum)
  healing by secondary intention, 264
  post-auricular artery island flap, 272
  post-auricular transposition flap, 275
  pre-auricular transposition flap, 280
  revolving door flap, 266
  skin grafts, 264
Cutler-Beard flap, 232
Cymba concha, 264–280

D

Deep temporal fascia
  deep layer, 74
  superficial layer, 74, 152
Dog-ear (standing cutaneous deformity), 67, 198, 364, 419, 439, 445

E

Ectropion, 39, 215, 343, 347, 355
External nasal nerve block, 12
Eyebrow, 7, 23, 27, 39, 120, 122–132, 134–142, 156, 159, 165, 172, 180, 207, 215, 222, 227, 251
Eyelid
  aesthetic subunits, 40
  aesthetic units, 39, 215
  anatomy, 39, 215
  medial canthus
    glabellar island flap, 487
    glabellar transposition flap, 172
    healing by secondary intention, 487
    skin graft, 174

F

Flaps
  Abbe-Estlander flap, 399, 437
  Abbe flap, 441
  advancement flap, 45, 46, 59, 110, 112, 130, 132, 150, 195, 290, 299, 343, 347, 395, 404, 415, 419, 424, 439
  apron flap, 190
  A-T flap, 128, 138
  bilateral advancement flap, 45, 46, 132
  bilateral fan flap, 411
  bilobed flap, 51, 104, 176, 184, 187, 198, 370
  bilobed flap (laterally based), 198

bilobed flap (medially based), 187, 200
cervical rotation flap, 154
cheek rotation flap, 154
Cutler-Beard flap, 232
fan flap, 411
forehead rotation flap, 152
Fricke flap, 222
glabellar advancement flap, 169
glabella island flap, 487
glabellar transposition flap, 172, 180, 227
helical rim advancement flap, 290
Hughes flap, 254
interpolated flap, 190
island advancement flap, 45, 334, 358
Karapandzic + Abbe flap, 401, 409
Karapandzic flap, 409, 411, 441
McGregor flap, 243, 247, 343
melolabial flap (two stage), 213–214
mucosal advancement flap, 387
multiple Limberg flap, 87
multiple rotation flap (pinwheel flap), 84
Mustardé flap, 249
nasolabial + Abbe flap, 441
nasolabial flap (inferiorly based), 202, 383, 386, 429, 441
nasolabial flap (superiorly based), 383–386, 429
O-Z flap, 462, 469, 477
paramedian forehead flap, 207
perialar cresentric advancement flap, 419, 439
pericranial flap, 93, 96, 100, 114
post-auricular flap (two stage), 302
post-auricular flap (inferiorly based), 302
post-auricular flap (superiorly based), 302
post-auricular island flap, 272
post-auricular transposition flap, 318
pre-auricular flap (superiorly based), 304
revolving door flap, 266
rhombic flap (Limberg flap), 63, 341, 352, 360, 370
rotation flap, 81, 114
rotation/transposition flap (inferiorly based), 347–349
rotation/transposition flap (laterally based), 364
Tenzel flap, 251
transposition flap, 51, 54
tripier flap, 235
unilateral advancement flap, 110, 130
V-T flap, 126, 142
Forehead
aesthetic subunits, 28
aesthetic units, 27
anatomy, 119
central defects
A-T flap, 138
bilateral advancement flap, 483
M excision, 161
primary closure, 483
rotation/transposition flap, 483
unilateral advancement, 483
V-T flap, 126, 142
W excision, 161
local anaesthesia, 5
nerve supply, 5
paramedian defects
A-T flap, 138
bilateral advancement flap, 136
primary closure, 161
rotation/transposition flap, 145
unilateral advancement flap, 136
V-T flap, 140, 142
temple/lateral forehead
primary closure, 161
rhombic flap, 147
rotation/transposition flap, 145
skin graft, 159
V-T flap, 142
Fricke flap, 222

G

Glabella advancement flap, 485, 486
Glabella island flap, 258
Glabella transposition flap, 213, 258, 485–487
Grafts
cartilage graft, 204, 232
skin graft (full thickness), 108, 174, 180, 211
skin graft (split thickness), 108
Great auricular nerve, 16, 20, 367, 370
Greater occipital nerve, 18

H

Haematoma, 9, 264
Helix, 9, 16, 280, 299, 304, 324
Hughes flap, 259, 488

I

Inferiorly based nasolabial flap, 202, 491, 492
Inferiorly based rotation/advancement flap, 347–349
Infraorbital nerves, 328
Infratrochlear nerve, 12, 13
Integra®, 484, 485

Interpolated flap, 190
Island advancement flap, 373, 486, 490
Island flap, 60, 224, 258, 272, 324, 487, 488

K
Karapandzic flap, 455
Karapandzic flap + Abbe flap, 455, 492

L
Labiomental fold, 23
Lamella
  anterior, 39, 215, 218, 235, 254, 258, 487–488
  middle, 39, 215
  posterior, 39, 215, 216, 247, 249, 251
Lateral canthotomy, 231, 243, 247, 251, 258, 259, 487, 488
Lateral cantholysis
Lateraly based rotation advancement flap, 343
Lesser occipital nerve, 16, 18, 20, 76
Lid retractors, 39, 215
Lines of maximum extensibility (LME), 23
Lips
  chronic ulcer/ atrophy
    nanofat injection, 492
  full thickness
    Abbe- Estlander flap, 456, 492
    Abbe flap, 397, 434, 492
    bilateral advancement flap + commissurotomy, 491, 492
    bilateral nasolabial flap + Abbe flap, 456, 492
    fan flap, 492
    Karapandzic flap, 456, 491, 492
    Karapandzic flap + Abbe flap, 455, 492
    primary closure (shield excision), 390, 432
    W excision, 393, 484, 491
  Lower lip defect, 397, 406, 411
  mucosa only
    mucosal advancement flap, 387–389
    primary closure, 387, 491
  skin only
    A-T flap, 128, 138, 380, 417, 484, 491, 492
    inferiorly based nasolabial flap, 456, 491, 492
    island advancement flap, 456, 492
    laterally based rotation/ transposition flap, 456, 492
    M closure, 491
    perialar cresentric advancement flap, 456
    primary closure, 312, 378, 413, 491, 492
    superiorly based nasolabial flap, 491
    W closure, 491
  upper lip defect, 401, 441
Lobule, 154, 280, 290, 322, 325, 343, 355, 367, 483
Local anaesthesia
  auricle/pinna, 17
  cheek, 29
  chin, 35
  external ear, 16
  external nose, 13
  forehead, 7–11, 27
  lower lip, 14, 378–411
  neck, 20
  scalp, 41
  temple, 9
  upper lip, 14, 375, 492
Lower eyelids
  anterior lamella defects
    advancement flap, 235
    McGregor flap, 247
    Mustarde flap, 249
    primary closure, 235
    tripier flap, 235
  full thickness defects
    Hughes flap, 254
    Mustardé flap, 249
    primary closure, 241
    primary closure with lateral canthotomy/cantholysis, 247
    Tenzel flap, 251

M
McGregor flap, 243, 247, 259, 488
Mental foramen, 14
Mental nerves, 387, 404
M excision, 484
Middle lamella, 39, 215
Mucosal advancement flap, 491
Multiple Limberg flap, 483
Multiple rotation flap, 84–86
Mustardé flap, 249

N
Nanofat injections, 453, 492
Nasolabial fold, 23, 33, 375, 383, 386, 401, 404, 411, 421, 429
Neck
  central defect
    O-Z flap, 469, 481, 493

primary closure, 474, 493
rhombic flap, 63, 493
lateral defect
O-Z flap, 493
primary closure, 493
rotation/transposition flap, 493
posterior defect
O-Z flap, 493
primary closure, 493
rotation/ transposition flap, 493
Nerves
accessory, 20
auricular branch of vagus, 16
auriculotemporal, 9, 10, 16
external nasal, 12, 13
facial, 9, 74, 120, 142, 147, 150, 152, 154, 222, 239, 249, 328, 339, 343, 350, 355, 360, 364, 367, 376, 457, 465
great auricular, 16, 20, 367, 370
infraorbital, 13, 14, 328
infratrochlear, 12, 13
lesser occipital, 16, 18
mental nerve, 14, 15
phrenic, 20
supraclavicular, 20
supraorbital, 7
supratrochlear, 7, 8
third occipital, 18, 76
zygomaticofacial, 10, 11
zygomaticotemporal, 9, 10
Nose
aesthetic subunits, 25
aesthetic units, 25, 33, 375
ala
apron flap, 211, 486
bilobed flap (laterally based), 198, 486
bilobed flap (medially based), 200, 486
island advancement flap, 195, 486
paramedian forehead flap, 207, 486–487
two stage melolabial flap, 204, 486
anatomy, 31, 163, 164, 375
columella
paramedian forehead flap, 214
skin graft, 211, 486
two stage melolabial flap, 204, 486
dorsum
glabellar advancement flap, 169, 485
glabellar transposition flap, 172, 485
paramedian forehead flap, 207, 486–487
primary closure (horizontal), 167, 485
primary closure (vertical), 165, 485
local anaesthesia, 13, 29
nasal tip
bilobed flap, 176, 486
glabellar advancement flap, 169, 486
paramedian forehead flap, 214, 486–487
primary closure, 174, 485
skin graft, 174
sidewall
apron flap, 190, 486
bilobed flap, 184, 187, 486
glabellar transposition flap, 180, 486
healing by secondary intention, 213, 486
paramedian forehead flap, 207, 486–487
primary closure (vertical), 180, 486
skin graft, 180, 486

O
Orbicularis oculi, 39, 207, 215, 231, 232, 241, 243, 247, 249, 251, 328
Orbital septum, 39, 215
O-Z flap, 462, 463, 469, 470, 477, 478, 481, 493

P
Paramedian forehead flap, 207, 486–487
Peri-alar crescentric advancememnt flap, 492
Pericranial flap, 100
Periosteum, 11, 74, 89, 132, 154, 224, 272, 275, 315, 318, 343, 355, 441
Philtrum, 23, 33, 413–429, 432–441
Pin wheel flap, 87, 483
Pinna, 16–18, 25, 29, 37, 249, 261, 262, 266, 272, 275, 286, 290, 299, 302, 312–320, 325, 327, 328, 489
Postauricular artery island flap
Postauricular transposition flap, 324, 325, 488, 489
Posterior lamella, 215, 216, 247, 249, 251

R
ReCell®, 108, 483
Relaxed skin tension lines (RSTL), 23, 29, 33, 35, 39, 43, 45, 51, 56, 69, 120, 165, 215, 218, 328, 341, 350, 352, 355, 358, 360, 364, 367, 370, 376, 383, 386, 429, 443, 445, 447, 449, 457, 460, 462, 467, 469, 471
Revolving door flap, 324, 488

Rhombic flap, 325, 373, 374, 456, 481, 490, 491, 493
Rotation flap, 67, 152, 456, 493
Rotation/transposition flap, 145, 258, 373, 374, 483–485, 490

S

Scalp
  anatomy, 41
  central defects
    bilateral advancement flap, 483
    healing by secondary intention, 483
    multiple limberg flap, 483
    multiple rotation flap, 483
    O-Z flap, 483
    primary closure, 483
    ReCell®, 483
    rotation/transposition flap, 483
    skin graft, 483
    skin graft with Integra®, 483
    skin graft with pericranial flap, 483
    unilateral advancement flap, 483
  lateral defects
    bilateral advancement flap, 484
    healing by secondary intention, 484
    O-Z flap, 484
    primary closure, 483
    rotation/ transposition flap, 484
    skin graft with Integra®, 484
    skin graft with pericranial flap, 96
  local anaesthesia, 7, 9, 16, 18
  loose area, 41, 42
  nerve supply, 76, 77
  tight area, 41, 42, 74
Scapha, 286, 299
Skin graft, 484, 486
Skin graft (full thickness), 108, 211, 264, 280, 282, 304, 312
Skin graft (split thickness), 108
Skin graft with pericranial flap, 483
Superficial layer of deep temporal fascia, 74, 152
Superficial musculoaponeurotic system (SMAS), 73
Superficial temporoparietal fascia, 73, 74
Superiorly based pre-auricular flap, 324, 489
Supraclavicular nerve, 20
Supraorbital artery, 76, 207
Supraorbital nerve, 7, 8, 18, 120, 126
Supratrochlear nerve, 7, 8, 18, 76, 120, 152, 224
Supra-trochlear nerve, 126

T

Tarsal plate, 39, 215, 231, 241, 243, 251, 254
Temporal branch of facial nerve, 9, 120, 142, 147
Temporalis muscle, 74
Tenzel flap, 251, 258, 259, 487, 488
Tips, 48, 51, 54, 56, 59, 63, 70, 78, 81, 84, 87, 89, 93, 96, 100, 104, 108, 110, 112, 122, 124, 126, 128, 130, 132, 134, 136, 138, 140, 142, 145, 147, 150, 152, 154, 156, 159, 165, 167, 169, 172, 174, 176, 180, 184, 190, 195, 198, 200, 204, 207, 211, 218, 220, 222, 224, 227, 231, 232, 235, 239, 241, 243, 247, 249, 251, 254
Tissue expansion, 159, 485
Tragus, 9, 16, 308–310
Transposition flap, 51, 54, 56, 63, 93, 104, 156, 159, 202, 213, 222, 235, 258, 324, 325, 373, 374, 462, 469, 471, 477, 479, 481, 483–485, 488–491
Transverse cervical nerve, 20
Triangular fossa, 299, 324, 489
Tripier flap, 235, 258, 488
Two-stage melolabial flap, 213, 214, 486
Two-stage postauricular flap, 324, 489

U

Unilateral advancement flap, 45, 456, 483–485, 492
Unilateral perialar crescentic advancement flap
Upper eyelid
  anterior lamella defects
    advancement flap, 220
    Fricke flap, 222
    primary closure, 218
    skin graft, 254
  full thickness defects
    Cutler-Beard flap, 232
    primary closure, 231
    primary closure with lateral canthotomy/cantholysis, 231
    Tenzel flap, 251
Upper lip, 11, 33, 375, 411

V

Vermillion border, 23, 33, 376, 378, 380, 383, 387, 390, 393, 397, 399, 406, 409, 413, 417, 424, 429, 432, 434, 437, 439, 453
V-T flap, 455, 456, 484, 485, 493

W
W excision, 455

Z
Z plasty, 247, 343, 347
Zygomatic subunit, 29, 328
Zygomaticofacial foramen, 11
Zygomaticofacial nerve, 10, 11
Zygomaticotemporal nerve, 9, 10

GPSR Compliance

The European Union's (EU) General Product Safety Regulation (GPSR) is a set of rules that requires consumer products to be safe and our obligations to ensure this.

If you have any concerns about our products, you can contact us on ProductSafety@springernature.com

In case Publisher is established outside the EU, the EU authorized representative is:

Springer Nature Customer Service Center GmbH
Europaplatz 3
69115 Heidelberg, Germany

Batch number: 10732031

Printed by Printforce, the Netherlands